Antireflux Surgery

Antireflux Surgery

Lee L. Swanstrom • Christy M. Dunst

Editors

Antireflux Surgery

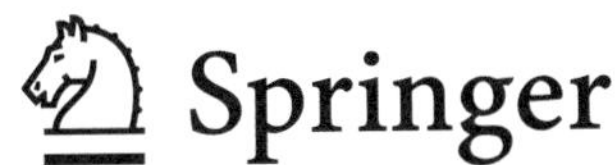 Springer

Editors
Lee L. Swanstrom
GI and MIS Surgery
The Oregon Clinic
Providence Portland Medical Center
Portland, OR, USA

Christy M. Dunst
GI and MIS Surgery
The Oregon Clinic
Providence Portland Medical Center
Portland, OR, USA

ISBN 978-1-4939-4329-6   ISBN 978-1-4939-1749-5 (eBook)
DOI 10.1007/978-1-4939-1749-5
Springer New York Heidelberg Dordrecht London

Springer is part of Springer Science+Business Media (www.springer.com)

I would like to dedicate this book to surgery of the esophagus:
This surgical specialty has rewarded me with a fabulous career, fascinating
research and peers around the world who are some of my best friends.
It has also helped thousands of my patients have a better quality of life—the
greatest reward I can imagine. Esophageal surgery has also given me two
of the best practice partners one could hope for: Christy Dunst and Kevin
Reavis, whose uncomplaining support makes my surgical practice
possible—thanks guys....

—Lee L. Swanstrom, MD

This book is dedicated to all those surgeons committed to excellence
in esophageal surgery. My sincerest thank you to my lovely husband Mark,
to my beautiful children Tyler and Hailey and to my cool partners who
supported me endlessly allowing this book to happen.

—Christy M. Dunst, MD, FACS

Foreword

Gastroesophageal reflux disease (GERD) is the most common foregut disease in the world and accounts for approximately 75 % of all esophageal pathology. The majority of afflicted patients have mild disease and are successfully managed with lifestyle modifications and acid suppression medication. However, the disease progresses in at least 10 % of patients leading them to seek surgical alternatives. For nearly 50 years, I have dedicated my career to the complex pathophysiology of this disease and its sequelae, which at its worst includes the progression to esophageal adenocarcinoma. Precise understanding of the functional and anatomical aspects of the reflux barrier is absolutely critical to successful surgical treatment.

The discovery of the lower esophageal high pressure zone, or LES as it was later named, leads to the realization that almost half of the patients with confirmed GERD have a normal LES on a motility study performed at rest, in the recumbent position, and after an overnight fast. The etiology of reflux in patients with a normal LES is transient openings of the LES when challenged by gastric distention or dilation. These events are called transient LES relaxations (TLESRs) and were first described by Dodds in 1982. Gastric distension occurs with overeating or excessive dry swallowing. Each dry swallow carries with it saliva and the 15 cc of air contained within the pharyngeal space. The swallowed food and air collect in the stomach and if excessive cause pressure generated gastric distension. Gastric dilation, on the other hand, is due to normal physiologic relaxation of gastric muscle with the ingestion of a meal and is termed adaptive relaxation. It should be noted that gastric dilation is not associated with an elevation of intragastric pressure.

There are two proposed explanations for the occurrence of TLESRs. One, favored mainly by gastroenterologists, proposes that TLESRs are due to a neuro-mediated reflex initiated by a pressurized gastric distension or gastric dilation from a meal induced adaptive relaxation. These conditions stimulate stretch receptors in the gastric fundus that in turn stimulate vagal afferents that relay the input from the receptors to the medulla. Medullary nuclei then orchestrate the efferent limb of the reflex via the vagal and phrenic nerves to elicit prolonged LES relaxation, crural diaphragm inhibition, and distal esophageal shortening. The second explanation, favored mainly by surgeons, proposes that TLESRs are due to transient shortening of the LES length with the effacement of the LES by pressurized gastric distension or dilation due to meal induced adaptive relaxation. Normally in the fasting state and resting recumbent position the median overall LES length is 3.6 cm and the intra-abdominal length is 2.2 cm. With gastric distension or dilation, the length of the LES shortens as the LES is effaced and taken up by the gastric fundus. When gastric distention or dilation is excessive, the length of the LES shortens to the point where the corresponding pressure of the LES can no longer maintain closure, the LES opens and gastroesophageal reflux occurs. This occurs predominately during the postprandial period. During shortening, the distal end of the LES is taken up by the fundus and exposed to gastric juice causing inflammation and ulceration of the distal LES. If the inflammation continues, it can permanently reduce the abdominal length to <1 cm and limit the ability of the LES to respond to intra-abdominal pressure challenges. Persistence of the inflammation can reduce the overall length of the LES to <2 cm and limits its ability to resist gastric distension or dilation. In both situations, a transient failure of the LES due to gastric distension or dilation has advanced to a permanent failure of the LES due to the loss of functional sphincter length and the development of axial hiatal hernias from chronic inflammatory injury. At this point, patients develop more severe volume reflux and atypical symptoms such as aspiration and cough. With a completely destroyed barrier, medication will no longer be able to mitigate the symptoms and surgical reconstruction is advised.

The impetus to identify and counsel patients with progressive disease regarding the need for surgical therapy is critical. This goes largely unheeded by the gastroenterologists due to their lack of confidence in the durability of a fundoplication and concern over the side effects of the operation. Consequently, the early referral of a patient with symptoms and signs of progressive disease for surgical therapy is resisted. Further, there is widespread concern that not all surgeons are sufficiently experienced in evaluating esophageal patients, many are not knowledgeable enough to select the proper anti-reflux procedure and some are not sufficiently trained to properly perform the procedures.

While these concerns are valid, I would argue that they are somewhat outdated, as major advances to individualize surgical treatments to the individual patient pathophysiology have evolved over the decades to improve outcomes. For example, we now know that performance of a complete fundoplication on a patient with a normal LES that transiently fails leads to excessive post-prandial symptoms. This occurs because the fundoplication prevents the shortening and opening of the sphincter to relieve post-prandial distension or excessive dilation. As would be expected, these patients complain of bloating, the inability to belch, and social problems associated with increased flatus. These side effects are less frequent and severe when a fundoplication is placed over a LES that has been partially or completely destroyed. Furthermore, it is generally accepted that a modified or partial fundoplication may be a better choice for patients with underlying esophageal body dysmotility or troublesome gas bloat symptoms. The recognition of the differences in side effects between a permanently failed LES and a LES that transiently fails has led to the development of surgical procedures specifically designed to prevent transient LES failure and block the progression to permanent LES failure with minimal surgical dissection and minimal to no side effects. It is hoped that the effectiveness and gentleness of these newer procedures will encourage their use earlier in the course of GERD, when the symptoms and signs of progressive disease first appear.

Overall, advancements in surgical techniques such as modified fundoplication and isolated sphincter augmentation have been made only through dedicated research efforts aimed at unveiling the intricate interaction between anatomy, physiology, function and symptoms of GERD. It is expected that these procedures will interrupt the progression of disease, avoid the complications of end stage GERD, and eliminate the risk of Barrett's esophagus. Armed with a genuine curiosity and fascination of the esophagus and the gastroesophageal reflux barrier similar to my own, editors Lee Swanstrom and Christy Dunst have structured this textbook as a comprehensive resource filled with contributions from the world's most recognized esophageal surgeons. "Antireflux Surgery" is a must-read for anyone performing antireflux surgery today.

Tom R. DeMeester, MD

Preface

Gastroesophageal reflux disease (GERD) is one of the most common medical disorders in the USA, and increasing worldwide, affecting approximately 40 % of the population. GERD may lead to Barrett's esophagus, which is a direct risk factor for esophageal adenocarcinoma of the esophagus. With the incidence of esophageal adenocarcinoma worldwide there is a growing interest in treatment options for gastroesophageal reflux disease. Over $40 billion is spent annually for the treatment of GERD.

The mainstays of GERD treatment include medications and surgery. Antireflux surgery has been an important part of GERD therapy since the 1950s but lost its popularity with the advent of potent antacid medications, specifically proton pump inhibitors. However, in the 1990s laparoscopy introduced a renaissance in the interest in surgical treatment leading to an increase in antireflux procedures. Nevertheless, antireflux surgery is not a "one size fits all" procedure. The various degrees of anatomic derangement of the antireflux barrier, the pathophysiology of reflux, and the complex patient population seeking treatment are complicated and often not understood well enough by the consulting surgeon. Furthermore, the technical difficulty of the operations has led to a lack of consistency in outcomes bringing criticism to the field. Still, with up to 40 % of patients reporting dissatisfaction with current medical therapy, it is imperative that quality surgical options are available.

"Antireflux Surgery" represents the only resource of its kind designed to provide a comprehensive and state-of-the-art overview of the major issues specific to the field compiled as one reliable resource. The book provides exceptional instructional detail as well as comprehensive discussions of relevant pathophysiology. The book includes a comprehensive list of topics important to anyone involved in the care of patients with GERD but is tailored purposefully to meet the needs of the antireflux surgeon with chapters written by recognized esophageal experts from around the world.

Portland, Oregon, USA

Lee L. Swanstrom, MD
Christy M. Dunst, MD

Contents

Contributors

Mehran Anvari, MBBS, PhD, FRCSC, FACS Department of Surgery, St. Joseph's Healthcare Hamilton, Hamilton, Ontario, Canada

Ralph W. Aye, MD, FACS Thoracic and Esophageal Surgery, Swedish Medical Center and Cancer Institute, Swedish Thoracic Surgery, Seattle, WA, USA

Astha J. Bhatt, MD Department of Surgery, St. Agnes Hospital, Baltimore, MD, USA

Luigi Bonavina, MD Division of General Surgery, Department of Biomedical Sciences for Health, IRCCS Policlinico San Donato, Milano, Italy

Nathan W. Bronson, MD Department of Surgery, Oregon Health and Science University, Portland, OR, USA

Dustin A. Carlson, MD Department of Medicine, Northwestern Memorial Hospital, Chicago, IL, USA

Parakrama Chandrasoma, MD, MRCP (UK) Department of Pathology, Los Angeles County – University of Southern California Medical Center, Los Angeles, CA, USA

Nathan Conway, MD Department of Surgery, Tacoma, WA, USA

Bernard Dallemagne, MD Digestive and Endocrine Surgery, NHC – University Hospital of Strasbourg, Strasbourg, France

Steven R. DeMeester, MD Department of Surgery, Keck School of Medicine of the University of Southern California, Los Angeles, CA, USA

Tom R. DeMeester, MD Department of Surgery, Keck Medical Center of USC, San Marino, CA, USA

Christy M. Dunst, MD, FACS Division of GI and MIS Surgery, The Oregon Clinic, Portland, OR, USA

Cecilia Engström, MD, PhD Department of Surgery, Sahlgrenska University Hospital, Goteburg, Sweden

Juan Guo, MD, PhD Department of Pathology, Los Angeles County – University of Southern California Medical Center, Los Angeles, CA, USA

Aditya Gupta, MD Swedish Thoracic Surgery, Swedish Medical Center and Cancer Institute, Seattle, WA, USA

Christina L. Greene, MD Department of Surgery, Keck School of Medicine of the University of Southern California, Los Angeles, CA, USA

Marcelo W. Hinojosa, MD Department of Surgery, University of Washington, Seattle, WA, USA

Toshitaka Hoppo, MD, PhD Department of Surgery, Institute for the Treatment of Esophageal and Thoracic Disease, West Penn Hospital (Allegheny Health Network), Pittsburgh, PA, USA

John G. Hunter, MD Department of Surgery, Oregon Health & Science University, Portland, OR, USA

Blair A. Jobe, MD Department of Surgery, Institute for the Treatment of Esophageal and Thoracic Disease, West Penn Hospital part of Allegheny Health Network, Pittsburgh, PA, USA

Philip O. Katz, MD Division of Gastroenterology, Department of Medicine, Einstein Medical Center, Philadelphia, PA, USA

Ashwin Antony Kurian, MBBS, MD SurgOne Foregut Institute, Englewood, CO, USA

Steven G. Leeds, MD Minimally Invasive Surgery Department, Baylor University Medical Center, Dallas, TX, USA

John C. Lipham, MD Division of Upper GI and General Surgery, Department of Surgery, Keck Medical Center of USC, Los Angeles, CA, USA

Renato A. Luna, MD, MS Servidores do Estado do Rio de Janeiro Hospital, Rio de Janeiro, Brazil

Lars Lundell, MD, PhD Gastrocentrum Surgery, Karolinska University Hospital, Stockholm, Sweden

Stefan Niebisch, MD Gerneral-, Viszeral- and Transplant-Surgery, University of Mainz Medical Center, Mainz, Germany

Brant K. Oelschlager, MD Division of General Surgery, Department of Surgery, University of Washington, Seattle, WA, USA

John E. Pandolfino, MD, MSCI Department of Medicine, Northwestern Memorial Hospital, Chicago, IL, USA

Silvana Perretta, MD Department of Digestive and Endocrine Surgery, NHC Strasbourg, Strasbourg, France

Radu Pescarus, MD Department of Surgery, Hopital Sacre Coeur, Montreal, QC, Canada

Jeffrey H. Peters, MD Department of Surgery, University of Rochester Medical Center, Rochester, NY, USA

Kevin M. Reavis, MD Division of Gastrointestinal and Minimally Invasive Surgery, The Oregon Clinic, Portland, OR, USA

Greta Saino, MD IRCCS Policlinico San Donato, University of Milano Medical School, San Donato Milanese, Italy

Benjamin D. Shogan, MD Department of Surgery, University of Chicago Medical Center, Chicago, IL, USA

Nathaniel J. Soper, MD Department of Surgery, Northwestern University, Chicago, IL, USA

C. Daniel Smith, MD, FACS Department of Surgery, Mayo Clinic Florida, Jacksonville, FL, USA

Lee L. Swanstrom, MD Division of GI and MIS Surgery, Providence Portland Medical Center, Portland, OR, USA

Ezra N. Teitelbaum, MD Department of Surgery, Northwestern University, Chicago, IL, USA

Michael Ujiki, MD, FACS Department of General Surgery, NorthShore University HealthSystem, Evanston, IL, USA

Jorge R. Uribe, MD Department of Medicine, Einstein Medical Center, Philadelphia, PA, USA

Vic Velanovich, MD Department of Surgery, University of South Florida, Tampa, FL, USA

David I. Watson, MBBS, MD, FRACS Flinders University, Department of Surgery, Flinders Medical Centre, South Australia, Australia

Stephanie G. Worrell, MD Department of Surgery, Keck Medical Center of USC, Los Angeles, CA, USA

Andrew S. Wright, MD Department of Surgery, University of Washington, Seattle, WA, USA

Joerg Zehetner, MD, MMM Department of Surgery, Keck School of Medicine of USC, Los Angeles, CA, USA

Part I

The Basics of GERD

Surgical Anatomy of the Esophageal Hiatus

Christy M. Dunst and Steven R. DeMeester

Introduction

The anatomy surrounding the esophageal hiatus is complex and having a clear understanding of the structural relationships in this area is crucial to the esophageal surgeon. This chapter will demonstrate the surgical anatomy of the esophageal hiatus.

The Gastroesophageal Junction

The normal gastroesophageal junction (GEJ) lies within the abdomen just below the esophageal hiatus of the diaphragm. The longitudinal and circular muscular fibers extend from the thoracic esophagus across the GEJ where they are joined by sling fibers that help create the Angle of His (Fig. 1.1). The lower esophageal sphincter (LES) is made up of prominent circular muscles that span the GEJ. The phrenoesophageal ligament (PEL) is an extension of the inferior diaphragmatic fascia and attaches to the esophagus at the GEJ. The PEL serves to seal the esophageal hiatus to maintain separation between the chest and abdominal cavities. The upper layers of the PEL extend into the mediastinum and attach the esophagus to the superior aspect of the diaphragmatic hiatus while the lower layers secure the bottom of the GEJ and proximal stomach to the inferior surface of the diaphragm (Fig. 1.2).

C.M. Dunst, MD, FACS (✉)
Division of GI and MIS Surgery, The Oregon Clinic,
4805 SE Glisan St #6N60, Portland, OR 97213, USA
e-mail: cdunst@orclinic.com

S.R. DeMeester, MD
Department of Surgery, Keck School of Medicine of the University of Southern California, 1510 San Pablo Street, Suite 514, Los Angeles, CA 90033, USA
e-mail: Steven.DeMeester@med.usc.edu

Anatomy of the Diaphragm

The diaphragm has three major openings: the esophageal hiatus, caval hiatus, and the aortic hiatus (Fig. 1.3) The inferior vena cava (IVC) runs posterior to the liver and through the diaphragm at the right side of the central tendon. Although the IVC is generally not encountered during routine antireflux surgery it can be very close to the margin of the right crus during paraesophageal hernia repair (Fig. 1.4). There have been reports of surgeons mistaking the IVC for the right crus or even the esophagus, leading to disastrous complications. The diaphragmatic crura tether the diaphragm to the vertebral column. These "legs" of the diaphragm split from the central tendon and extend around the esophagus to create the hiatus. The area where the legs cross inferiorly to the esophagus and across the aorta is known as the crural decussation and median arcuate ligament. The right crus is typically straight at the hiatus while the left crus tends to bow out towards the left. This has implications when closing the crural defect in hiatal hernia repair as one often must travel farther on the left crus than the right for a symmetric closure.

Exposing the Esophageal Hiatus

Most esophageal surgeries begin with gaining exposure to the esophageal hiatus. The gastrohepatic ligament (GHL) is divided to gain access to the right crus (Fig. 1.5). Typically, the anterior esophageal fat pad is retracted laterally to the left to maximize exposure and the GHL is divided leaving sizable accessory or replaced left hepatic arteries along with the hepatic branch of the vagus nerve intact. This maneuver will expose the right crus so that the PEL can be identified and divided to access the mediastinum and mobilize the GEJ. The left crus is more simply accessed by adjusting the fat pad retraction to the right and rotating the angled camera towards the left (Fig. 1.6). In cases of paraesophageal hernia (PEH),

L.L. Swanstrom and C.M. Dunst (eds.), *Antireflux Surgery*,
DOI 10.1007/978-1-4939-1749-5_1, © Springer New York 2015

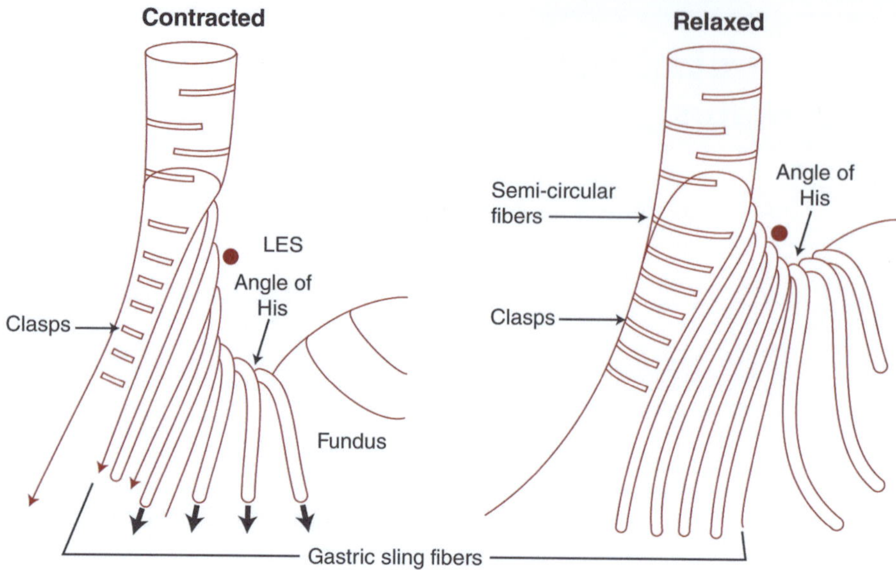

Fig. 1.1 The clasp and sling muscle fibers that make up the lower esophageal reflux barrier in the contracted and relaxed state

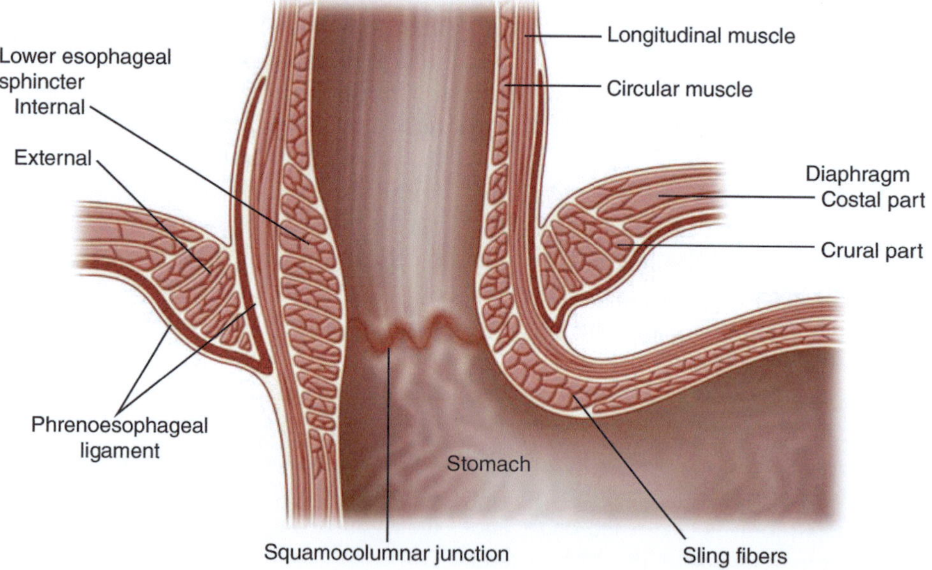

Fig. 1.2 The anatomic relationship of the gastroesophageal junction, the phrenoesophageal ligament, and the diaphragm at the esophageal hiatus

the hiatus is generally exposed and the PEL are elongated and loose (Fig. 1.7). In contrast to the division of the PEL in normal anatomy, this maneuver is actually much easier in a PEH surgery. A typical dissection begins at the 12 o'clock position at the hiatal margin far away from the esophagus (Fig. 1.8).

The posterior vagus nerve will often remain on the base of the right crus with anterior retraction of the esophagus. Care must be taken to make sure that all tissue in front of the decussation is mobilized with the GEJ to avoid injury to the posterior vagus nerve during mobilization of the GEJ (Fig. 1.9). The anterior vagus nerve is typically more embedded into the esophageal wall located at the 12–1 o'clock position at the hiatus. Injury can be avoided with gentle downward traction of the anterior fat pad and careful dissection of this area.

Vascular Anatomy for Foregut Surgery

During routine antireflux surgery, particularly a first time procedure, the risk of a vascular injury or significant bleeding is very low. Apart from difficulty during division of the short gastric vessels the major potential for injury is the

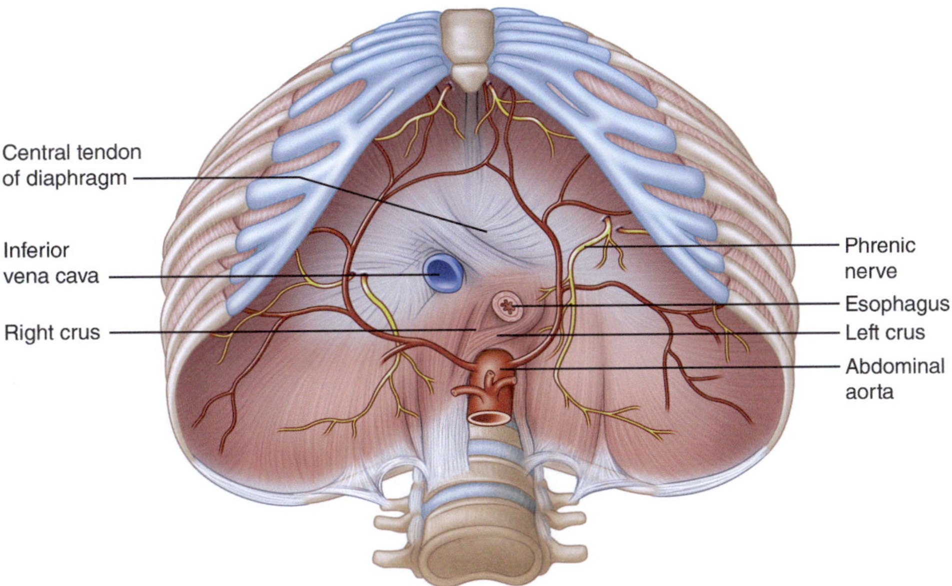

Fig. 1.3 Anatomy of the inferior diaphragm showing the relationships between the esophageal, aortic and inferior vena caval hiatus as well as the central tendon and phrenic nerves

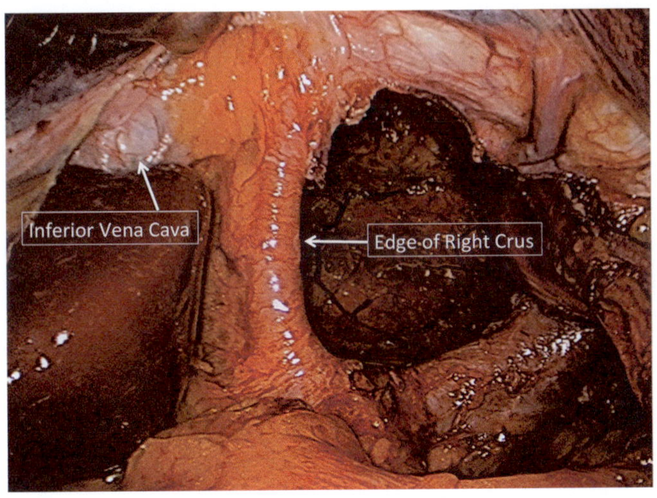

Fig. 1.4 The enlarged diaphragmatic hiatus following paraesophageal hernia reduction surgery. Note the location of the inferior vena cava in relation to the right crus

progressively anteriorly from the hiatus to the aortic arch. Consequently the dissection along the aorta must not be done in a horizontal plane, but instead should always move anteriorly as the dissection is continued upwards into the mediastinum. During this aortic dissection the esophageal perforators should be identified and carefully ligated with an energy device or clips at a slight distance from the aortic wall to prevent the significant aortic bleeding that can occur should one of these be sheared off flush with the aorta. Another reason to identify the aorta in the mediastinum is that it facilitates safe crural closure particularly during the first several sutures at the decussation of the right and left crura. A sudden hematoma near the aorta after suture placement may indicate that the suture needle hit or traversed the aorta, but it can also occur secondary to bleeding from a crural artery, particularly on the left crus. However, if there is any suspicion that the suture went into the aorta it must be removed to prevent the development of a pseudoaneurysm that can have potentially lethal consequences. Usually, holding pressure is all that is necessary after removal of the needle, but if not the injury will have to be suture repaired.

During PEH repairs dissection in the mediastinum will commonly encounter the azygous vein (Fig. 1.12). This is particularly true when the pleura is firmly adherent to the hernia sac and the right pleural space is entered. Further, in some patients the aorta is quite far to the left and upward dissection in the mediastinum, in an area where the aorta should be located, reveals the azygous instead. Injury is rare, but the significant low pressure bleeding can be challenging to control.

Another potential source of bleeding is the left gastric vessels. During PEH repair when ½ or more of the stomach is

aorta. Particularly in thin patients the aorta can be very close to the right and left crus. Care must be exercised when initially developing the plane between the right crus and esophagus to not go too far posterior and encounter the aorta. Similarly when mobilizing the left side of the esophagus it is critical to have the aorta in sight as the tissues between the esophagus and left crus are separated (Fig. 1.10). This is facilitated by identifying the aorta early in the mediastinal dissection during mobilization of the esophagus (Fig. 1.11). During PEH repairs it is also important to remember that many of these patients are kyphotic and the aorta moves

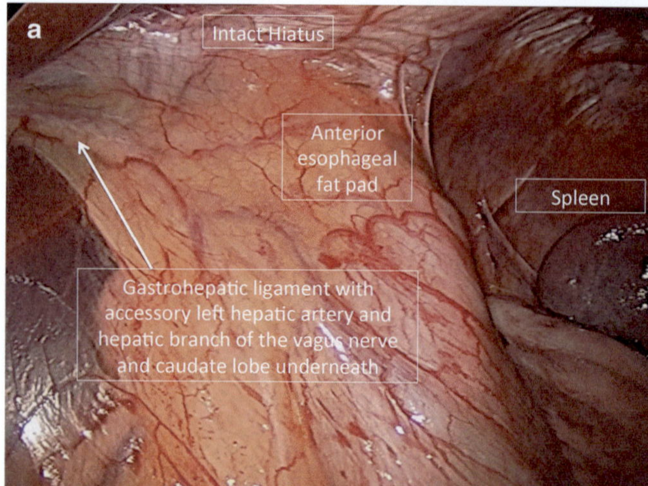

Fig. 1.5 Division of the gastrohepatic ligament provides access to the right crus. (**a**) Anatomy at the beginning of an esophageal surgery with normal anatomy. (**b**) Division of the gastrohepatic ligament, leaving the accessory left hepatic artery and hepatic branch of the vagus nerve intact, provides exposure to the right crus

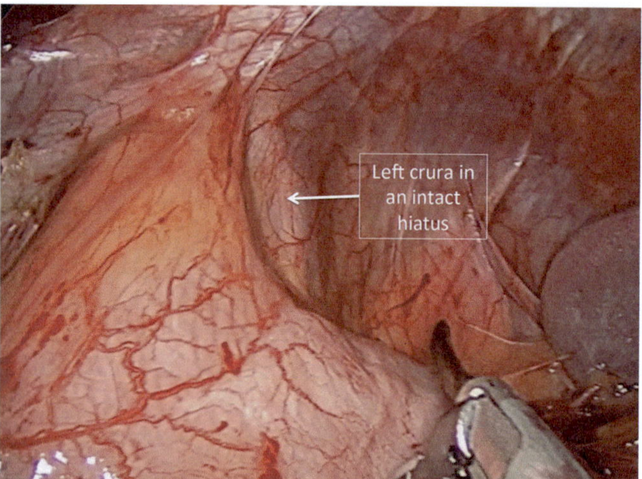

Fig. 1.6 Identifying the left crus

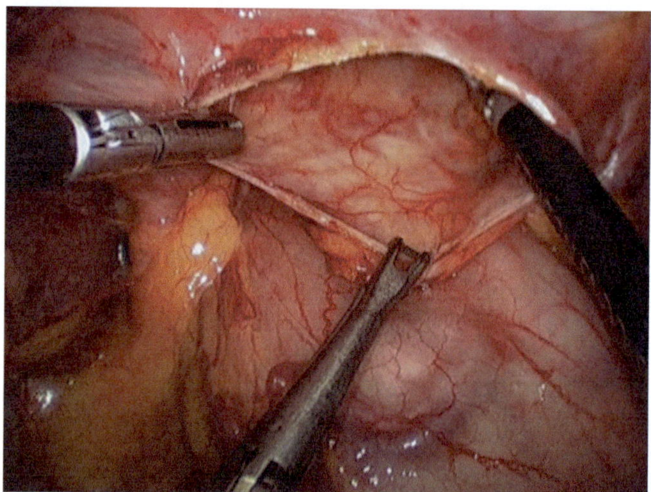

Fig. 1.8 The PEL is divided at the 12 o'clock position and the dissection plane developed to reduce the hernia sac from the mediastinum. The PEL is then divided circumferentially as the hernia is reduced

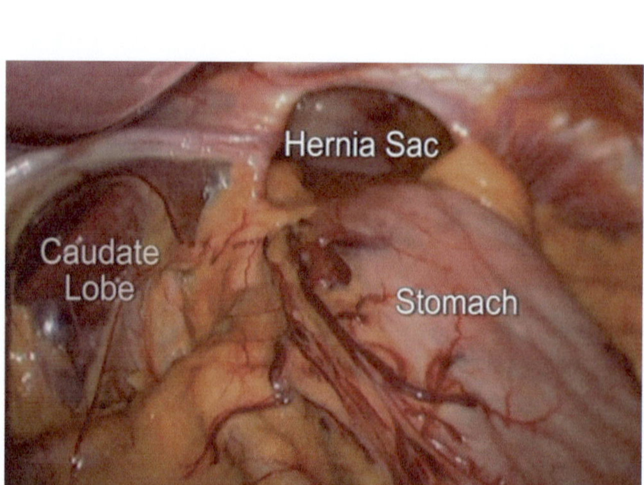

Fig. 1.7 Typical anatomy in a paraesophageal hernia

intra-thoracic it is a virtual certainty that the left gastric vessels have migrated up into the chest (Fig. 1.13). Initial dissection along the right crus as is done for a routine laparoscopic fundoplication is therefore ill-advised. Instead, the safest way to approach a PEH is with initial sac dissection starting at the 12–2 o'clock position on the hiatus. After the sac is sufficiently mobilized and collapsed there should be almost no resistance when reducing the intra-thoracic contents, including the left gastric vessels, back into the abdomen (Fig. 1.14). This then allows safe dissection of the sac off the right crus. Injury to the left gastric vessels is usually controllable but can compromise the perfusion of the GEJ and especially of a Collis gastroplasty if one is necessary. Although uncommon, the splenic artery can also migrate upward towards or even

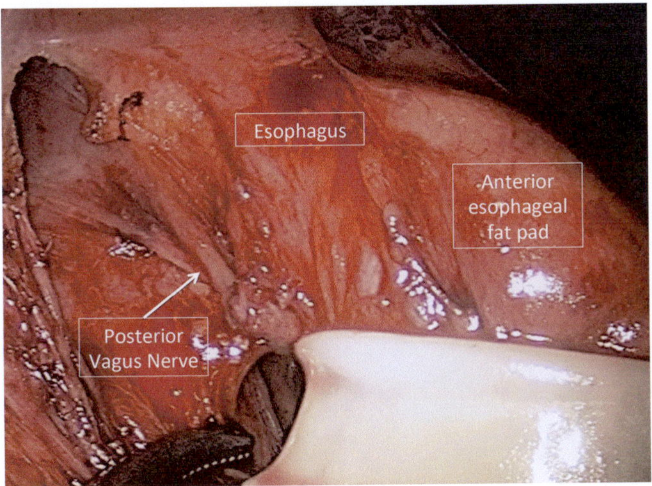

Fig. 1.9 Mobilization of the GEJ during a LINX procedure leaving the PEL intact and identifying the posterior vagus nerve

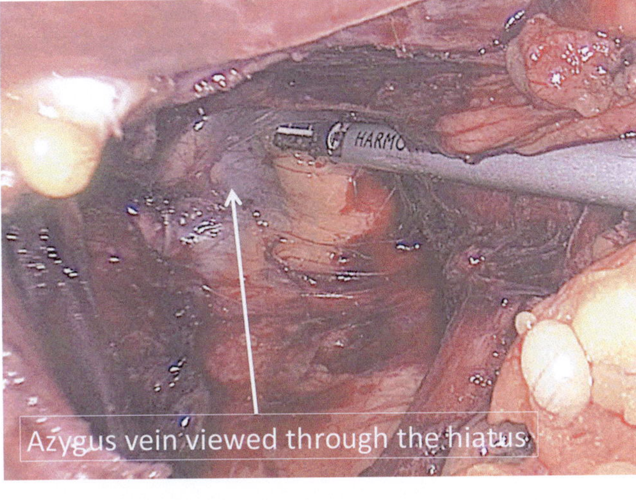

Fig. 1.12 The azygus vein is exposed during excision of the hernia sac and esophageal mobilization in a patient with a large paraesophageal hernia. The aorta is seen just below the left crus

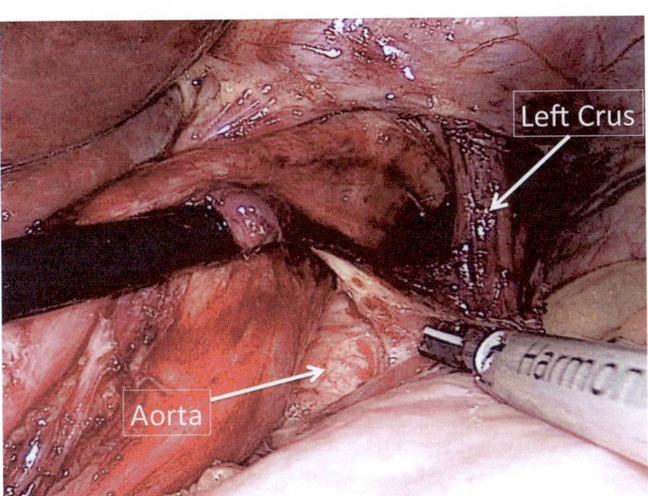

Fig. 1.10 The aorta is typically very close to the base of the left crus, and when working inside the left crus it is critical that the aorta has initially been exposed from the right side to avoid inadvertent injury

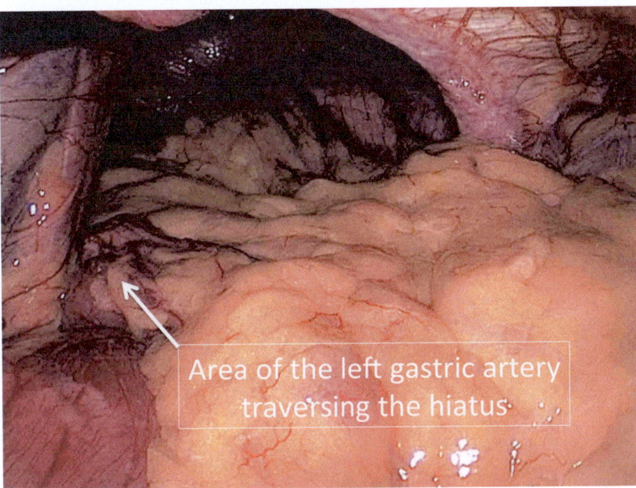

Fig. 1.13 In this patient with intra-thoracic volvulized stomach the left gastric vessels are up in the chest. Starting the sac dissection along the right side can lead to injury of these vessels. There is no need to reduce the stomach at all at this point. Instead, the sac dissection should commence at the readily visible 2 o'clock position. Inferiorly along the left crus the splenic artery must be identified since it may have moved up into the chest in patients with a very large hiatus like this

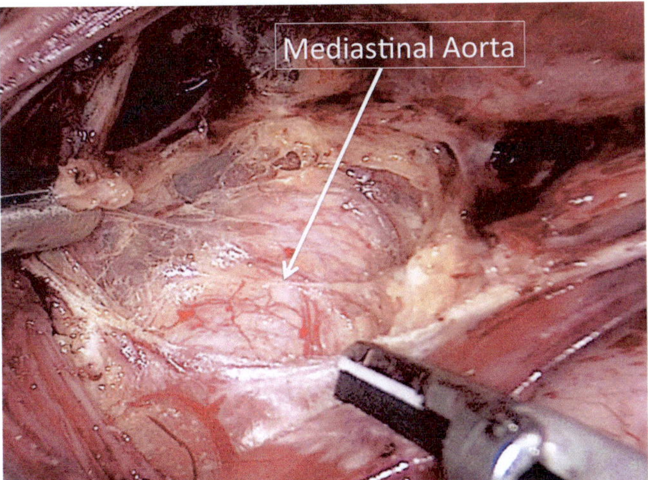

Fig. 1.11 Exposure of the aorta from the right side with the esophagus elevated using a penrose drain. The crural decussation is visible at the bottom of the image. Clear exposure of the aorta facilitates safe placement of the crural closure sutures

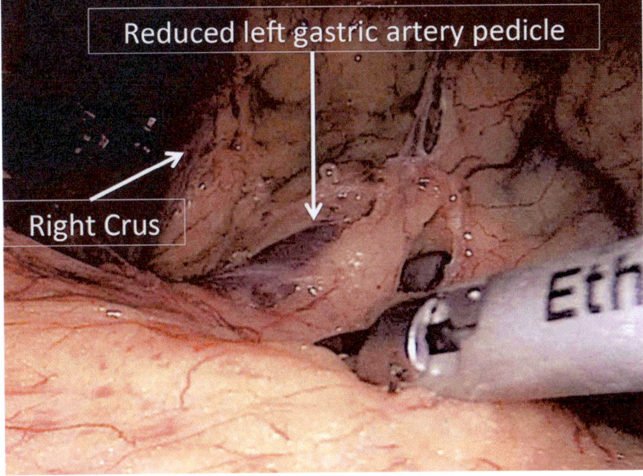

Fig. 1.14 The stomach and hernia sac have been reduced and now the left gastric vessels are clearly visible in the abdomen below the right crus

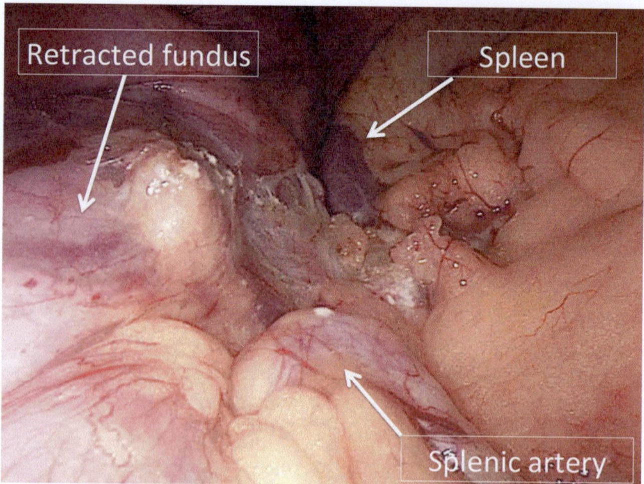

Fig. 1.15 The splenic artery visible along the posterior border of the stomach when viewed inside the lesser sac. In patients with a large PEH it can be next to or up inside the left crus

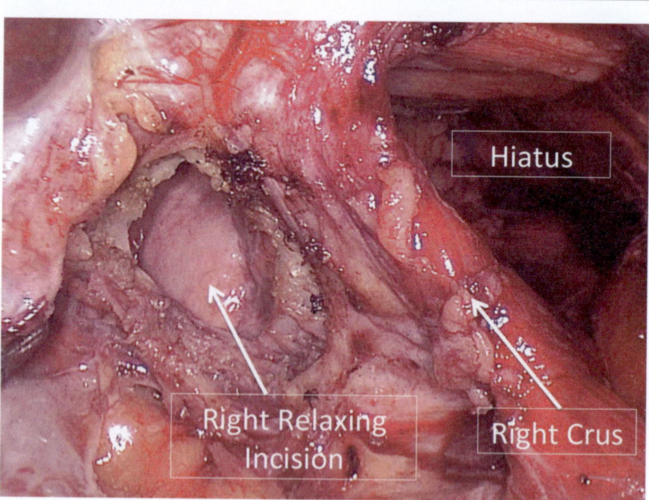

Fig. 1.17 Location of a right relaxing incision

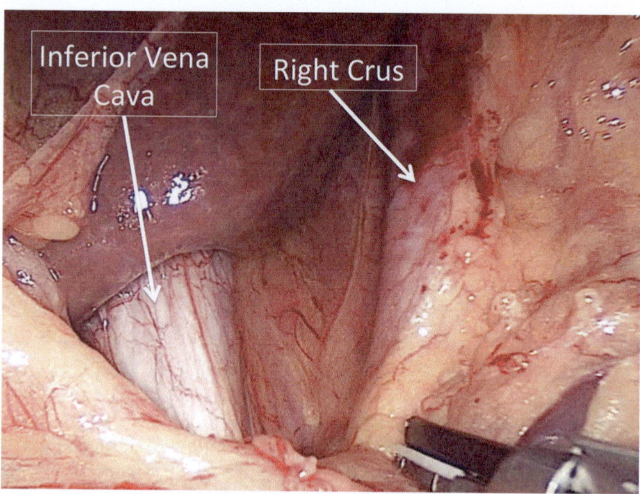

Fig. 1.16 The inferior vena cava is normally protected by the caudate lobe of the liver but on redo operations it may be adhered to the right crus

above the hiatus into the chest in patients with a large PEH. It is important during mobilization of the greater curve and fundus that the splenic artery is identified to avoid inadvertent injury as it can sometimes curl up close to the left crus (Fig. 1.15). Division of the short gastric vessels is typically easy in patients with a PEH since they are quite elongated.

Lastly, the inferior vena cava can be in the vicinity of the dissection of the right crus, particularly during a redo procedure with extensive adhesions (Fig. 1.16). It also must be watched along with the intra-thoracic vena cava during a right-sided crural relaxing incision (Fig. 1.17). The right crus should be at least 1 cm in width to allow sufficient tissue for secure crural closure with a relaxing incision. At the most superior aspect of the right crural dissection one encounters the left hepatic vein where it empties into the vena cava. If injury to these major venous structures happens pressure should be applied while deciding whether to perform the repair laparoscopically or by converting to open.

During a standard laparoscopic Nissen or PEH repair these are the major relevant vascular structures. If a right crural relaxing incision is necessary to allow primary crural closure with minimal tension then two other structures come into play. The first is the thoracic duct, which traverses with the aorta through the aortic hiatus. Since the release gained with a right crural relaxing incision is most needed anteriorly, there should be no reason to be down near the crural decussation and in a position to injury the thoracic duct. A more legitimate concern is injury to the intra-thoracic vena cava by excessive upward or anterior extension of the relaxing incision. This injury must be avoided by staying inferior to the anterior crural vein which typically runs across the diaphragm just above the apex of the hiatus and delineates the anterior extent of a right relaxing incision. Staying below this vein during a right crural relaxing incision typically avoids the intra-thoracic vena cava.

Conclusion

Understanding of the structural relationships of the esophageal hiatus is essential to the esophageal surgeon. While significant bleeding from injury to a major vascular structure is rare during a routine foregut surgery, it is important to identify the anatomy sufficiently to visualize the areas of potential trouble. Having a clear understanding of this complex area will promote surgical efficiency and will go a long way towards preventing injury during foregut surgery.

Parakrama Chandrasoma and Juan Guo

Introduction

The entire esophagus is lined by stratified squamous epithelium from its proximal cricopharyngeal end to its distal limit at the gastroesophageal junction. In the normal person, the squamous epithelium is protected from exposure to gastric contents by the lower esophageal sphincter.

The cellular changes of reflux occur when the lower esophageal sphincter fails to protect the esophageal squamous epithelium and allows it to become exposed to gastric contents. Reflux is like a battle to attack a target (the esophageal squamous epithelium) with the lower esophageal sphincter being the defense and gastric juices the offense.

Exposure of esophageal squamous epithelium occurs when there is free reflux of gastric contents into the esophagus as a result of temporary sphincter relaxation or permanent sphincter destruction. The latter is the primary cause and sine qua non of chronic gastroesophageal reflux disease. When the barrier of adequately high sphincter pressure is removed, reflux tends to occur because there is a pressure gradient from positive in the gastric lumen to negative in the intra-thoracic esophagus. Such free reflux can be measured by an abnormal 24-h pH test where a pH sensitive electrode placed in the distal esophagus detects acid exposure, which is a marker of exposure of the esophagus to gastric contents.

Exposure of the squamous epithelium to gastric juice may occur during the post-prandial period if the stomach becomes over-distended without there being free reflux into the esophagus. Gastric over-distension and increased intra-gastric pressure put pressure on the sphincter, causing it to shorten. As the sphincter is effaced, there is an effective downward movement of the squamo-columnar junction, causing the squamous epithelium to be progressively exposed to the environment of the stomach and thus the gastric juice. This mechanism of the descent of the squamo-columnar junction into the stomach can be simulated and observed when the stomach is insufflated with air during endoscopy.

The changes caused by reflux in the esophageal mucosa must initially be limited to changes in the squamous epithelium because there is no other epithelium in the normal esophagus. However, one of the consequences of chronic reflux disease is columnar metaplasia of the squamous epithelium. This appears to occur early in the course of reflux disease and is seen at a microscopic level in the vast majority if not all patients with chronic reflux disease [1, 2]. Once columnar metaplasia has occurred in the esophagus the gastric contents cause a range of pathologic changes in this metaplastic columnar epithelium that is very different than in the native squamous epithelium.

Present management algorithms of reflux disease are directed towards control of symptoms and of erosive esophagitis. Symptoms and erosive esophagitis are largely the result of acute damage to the squamous epithelium caused by acid exposure. These acute squamous epithelial changes are reversible and largely curable with acid suppressive drug therapy. The metaplastic columnar epithelium of patients with reflux disease is more resistant to acid and less sensitive than squamous epithelium. Acid suppressive drug therapy is, however, not aimed at addressing the pathologic changes in metaplastic columnar epithelium.

Management guidelines that single-mindedly emphasize acid neutralization and acid suppressive drug therapy to treat patients with reflux disease have been in place for five decades. The increasing effectiveness of acid suppression in this time frame has resulted in better control of symptoms, improved healing of erosive esophagitis, and prevention of chronic squamous epithelial complications such as deep intractable ulcers and strictures. Alkalinization of gastric contents is powerful in protecting and healing the esophageal squamous epithelium in a patient with reflux [3].

P. Chandrasoma, MD, MRCP (UK) • J. Guo, MD, PhD (✉)
Department of Pathology, Los Angeles County –
University of Southern California Medical Center,
1100 N. State Street, Room CT7A120,
Los Angeles, CA 90033, USA
e-mail: ptchandr@usc.edu; juanguo9999@gmail.com

L.L. Swanstrom and C.M. Dunst (eds.), *Antireflux Surgery*,
DOI 10.1007/978-1-4939-1749-5_2, © Springer New York 2015

During the past five decades, however, there has been an explosion in the incidence of Barrett esophagus and esophageal adenocarcinoma which are columnar epithelial complications of reflux disease. We will explore the possibility that Barrett's esophagus and adenocarcinoma may be promoted by the alkalinization of gastric contents that result from acid suppression.

The Offense: Gastric Contents

The composition of gastric contents represents the offensive side of the equation of the pathology of reflux. If gastric contents were not noxious to esophageal squamous epithelium, there would be no "reflux disease" even if reflux were to occur. Gastric contents include gastric secretions which contains acid and pepsin, ingested food and saliva, and duodenal contents if the patient has duodeno-gastric reflux. Duodenal contents include bile and proximal small intestinal enzymes.

Present management with acid suppressive drugs is based on the premise that neutralizing or suppressing secretion of acid in the stomach converts the gastric contents from being noxious to esophageal mucosa to being innocuous. The single minded emphasis on acid suppression in the medical treatment of reflux disease only makes logical sense because the medical community believes that acid is the cause of every pathologic change that occurs in esophageal mucosa. This is likely to be close to the truth for esophageal squamous epithelium, but not for metaplastic columnar epithelium.

In contrast, surgical treatment of reflux disease with some type of repair or augmentation of the function of the lower esophageal sphincter aims at decreasing or preventing reflux. If successful, exposure of both squamous and metaplastic columnar esophageal epithelia to all gastric molecules is prevented.

Converting the strong acid milieu of gastric contents to an alkaline milieu has unintended consequences that are recognized complications of long-term proton pump inhibitor use. Decreased absorption of minerals results in decreased bone density and hip fractures [4]; bacterial infections are increased, notably *Clostridium difficile* colitis [5]. Little attention has been paid, however, to assessing whether gastric alkalinization promotes intestinal metaplasia (i.e., Barrett esophagus) and progression to adenocarcinoma in metaplastic esophageal columnar epithelia.

The stomach in its resting state between meals and after it has emptied completely contains the low volume of resting acid secretion by the parietal cells. In the normal individual, the resting state gastric juice has a pH of 1–2. The empty stomach is collapsed, with the mucosal rugae being maximally folded.

With food ingestion the stomach distends, slowly flattening the mucosal rugal folds and the gastric glands are stimulated to rapidly increase acid and enzyme secretion. The secreted acid mixes with the food, which tends to be near the neutral pH range, and results in a pH of the gastric contents that varies with the type and volume of the meal. It has been shown that the gastric pH in the stomach that contains food is not constant throughout the column of food. In particular, there appears to be a very low pH pocket (the "acid pocket") at the top of the food column [6]. When the stomach is full after a heavy meal, this acid pocket is in the proximal stomach, very close to the distal end of the LES and squamous epithelium of the esophagus.

This normal condition of gastric contents can be altered significantly by three relatively common situations that may exist in a large percentage of patients in different populations:

Helicobacter pylori Infection

Helicobacter pylori infection varies greatly in incidence in different populations. It is interesting that in those populations where *H. pylori* is prevalent, such as South Korea and Japan, the incidence of gastric adenocarcinoma is high and that of Barrett esophagus and esophageal adenocarcinoma is low. This has led to the suggestion that *H. pylori* infection is protective against reflux disease. The reason why this could be true is that chronic *H. pylori* gastritis is often associated with atrophic gastritis and hypochlorhydria. The low acid secretion in the stomach acts as a natural acid suppressant.

In populations where *H. pylori* has a high prevalence, infection likely occurs early in life and the hypochlorhydric state prevents squamous epithelial damage and columnar metaplasia.

In populations where *H. pylori* is uncommon such as the USA and Western Europe, reflux usually occurs without the natural acid suppression associated with the infection and results in columnar metaplasia. *H. pylori* infection occurring after columnar metaplasia has been generated can limit further squamous epithelial damage but will not prevent damage to the already established columnar mucosa in the esophagus.

Duodeno-Gastric Reflux

Duodeno-gastric reflux is characterized by alkaline duodenal contents that contain bile salts and acids, bilirubin and duodenal enzymes refluxing into the stomach. Duodeno-gastric reflux is a relatively common phenomenon. Reflux of duodenal contents neutralizes gastric acid to an extent that depends on the volume and frequency of entry of duodenal contents into the stomach. It therefore effectively increases gastric pH.

When duodeno-gastric reflux is present in a patient who has gastroesophageal reflux, the term duodeno-gastro-esophageal reflux is sometimes used. The presence of duodenal admixture in the refluxate can be measured by placing a sensor in the lower esophagus that recognizes a unique duodenal molecule such as bilirubin. Bilitec is such a probe that was used in the past and provided excellent data on the effect of duodenal admixture in the refluxed gastric contents.

The presence of duodenal elements in gastric contents significantly influences the pathologic changes seen in the esophageal mucosa in reflux disease. The damage to squamous epithelium resulting from a mixture of gastric and duodenal material is greater than gastric material alone. The prevalence of Barrett's esophagus is significantly associated with a positive Bilitec test [7]. Bile salts/acids have been shown in vitro to suppress genes that maintain squamous epithelium and activate genes that promote columnar metaplasia of squamous epithelial cells, intestinal metaplasia in columnar epithelium, and carcinogenesis [8, 9].

Evidence has also been presented that suggest that bile salts/acids entering the stomach have different activity at different gastric pH. In a strong acid milieu, the bile salts/acids become inactivated by precipitation. At a pH above 6, they remain ionized, in solution, and do not produce oncogenic mutations in animals. At a gastric pH of 3–5, the bile salts/acids become un-ionized and capable of producing oncogenic mutations in the esophageal epithelial cells. The typical gastric pH achieved with medical treatment of reflux disease with acid suppressive drugs is also 3–5.

Based on these data, many authorities believe that some derivative of bile salts/acids is the most likely agent involved in the genesis of adenocarcinoma in the esophageal mucosa in patients with reflux. There is no doubt that the carcinogen is present in the gastric contents and delivered to the esophageal mucosa by reflux. A recent radical surgical treatment for Barrett esophagus proposed by Csendes et al. [10] separates the duodenum from the stomach, precluding bile entry into the stomach. In his series with significant follow-up, no patients so treated progressed to adenocarcinoma, suggesting that bile in the refluxed gastric contents plays an important role in carcinogenesis.

Acid Suppressive Drug Therapy

Acid suppressive drug therapy aims to control gastric pH. There is good evidence that maintaining the gastric pH above 4 for greater than 12 h is an effective method of controlling heartburn and causing erosions to heal [3]. When the gastric pH is maintained above this level, symptoms and erosions are effectively prevented in the majority of patients with reflux. Proton pump inhibitors used in adequate dosage have the capability of suppressing acid secretion to a level that maintains pH for 12–18 h of the day [11]. Histamine-2 receptor antagonists are less effective and acid neutralizing agents have only a temporary effect in alkalinizing gastric contents.

The Defense: The Lower Esophageal Sphincter

The lower esophageal sphincter is a high-pressure zone that occupies the distal 3–5 cm of the esophagus, including the entire extent of the abdominal part of the esophagus. Competence of the sphincter depends on its resting pressure, total length, and abdominal length [12]. In the normal person, the sphincter relaxes to permit venting of intra-gastric gas, resulting in belching.

Whenever the lower esophageal sphincter fails to function normally, either because of permanent damage or transient relaxation, free reflux of gastric contents into the esophagus occurs when there is a sufficient pressure gradient from stomach to esophagus that overcomes any residual sphincter function.

Reflux is a dynamic event. It can be likened to a jet of water issuing from a vertically held hose when the tap is opened. In a patient with a mildly damaged sphincter and high-pressure gradient, reflux will have a jet-like form with a low volume and higher progression into the esophagus. With a severely damaged sphincter and a low pressure gradient, the flow will be higher in volume with a lower retrograde propulsive force. The entry of gastric contents into the esophagus results in a response from the esophagus designed to clear the refluxed contents back into the stomach, probably by a stimulation of secondary peristalsis. The effectiveness of this clearing also varies, depending on the structural integrity of the esophageal muscle wall. Variations in the nature of the column of reflux, volume of reflux, and efficiency of clearing greatly influences the time of contact of the refluxed molecules with the esophageal epithelium. Impedance technology permits measurement of the rate of flow and height of the refluxed column. There is no ability to accurately measure volume of reflux.

Whatever the form of reflux, it creates a volume and pressure gradient in the esophagus. In the normal state, the esophagus is empty and at an approximately neutral pH 7. Immediately beyond the distal end of the sphincter the pH is strongly acidic. In both resting stomach and in the full stomach with its acid pocket, the pH immediately distal to the gastroesophageal junction is highly acidic (pH 1–2). The intra-gastric volume near the junction varies with the degree of gastric filling. When reflux occurs, a volume gradient is created in the esophagus as the refluxate is propelled upward. The exposure of the esophageal epithelium to every molecule in gastric juice is highest in the most distal esophagus and lowest at the top of the column of refluxed material, where it is zero (the normal state of the esophagus). This includes hydrogen ions; which means that a pH gradient is created that equals the baseline pH of gastric juice in the most distal esophagus and equal to the neutral esophageal pH at the height of the column. The amount of exposure of the esophageal epithelium to molecules in the refluxate is dependent on the volume of refluxed material and the efficiency of esophageal clearing, factors that are largely unmeasurable today.

Understanding this pathophysiology of reflux is critical to elucidating the reasons behind the observed pathologic changes that occur in the esophageal epithelium in patients with reflux. The lower esophageal sphincter is a physiological valve. Like any valve, it maintains zero volume and pH 7 on the esophageal side and higher volume (which increases during gastric filling) and a strong acid pH on the gastric side. Like any valve, the result of failure is an obliteration of these sharp gradients [13].

The Target: The Esophageal Squamous Epithelium

Squamous epithelium lining the normal esophagus is a non-keratinizing stratified squamous epithelium. This consists of a basal layer of cells containing stem cells. Above this is a proliferative basal zone consisting of 2–3 layers of cells. In the normal steady state, the basal cell layer is less than 30 % of the thickness of the epithelium. The proliferative cells undergo mitotic division to continually replace cells lost from the surface. A newly produced daughter cell in the proliferative zone is shed 4–6 days later at the surface [14].

The normal differentiation of the squamous epithelium is under the direction of a genetic signal which is most likely a gene in the Wnt complex. The presence of this signal in the dividing cells causes the daughter cells of mitotic division to differentiate towards keratinocytes and move towards the surface.

In addition to the epithelium, the mucosa of the esophagus contains the lamina propria and the muscularis mucosae. The lamina propria of the normal esophagus is scanty and consists largely of collagen with few inflammatory cells. The muscularis mucosa is a thin bi-layered smooth muscle layer. Mucous glands are present in the mucosa and submucosa. The ducts of these mucous glands pass through the mucosa and traverse the squamous epithelium to open at the surface. The mucin secreted by these glands serves to lubricate the squamous epithelium.

Neural elements present in the mucosa are so fine that they are not visible in routine sections. There are nerve endings in the stratified squamous epithelium that are largely afferent sensory nerves. Some of these are pain-sensitive. Others may be involved in local reflex arcs with the neurons in the submucosa and myenteric plexus that probably coordinate peristalsis and maintain sphincter tone. The vagus nerve innervates the esophagus and influences local neural pathways but are not essential to motor or sphincter function which persist even after complete denervation.

The normal stratified squamous epithelium of the esophagus consists of cells that are bound to each other by tight cell junctions in the cell membranes. This results in an epithelium that is impermeable to molecules in the lumen. The surface epithelium is exposed to luminal molecules during swallowing and if the esophagus is exposed to gastric contents. One function of the normal squamous epithelium is to prevent entry of these luminal molecules into the epithelium; the deep proliferative zone and stem cells are therefore protected.

The stage for epithelial battle with gastric contents when reflux occurs due to failure of the lower esophageal sphincter is now set. There are two epithelia in the normal person's upper digestive tract: normal stratified squamous in the esophagus and normal gastric oxyntic in the stomach. Normal gastric oxyntic mucosa is immune to damage by gastric contents. Esophageal squamous epithelium undergoes damage when exposed to gastric contents.

Definition of Normal Esophagus and Gastroesophageal Junction

The accurate definition of the gastroesophageal junction is critical in understanding the pathologic changes in the mucosa as a result of GERD. At present, the gastroesophageal junction is defined endoscopically as the proximal limit of the rugal folds [15]. It is well known that the inter-observer variability is high amongst clinicians asked to define the gastroesophageal junction using this definition. The American Gastroenterological Association consensus workshop recommended using this definition despite the fact that there was little or no evidence to support it; this was an opinion-based definition [16].

In 2007, Chandrasoma et al. [17], in a study of esophagectomy specimens, proposed that the definition of the true gastroesophageal junction was not possible by endoscopic criteria. The reason for this was that early damage to the abdominal segment of the lower esophageal sphincter and the associated columnar metaplasia results in dilatation of the damaged lower esophagus [2]. The GERD-damaged dilated distal esophagus became part of the gastric reservoir distal to the intact tubal esophagus, eventually developing rugal folds. The dilated distal esophagus has long been mistaken for proximal stomach at endoscopy because it was distal to the proximal limit of rugal folds. This study showed that there exists a variable length of metaplastic columnar epithelium distal to the proximal limit of rugal folds and the end of the tubal esophagus. In full thickness sections, this segment of metaplastic columnar epithelium was concordant with the presence of esophageal submucosal glands, proving that this was dilated distal esophagus rather than proximal stomach. Chandrasoma et al. proposed that the true definition of the gastroesophageal junction was the proximal limit of

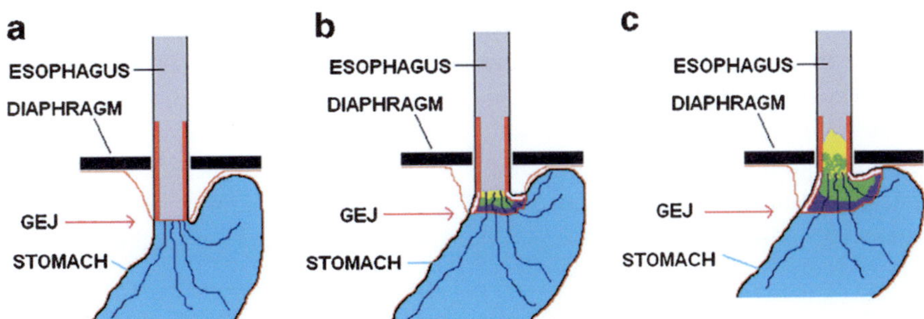

Fig. 2.1 Anatomy and histology in normal and increasing severity of chronic reflux disease. (**a**) In the normal patient, the esophagus is lined by squamous epithelium (*gray*) and the stomach is lined by gastric oxyntic mucosa with rugal folds (*blue*). There is no separation of squamous and oxyntic mucosa. (**b**): In mild reflux disease, the lower esophageal sphincter is shortened permanently and this is concordant with a dilated distal esophagus that is lined by metaplastic columnar epithe- lium (shown here as three types—*yellow*=intestinal metaplasia; *green*=cardiac mucosa; *purple*=oxyntocardiac mucosa). Note the partial loss of the acute angle of His and the presence of rugal folds in the dilated distal esophagus. (**c**): In severe reflux disease, the sphincter damage is greater, the dilated distal esophagus is larger, and there is columnar metaplasia in the distal tubal esophagus. Note the further decrease in the angle of His

gastric oxyntic mucosa, defined histologically. Because it is not possible to distinguish gastric oxyntic mucosa from metaplastic esophageal columnar epithelium in the dilated distal esophagus at endoscopy, it is also not possible to accurately define the true gastroesophageal junction at endoscopy. Submucosal glands are rarely seen in endoscopic mucosal biopsies. However, biopsies from metaplastic columnar epithelium of the esophagus may show the glandular ducts of these glands as they penetrate the mucosa [18].

If this new evidence-based histologic definition of the gastroesophageal junction is accepted over the present opinion-based endoscopic definition, the pathologic changes in the esophagus in early reflux disease become clear [2]. The squamous epithelium normally extends to the end of the esophagus where it transitions to gastric oxyntic mucosa which lines the proximal stomach (Fig. 2.1). This transition point is the gastroesophageal junction. Histologically, there is no other type of epithelium between esophageal squamous epithelium and gastric oxyntic mucosa in the normal gastroesophageal junction, i.e., the squamo-oxyntic gap is normally "zero" [1, 19].

The presence of cardiac mucosa, or non-intestinalized columnar mucosa, as a normal phenomena between the normal epithelium of the proximal stomach and squamous esophagus is a false dogma. This falsehood, based on observations made in the 1960s [20], is still accepted by the medical community despite powerful evidence against it, and prevents correct interpretation of histologic changes in reflux [21]. The new histologic definition of the gastroesophageal junction explains why pathology in the endoscopically defined "gastric cardia" such as intestinal metaplasia and adenocarcinoma has an association with GERD and not with distal gastric pathology. Intestinal metaplasia and adenocarcinoma of the gastric cardia are in reality intestinal metaplasia and sometimes adenocarcinoma of the dilated distal esophagus.

Reflux-Induced Damage to Esophageal Squamous Epithelium

Structural Cellular Changes

Exposure of esophageal squamous epithelium to gastric contents causes damage. It is almost certain that acid is the main cause of squamous epithelial damage although suggestion has been made that a combination of acid and bile and/or pepsin is more potent in producing damage than acid alone.

The first change in the squamous epithelium induced by acid is likely to be intraepithelial edema, referred to as "dilated intercellular spaces [22]" and an increase in the rate of loss of surface keratinocytes from the epithelium as a result of direct damage to the surface cells. This results in a more rapid turnover of the squamous cells. Increased surface loss stimulates the proliferative zone cells to increase in number as well as proliferative activity in order to maintain the structural integrity of the epithelium. This is seen morphologically as an increased thickness of the basal cell zone of the epithelium to greater than 30 % of epithelial thickness. This basal cell hyperplasia is associated with elongation of the papillary processes between the rete pegs; these papillary processes become highly vascularized. Staining of the epithelium with Ki67 shows that the proliferative zone has expanded considerably.

Damage to superficial keratinocytes by acid also results in the release of cytokines. These diffuse across the epithelium into the lamina propria where they have many potential effects. One of these is that many of these cytokines are chemo-attractive to eosinophil leukocytes which migrate into the epithelium, usually in small numbers.

With severe damage to the epithelium, superficial erosions may occur in the epithelium and can progress to ulcers that involve the full thickness of the mucosa. Healing associated with these ulcers can induce fibrous strictures in the esophagus.

It is important to note that reflux disease is not associated with an increased incidence of *squamous* carcinoma of the esophagus. This is fortuitous and implies that gastric contents do not contain molecules that can interact with cell receptors in squamous epithelium and induce mutational changes that result in oncogenic transformation of squamous epithelial cells to squamous dysplasia and carcinoma.

Endoscopic Features

Endoscopic examination of the squamous epithelium is relatively insensitive for the diagnosis of reflux disease. Hyperemia and gross erosions are used as the main diagnostic criteria. The extent of erosions has been used to classify erosive esophagitis into increasing grades of severity (A–D) in the Los Angeles classification [23].

Unfortunately, erosive esophagitis is present in only a minority of patients with symptomatic reflux disease, making it a relatively insensitive endoscopic diagnostic criterion. The presence of erosions is also not specific for reflux disease; erosions may occur in many other esophageal diseases such as infections and pemphigus vulgaris. However, in a patient with clinical reflux disease, the presence of erosions is useful to separate patients into those with and without erosive disease. Patients with erosive esophagitis tend to have more complications and their symptoms are less easily controlled by medical therapy. Patients with clinical reflux disease who have no visible endoscopic abnormality fall into a designation of "non-erosive reflux disease" or NERD.

Biopsy Diagnosis of Reflux Esophagitis

The microscopic changes of squamous epithelial damage represent the presently used criteria for the biopsy diagnosis of reflux disease. A combination of dilated intercellular spaces, basal cell hyperplasia with increased expression of Ki67 by immunoperoxidase staining, increased height of papillary ridges and the presence of intraepithelial eosinophils are histologic features that are associated with reflux esophagitis.

Unfortunately, these morphologic changes in squamous epithelium are of little value in the practical diagnosis of reflux disease. All of these are relatively nonspecific general features of tissue injury rather than specific changes due to reflux. All of these can be seen in esophageal disease other than reflux, notably allergic (eosinophilic) esophagitis [24]. These diagnostic criteria are also not very sensitive; approximately 50 % of patients with symptomatic reflux will not have significant changes on biopsy of their squamous epithelium.

In essence, biopsy of the squamous epithelium has a very low predictive value for the diagnosis of reflux when positive histologic criteria are present. The absence of histologic criteria for reflux also has a very low predictive value for the absence of reflux. Therefore, in and of itself, biopsy of the squamous epithelium is therefore of little value in the evaluation of the patient with reflux disease.

Pathophysiologic Changes

An elegant series of in vitro studies by Tobey et al. [25] has provided excellent evidence of the cellular mechanism involved in acid-induced damage of the squamous epithelium. When the squamous epithelium is exposed to acid in high enough concentration for a sufficient length of time, damage occurs in a highly predictable and progressive manner. The severity and rate of progression of damage is dose-related.

The first visible morphologic change is a separation of the squamous cells due to disruption of the tight junctions between the cells. This is seen electron microscopically as "dilated intercellular spaces" as the earliest morphologic evidence of reflux. With increasing damage, the separation of the squamous cells increases and can easily be recognized by light microscopy in routine sections. The severity of the dilated intercellular spaces correlates with the severity of reflux.

The separation of squamous cells increases the permeability of the epithelium. As reflux-induced damage increases, the normally impervious epithelium becomes increasingly permeable. Luminal molecules of increasing size penetrate the squamous epithelium to an increasing depth [25]. Increased infiltration of luminal molecules into the squamous epithelium has the potential to produce numerous additional effects in the squamous epithelium apart from the morphologic injury.

(a) Pain: With even mild damage, small molecules like acid (hydrogen ions/protons) can enter the epithelium and stimulate pain-sensitive nerve endings in the epithelium, resulting in "heartburn." While acid is an extremely powerful pain inducer, other luminal molecules may also enter the damaged squamous epithelium and stimulate nerve endings resulting in discomfort. These other molecules are less effective than acid in causing pain because they are less noxious and larger in size. However, they may be the cause of continuing discomfort in the patients whose symptoms are not completely controlled with acid suppressive drug therapy.

(b) Eosinophilic esophagitis: The entry of eosinophils into the epithelium is part of the usual pathologic change in reflux disease. This is likely the result of cell damage caused by acid, causing release of chemotactic cytokines by the damaged cells which causes eosinophil migration into the epithelium [24, 26]. However, the absolute number of eosinophils in patients with reflux is usually small.

Eosinophilic esophagitis is considered to be an atopic type I hypersensitivity reaction of esophageal squamous epithelium to ingested allergens. In this condition, the squamous epithelium typically shows severe damage associated with numerous intraepithelial eosinophils. Atopy results from interaction of ingested allergens with sensitized IgE containing mast cells that are usually found in the lamina propria under the squamous epithelium. In normal epithelium, ingestion of allergens does not evoke the atopic response even in the sensitized individual because the allergen does not penetrate the squamous epithelium and is therefore sequestered from the effector mast cell. When the squamous epithelium is damaged by reflux, the allergen can enter and traverse the epithelium and interact with the mast cell. This causes mast cell degranulation and release of histamine and other cytokines that are extremely chemo-attractive to eosinophils, resulting in the massive intraepithelial eosinophil infiltrate that is typical of eosinophilic esophagitis [26].

As expected from this pathophysiology, eosinophilic (atopic) esophagitis can be treated effectively in many patients with acid suppressive drug therapy. PPIs have anti-inflammatory properties in addition to potent acid suppression and are highly effective in reversing the squamous epithelial damage caused by reflux and restoring the impermeable status of the normal esophageal epithelium. The allergen is therefore prevented access to the effector mast cell, preventing the atopic reaction.

(c) Columnar metaplasia: Entry of large molecules in the gastric juice into the esophageal squamous epithelium because of its increased permeability is the basic reason for columnar metaplasia. These large molecules, when they reach the proliferative and stem cell zone in the deeper part of the epithelium, can interact with cell surface receptors and have the potential to induce alterations in the genetic control mechanisms of the cells.

Cell surface and cytoplasmic receptors usually have complex tertiary structures that require complex complementary molecules for reaction. It is highly unlikely that receptors exist for simple particles like hydrogen ions (protons); acid is not a molecule that is likely to have the capability to cause cell receptor interactions that can result in genetic changes in the cell.

Columnar metaplasia of the esophagus results from the interaction of an unknown molecule in gastric contents that penetrates the damaged squamous epithelium, interacts with the basal region proliferative cells, and causes a switch in the genetic differentiating signal. This switch from the normal signal that dictates squamous differentiation to a new signal that includes BMP-4 (bone morphogenesis protein 4) induces columnar differentiation [27]. The proliferating cell in the deep part of the squamous epithelium, under the BMP-4 signal, differentiates into a columnar epithelium.

There is strong evidence that columnar metaplasia occurs early and is actually seen in most patients with chronic reflux disease [28].

Columnar metaplasia first occurs in the most distal esophagus where the damage to the esophagus is highest in reflux disease. This metaplastic columnar epithelium separates the esophageal squamous epithelium from the normal oxyntic mucosa that lines the proximal stomach, creating a histologic squamo-oxyntic gap [1]. The presence of this metaplastic columnar epithelium and the gap is an absolutely specific and an extremely sensitive marker for reflux disease.

With increasing reflux-induced damage of esophageal squamous epithelium, the amount of columnar metaplasia progressively increases and the squamo-oxyntic gap increases in length as the squamo-columnar junction (Z-line) moves cephalad. In the vast majority of patients with chronic reflux disease, a microscopic squamo-columnar gap with endoscopically invisible columnar metaplasia exists [1, 2]. The length of the squamo-oxyntic gap is lowest in autopsy specimens in patients without a history of reflux disease during life [19, 29]. When the disease becomes severe, the squamo-oxyntic gap becomes visible at endoscopy and is recognized as a visible columnar lined esophagus.

In almost all patients with chronic reflux disease, there are two epithelial types in the esophagus: normal squamous epithelium and metaplastic columnar epithelium. The extent (length) of the latter is directly proportional to the severity of cumulative life-long damage to the esophageal squamous epithelium by reflux [30]. The response of these two epithelial types to reflux is different.

As we treat reflux by altering the composition of the offensive agent (gastric contents) with acid suppressive drug therapy, we must be cognizant about how alkalinization of gastric contents impacts both squamous and columnar epithelia in the esophagus. At present, we do not do this; we concentrate on the great benefit produced in controlling squamous epithelial damage and completely ignore changes that result in the columnar epithelium.

One reason for this is that most physicians harbor the notion that columnar metaplasia does not exist until they can recognize it at endoscopy. This is false. The resolution of endoscopes, even with narrow band imaging and magnification, is too low to see the microscopic columnar epithelium that is present in all patients with chronic reflux disease. What the eye does not behold at endoscopy exists in the patient under the microscope [2]. To not recognize this is a fundamental error.

Effect of Acid Suppressive Drug Therapy on Squamous Epithelium

Acid in gastric contents is responsible for most if not all of the reflux-induced damage produced in the squamous epithelium of the esophagus.

It is probably true that if there was no acid in the stomach, reflux would not cause any damage. At lectures, we have been asked whether the use of acid suppressive agents from birth would prevent reflux-induced damage in the esophageal epithelium. The answer to this is probably affirmative.

Populations who have a high prevalence of *H. pylori* infection have a very low prevalence of reflux disease and GERD-induced adenocarcinoma [31]. This is most likely because the infection causes gastritis with atrophy with achlorhydria early in life and this protects the infected population against reflux disease. Unfortunately, there is a price that is paid in these populations; they have a high incidence of *H. pylori* induced gastric adenocarcinoma.

It is also not feasible to use acid suppressive drugs from early life to prevent reflux disease because gastric acid also has a vital function. In fact, the present long-term use of proton pump inhibitors for treatment of reflux disease has been reported to have significant side effects. Acid suppression with long-term proton pump inhibitor therapy has been reported to increase infections, notably *C. difficile* colitis [5], pneumonia; cause malabsorption of minerals like magnesium and calcium (increased risk of decreased bone density and hip fracture [4]); and produce drug interactions.

Suppressing gastric acid secretion is a highly effective method of treating squamous epithelial damage caused by reflux. In adequate dosage, proton pump inhibitors can maintain gastric pH above a pH of 4 for 12–14 h of the day [11]. At this level of alkalinization of gastric contents, the most potent molecule in the offensive agent in the causation of reflux damage of the squamous epithelium is effectively neutralized.

The most reliably reproducible effect of effective acid suppression in patients with reflux disease is healing of erosive esophagitis in over 90 % of patients, usually within a month of initiation of therapy. Continued acid suppression also prevents recurrence of erosive esophagitis, prevents progression of erosions to deeper ulcers, and markedly decreases the incidence of complex strictures of the esophagus. The practical effect of this change has been obvious; deep and intractable ulcers and fibrous strictures of the esophagus have become rare complications of GERD. This is a dramatic change from five decades ago when these complications were common and very difficult to treat.

The second positive effect of alkalinizing gastric contents with proton pump inhibitors is that it controls pain. Heartburn is reduced significantly in most patients because suppression of acid removes the most potent stimulator of pain-sensitive nerve endings. Control of heartburn improves the quality of life for most patients with reflux disease. The availability of proton pump inhibitors for treating reflux disease has in fact, dramatically decreased the misery index of reflux disease in the past five decades.

When investigated carefully however, acid suppression does not completely eradicate pain in many patients with reflux.

Approximately 30 % of patients continue to have significant pain and few are completely symptom free even with maximum and long terms proton pump inhibitor therapy.

This can be understood by the fact that proton pump inhibitor therapy does not actually stop or decrease reflux [32, 33]. Patients on PPIs continue to have reflux at the same frequency as before. The squamous epithelium is exposed to all the molecules in the refluxate except acid. In many patients whose symptoms persist despite adequate dosage of acid suppressive drugs, the continuing "weak-acid (pH 4–6)" reflux can still cause pain [34].

Effective control of pain in patients with reflux disease is probably most dependent on restoring the normal impermeable state of the squamous epithelium. It is only when this is achieved that the refluxed material in the lumen of the esophagus is kept completely away from the pain-sensitive nerve endings in the esophagus. The fact that some pain and discomfort frequently occurs despite acid suppression can be explained if the squamous epithelial permeability is not fully reversed. Non-acid molecules in the refluxate can also penetrate the epithelium and stimulate nerve endings to cause pain. While this may be at a lower level than acid-induced pain that was present before treatment was instituted, it is often still a source of significant discomfort. It is interesting that studies of symptomatic patients with "weak-acid reflux" show that successful antireflux surgery eradicates their pain [35].

Acid suppressive drug therapy is only directed against the acid in the offensive mixture of reflux disease. It does not address the fact that other molecules in the refluxate may continue to cause both symptoms and pathologic changes in the esophageal epithelium. It also does not correct or improve the damaged lower esophageal sphincter or decrease the number or frequency of reflux events [32, 33].

Study of patients treated with acid suppressive drug therapy will therefore show those elements of reflux disease that are poorly controlled: these include symptoms resulting from exposure of the epithelium to weak-acid reflux, regurgitation, and the progression of pathologic changes in the metaplastic columnar epithelium.

Effect of Acid Suppressive Drug Therapy on Metaplastic Esophageal Columnar Epithelium

Gastroesophageal reflux disease has changed its character over the past six decades. In the 1950s, reflux disease was defined almost entirely by its effects on squamous epithelium. The inability to control pain, ulceration, and strictures were the main problems. Approaches to address these issues sometimes require even esophagectomy. The pharmaceutical industry subsequently stepped up to the plate, developing increasingly potent drugs to control acid secretion, which have proved to be highly successful in controlling pain, ulcers, and strictures.

Columnar metaplasia of the esophagus was common in the 1950s. Examination of detailed descriptions of columnar lined esophagus by Barrett [35, 36] and Allison and Johnstone [37] shows that many patients had extremely long segments of columnar lined esophagus. In fact, evidence suggests that the very long segments of columnar lined esophagus that were common in the 1950s are increasingly rare today. It would be expected that effective acid suppression used early in patients with symptomatic reflux disease would decrease columnar metaplasia of squamous epithelium.

The biggest and most dramatic change in the last six decades has been the explosion in the incidence of intestinal metaplasia and adenocarcinoma within the columnar lined esophagus. In the 1950s, histologic descriptions of the epithelium show that intestinal metaplasia defined by the presence of goblet cells was very uncommon even in very long segments of columnar lined esophagus [35, 37]. Adenocarcinoma was so rare that single cases were reported. The first case was reported in 1952 by Morson and Belcher [38]. Allison and Johnstone's 1953 paper had the second case [37].

Today, Barrett's esophagus, defined as intestinal metaplasia in a biopsy taken from visible columnar lined esophagus, is present in an estimated 5–10 % of adults in the population [39]. If symptomatic patients with normal endoscopy are biopsied, intestinal metaplasia is found in up to 25 % of patients in some studies [40]. The increase in the prevalence of intestinal metaplasia in the population from 1950 to 2012 has been astounding.

Similarly, the incidence of esophageal adenocarcinoma has shown an increase not seen for any other human cancer type in human history over such a short period. From the first reported case in 1952, the incidence has increased exponentially. In 1982, Rodger Haggitt declared esophageal adenocarcinoma "an epidemic" [41]. From 1975 to 2003, the incidence of esophageal adenocarcinoma increased six-fold [42]. In 1995, the incidence of adenocarcinoma of the esophagus overtook that of esophageal squamous carcinoma in the USA [42]. Today, I see adenocarcinoma of the esophagus ten times more frequently than squamous carcinoma. Of the 16,000 patients who developed esophageal carcinoma in 2010, it is likely that 90 % (over 14,000) were adenocarcinomas. When adenocarcinoma of the gastroesophageal junctional region and gastric cardia (which are, in reality adenocarcinomas of the distal esophagus [43] and so classified by the AJCC 7th edition [44]) are added to this number, an astonishing 20,000 people in the USA developed adenocarcinoma in 2010. The number is still increasing in an incidence curve that is still upward. A sobering thought is that, with an overall mortality of 85 %, esophageal adenocarcinomas are responsible for the death of nearly 17,000 people every year in the USA alone.

Barrett's esophagus and esophageal adenocarcinoma are solely the result of gastroesophageal reflux disease. There is no other cause for either of these entities despite some associations with obesity and smoking.

Despite what must be the most dramatic increase in the mortality from a single cancer type in the history of medicine, there has been little or no attempt to address this problem by the medical community at large. The treatment of reflux disease is still aimed at controlling heartburn and healing erosive esophagitis with acid suppressive drugs. While this goal has been met and the medical community declares self-satisfied success at the wonder of their drugs and their ability to control reflux disease and improve quality of life, the number of people dying from cancer that is the complication of reflux disease is increasing exponentially.

As pathologists, we tend to view every disease from a different viewpoint. To us, the criterion of success of treatment of any disease is the mortality rate from that disease. By that criterion, the treatment of reflux disease rivals the worst failures in the history of medicine. From having an occasional death resulting from intractable ulceration or hemorrhage in the 1950s, reflux disease in 2010 is responsible for approximately 17,000 deaths from adenocarcinoma in the USA and many more in Europe.

The goal of a treatment of a disease should be to prevent death at all costs; everything else is secondary. The present treatment algorithms for reflux disease have as their goal the improvement of the quality of life of millions of people who have heartburn caused by reflux. This is an easy goal to achieve but should not be mistaken for an attempt at preventing cancer in the many thousands of patients every year. It is merely the treatment of the squamous manifestations of the disease when the development of cancer is in fact a disease of the columnar metaplastic epithelium.

We need to set a new goal for patients with reflux disease. We need to tell ourselves that our primary goal in this disease is to prevent cancer and death. When we do this, we will stop ignoring the columnar lined esophagus; rather we will focus on it with all the technology that is available.

Metaplastic Esophageal Columnar Epithelial Types

The change in the differentiating genetic signal from the postulated Wnt to BMP-4 in the proliferating cells of the esophageal epithelium results in the transformation of the stratified squamous epithelium to a columnar epithelium composed entirely of undifferentiated mucous cells. These cells line the surface and form a foveolar pit and glands, all composed of morphologically similar mucous cells. This is *cardiac epithelium* which is defined as an epithelium composed entirely of mucous cells without parietal or goblet cells [45].

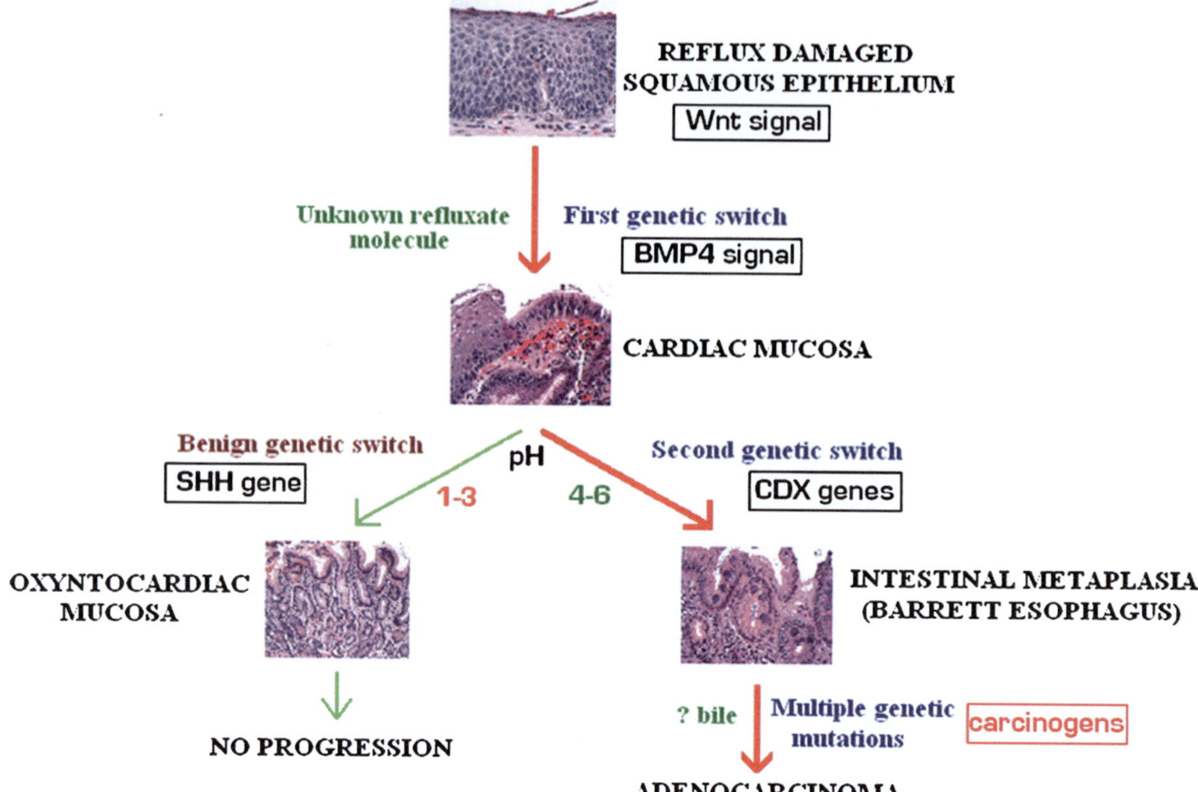

Fig. 2.2 Sequence of epithelial changes in the esophagus caused by reflux disease. In the initial step, squamous epithelium undergoes columnar metaplasia to cardiac mucosa. The cardiac mucosa then evolves in one of two directions: (**a**) in a strong acid milieu, Sonic Hedgehog gene is activated leading to parietal cells and oxyntocardiac mucosa. This is a stable epithelium that does not progress to cancer. (**b**) In a weaker acid milieu, CDX2 is activated and intestinal metaplasia results

Cardiac epithelium has also been called "junctional epithelium" and "mucous-cell only epithelium."

Cardiac epithelium is subjected to attack by gastric contents as a result of continuing reflux disease. As a result, it has the potential to evolve into two other significant epithelial types within the columnar lined esophagus—oxyntocardiac and intestinal epithelia [46]. These are defined by the presence of parietal cells and goblet cells. Figure 2.1 Many other differentiated cell types can be seen in metaplastic esophageal columnar epithelium—neuroendocrine cells, pancreatic cells, chief cells, Paneth cells, ciliated cells. At present, these cell types have no known significance and are pretty much ignored in the definition of the three basic types of metaplastic epithelia.

The first type of change in cardiac mucosa occurs as a result of development of parietal (oxyntic) cells within its glands (Fig. 2.2). The presence of parietal cells in cardiac mucosa converts the epithelium to *oxyntocardiac epithelium*. This is defined as a columnar epithelium where the glands contain a mixture of mucous cells and parietal cells. It does not have goblet cells. Like the cardiac metaplasia of squamous epithelium resulted from a genetic switch, oxyntocardiac mucosa is generated in cardiac mucosa by activation of a different differentiating genetic signal—possibly a combination of BMP-4 and the Sonic Hedgehog gene [47]. Sonic hedgehog gene is the usual genetic signal in the gastric oxyntic mucosa and is required for development of parietal cells in gastrointestinal columnar epithelia [48]. Oxyntocardiac epithelium has also been called "gastric fundic-type epithelium" and "mixed mucous and parietal cell epithelium."

The second type of change in cardiac epithelium occurs as a result of development of goblet cells which can appear in the surface, foveolar region, or in the glands. This is *intestinal metaplastic epithelium* (Fig. 2.2). Intestinal epithelium is generated in cardiac mucosa by activation of yet another different differentiating genetic signal—the homeobox gene complex that includes CDX2 [8, 49]. CDX2 is the usual genetic signal in the intestine with CDX2 being dominant for colonic differentiation [50]. Intestinal epithelium in the esophagus has also been called "specialized columnar epithelium" or "Barrett's Esophagus."

These three columnar epithelia are the only significant columnar epithelial types that occur in the esophagus. Because the criteria for their definition are simple (based on the presence or absence of three easily recognizable cell type: mucous cells, parietal cells, and goblet cells), their identification in biopsies is easy, precise, and accurate with little inter-observer variation after minimal training.

Together, various combinations of these three columnar epithelial types comprise the entire pathologic metaplastic gap that results from columnar metaplasia of squamous epithelium [1, 40]. Because this process requires two steps (damage to squamous epithelium with increased permeability *and* a cellular reaction between molecules in gastric contents and esophageal epithelium that produces highly specific changes in differentiating genetic signals), the presence of any or all these epithelia are absolutely specific for reflux disease.

We therefore have a new definition of reflux disease at a cellular level: *Reflux disease is the presence of a gap between esophageal squamous epithelium and gastric oxyntic mucosa composed of any combination of cardiac, oxyntocardiac and intestinal epithelia.* This is the squamo-oxyntic gap [1]. This definition is 100 % specific for reflux disease; columnar metaplasia does not occur in any other esophageal disease. Having a precisely reproducible definition of reflux disease based on examination of routine biopsy specimens taken at endoscopy has enormous value.

Of the three types of metaplastic columnar epithelium in the esophagus, the only epithelium that is at risk for progression to dysplasia and adenocarcinoma is intestinal epithelium [51]. This defines Barrett esophagus. Patients who have intestinal metaplasia in a biopsy taken from a visible columnar lined esophagus are estimated to have a risk of future cancer of ~0.5 % per year.

Present guidelines for biopsy at endoscopy do not emphasize a complete examination of the epithelium between the Z-line and gastric oxyntic mucosa. Biopsies are not recommended for patients who do not have a visible columnar lined esophagus. This results in early changes of GERD limited to the dilated distal esophagus being ignored [2]. In patients with a visible columnar lined esophagus, biopsies stop at the proximal limit of rugal folds, thereby missing the pathology in the dilated distal esophagus.

The Amount (Length) of the Squamo-Oxyntic Gap

From its normal length of zero cm, the squamo-oxyntic gap progressively increases in length in patients with reflux disease due to increasing amounts of columnar metaplasia of their squamous epithelium. Columnar metaplasia is usually a "permanent" change. Once it has occurred, reversal will not usually occur unless there has been a significant treatment induced alteration such as ablation of the epithelium. Although minor decreases in the presence of goblet cell metaplasia have been reported with therapy, neither acid suppressive drug therapy nor successful anti-reflux surgery reliably reverses

columnar metaplasia. As such, the squamo-oxyntic gap changes in only one direction—increase in length.

In autopsy studies of people who have died without symptoms of reflux disease during life, the squamo-oxyntic gap varies from zero to less than 1 cm [19, 29]. If assessed by measured biopsies distal to the endoscopic gastroesophageal junction in patients with heartburn undergoing endoscopy, the gap is usually also less than 1 cm. This gap is limited to *the dilated distal esophagus* that is often mistaken for proximal stomach by present endoscopic criteria [2]. When a visible columnar epithelium is present, the squamo-oxyntic gap is equal to the length of the endoscopically visible columnar segment (measured by the Prague criteria [52]) *plus* the endoscopically invisible area within the dilated distal esophagus [1, 17].

The measured length of the squamo-oxyntic gap is an accurate measure of cumulative reflux damage to squamous epithelium during life. Because further metaplasia is prevented by acid suppression, the length of the gap usually remains constant after the first endoscopy because patients who have a visible columnar lined esophagus are almost invariably placed on acid suppressive drug therapy.

The length of the squamo-oxyntic gap at first presentation is an exquisitely accurate measure of the severity of reflux. Oberg et al. [53] from our unit showed that the presence of cardiac and/or oxyntocardiac mucosa in biopsies of endoscopically normal patients compared with their absence correlated significantly with a greater likelihood of an abnormal 24-h pH test and lower esophageal sphincter abnormalities. In a study of pediatric patients at Harvard, Glickman et al. [54] showed that children who had greater than 1 mm of measured cardiac mucosa between the squamous epithelium and the first observed parietal cell had significantly greater evidence of reflux than those with less than 1 mm of cardiac mucosa. The presence of cardiac mucosa is therefore sensitive to within a measurement of 1 mm. Chandrasoma et al. [30] showed that there was a hugely significant difference in the amount of reflux as measured by a 24-h pH test in patients with a squamo-oxyntic gap that was greater than 20 mm (2 cm) compared with lengths less than 20 mm.

Based on this evidence we can now accurately define the severity of chronic life-long reflux in a patient by pathologic criteria. *Severity of reflux disease is defined by the length of the squamo-oxyntic gap.* Based on this, we recognize the following grades of severity of reflux disease:

Mild reflux disease: Endoscopically normal; squamo-oxyntic gap less than 1 cm limited to the dilated distal esophagus; with heartburn (mild symptomatic reflux disease) or without heartburn (asymptomatic reflux disease).

Moderate reflux disease: Endoscopically visible columnar lined esophagus; squamo-oxyntic gap of 1–2 cm; with heartburn (moderate symptomatic reflux disease) or without heartburn (asymptomatic moderate reflux disease).

Severe reflux disease: Endoscopically visible columnar lined esophagus; squamo-oxyntic gap of greater than 2 cm; with heartburn (severe symptomatic reflux disease) or without heartburn (asymptomatic severe reflux disease).

This new grading system is of great value because it rates reflux disease by chronic, irreversible changes in columnar epithelium that may ultimately result in adenocarcinoma. Unlike the present Los Angeles system for grading the severity of reflux disease which is based on reversible squamous epithelial changes, this system uses chronic changes in GERD and will demonstrate an uncomfortable truth: *reflux disease defined by the squamo-oxyntic gap is a chronic irreversible change that is not improved by medical therapy.*

Distribution of Columnar Epithelia in the Squamo-Oxyntic Gap

The three types of columnar epithelium in the squamo-oxyntic gap show infinite variation. Oxyntocardiac epithelium is present in all people. At autopsy in people without reflux and in patients with an oxyntic gap of less than 1 cm, oxyntocardiac epithelium is often the only columnar epithelium in the gap [19]. In patients with an oxyntic gap that is 1–2 cm (moderate reflux disease), cardiac epithelium is almost always present in the gap [40].

Intestinal metaplasia is present in the squamo-oxyntic gap in a minority of patients. The prevalence of intestinal metaplasia varies with the length of the squamo-oxyntic gap; the longer the gap, the greater the prevalence of intestinal metaplasia [40]. In the new millennium, intestinal metaplasia is present in 90 % of patients with a gap exceeding 3 cm and 100 % of patients when the gap exceeds 5 cm [1, 40].

The most dramatic historical change in reflux disease is in the prevalence of intestinal metaplasia in the squamo-oxyntic gap. In the 1950s intestinal metaplasia was rare even in long segments of columnar lined epithelium [35, 37]. In Paull et al.'s mapping study of 1976 [55], intestinal metaplasia was more prevalent than in the 1950s, but much less than at the present time. In 1994, Spechler et al. [56] reported a prevalence of 19.4 % of intestinal metaplasia in patients with visible columnar lined epithelium less than 2 cm in length. In our study from 2003, intestinal metaplasia was present in 70 % of patients with a squamo-oxyntic gap of 1–2 cm [40]. It should be noted that endoscopically visible columnar epithelium in the esophagus is shorter than the actual histologic squamo-oxyntic gap, making this difference highly significant. These data provide powerful evidence that the prevalence of intestinal metaplasia in columnar epithelium has increased greatly in the past 60 years. This increase is very likely to be

the most likely basis for the increased incidence of adenocarcinoma in patients with reflux disease.

Mapping studies of the squamo-oxyntic gap shows that the three epithelia are distributed in a remarkably non-random and constant manner [57]. Oxyntocardiac epithelium dominates the distal part of the gap. If intestinal metaplasia is present, it is almost always present in the most proximal region of the gap immediately adjacent to the squamo-columnar junction. When present, the amount of intestinal metaplasia varies greatly in different patients. In some patients intestinal metaplasia is limited to the most proximal region of the gap; in others, the intestinal metaplasia extends distally to involve an increasing part of the gap. The involvement is usually contiguous without skip areas. In a few patients, intestinal metaplasia is present in the entire gap but there is usually non-intestinalized cardiac and oxyntocardiac mucosa in the most distal part of the gap separating intestinal from gastric oxyntic mucosa.

Cause of Intestinal Metaplasia in Columnar Epithelia

The distribution of intestinal metaplasia in the columnar epithelium provides insight as to its causation (Fig. 2.3).

All changes that occur in the esophagus except intestinal metaplasia tend to be maximal in the distal esophagus. The reason for this is easy to understand; the concentration of all injurious molecules is greatest in the distal esophagus and decreases from distal to proximal. For this reason, most injuries like erosions and columnar metaplasia are maximal distally.

The only thing that increases from distal to proximal in the esophagus is the pH (i.e., the concentration of hydrogen ions decreases from distal to proximal). Reflux of acid gastric contents into the esophagus creates a pH gradient from baseline gastric pH (normally 1–2) in the most distal esophagus to neutral (pH 7) at the height of the column of reflux.

The fact that the prevalence of intestinal metaplasia increases as the length of columnar lined esophagus increases and the fact that intestinal metaplasia always begins in the proximal region adjacent to the squamous epithelium is powerful evidence that intestinal metaplasia is favored in a pH environment that is closer to neutral (pH 4–7) (Fig. 2.3). Stated in another way, CDX2 activation is favored in a higher than lower pH milieu [49].

In contrast, the fact that oxyntocardiac epithelium occurs in the most distal region of the squamo-oxyntic gap suggests that Sonic Hedgehog gene activation and development of parietal cells in cardiac mucosa is favored by a strong acid milieu.

The concept of evolution of cardiac epithelium in two directions based on the pH milieu of the esophagus has logic in its favor [47]. In the gastrointestinal tract, CDX genes are normally expressed in the small and large intestine which are

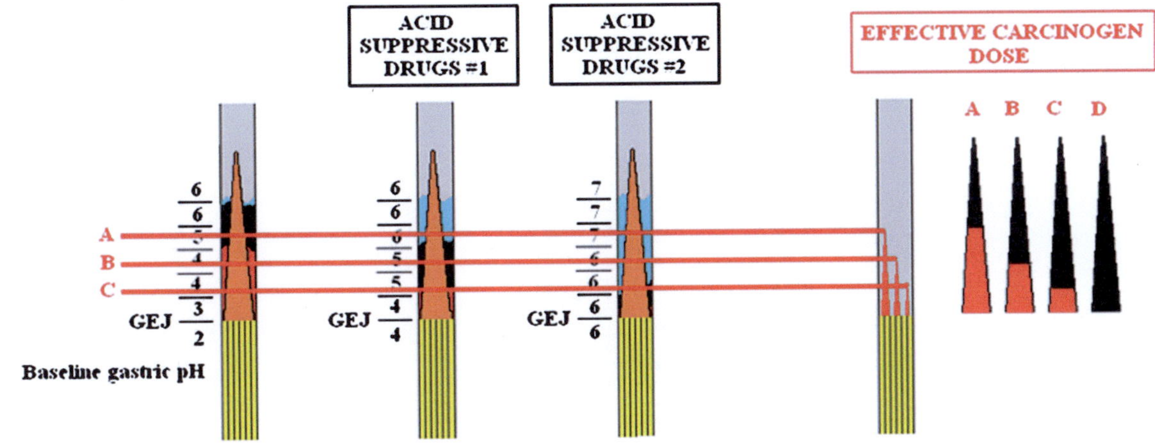

Volume of Reflux	HIGH	REMAINS HIGH	REMAINS HIGH
Time of Exposure	LONG	REMAINS HIGH	REMAINS HIGH
Amount of IM	SMALL	INCREASED	MORE INCREASED
Amount of OCM	MODERATE	LESS	STILL LESS
CANCER RISK	ZERO	LOW	HIGH

Fig. 2.3 Theoretical representation of a patient with severe reflux disease. During a reflux episode, a column of gastric contents is propelled into the esophagus, setting up a gradient of decreasing volume and increasing pH in the esophagus. The reflux has caused columnar metaplasia in the esophagus. If one assumes that intestinal metaplasia occurs in cardiac mucosa at pH 6, it can be seen that the extent of intestinal metaplasia progressively increases from normal (*left*) to partially acid suppressed with baseline gastric pH 4 (*center*) to severely acid suppressed with baseline gastric pH 6 (*right*). The three horizontal *red lines* indicate the effective carcinogen dose delivered to the esophagus by reflux in three patients with different carcinogen levels. It can be seen that the risk of carcinoma increases with increasing acid suppression because the interaction between the target epithelium (intestinal metaplasia) and carcinogen increases

high pH environments [50]. In the normal stomach, a low pH environment, Sonic Hedgehog gene is active [48]. In patients with atrophic chronic gastritis, a disease process that destroys parietal cells and decreases gastric acidity (i.e., increases pH), CDX2 is activated and results in intestinal metaplasia [58].

The fact that intestinal metaplasia in columnar lined esophagus is promoted by a pH in the 4–7 range has profound implications. The therapeutic goal of treating reflux disease with acid suppressive drugs is to alkalinize gastric contents to the pH 4–7 range over a large part of the 24 h period [3, 11]. The alkalinization of gastric juice in patients on acid suppressive drug therapy means that the esophageal pH gradient that is produced when reflux occurs is shifted. Instead of the gradient ranging from pH 1–2 in the distal esophagus to 7 at the height of the reflux column, the distal esophagus in the patients on proton pump inhibitor therapy is the altered baseline gastric pH which is over 4. The entire esophagus is now at a pH of 4–7.

This may well explain the greater extent of intestinal metaplasia today than existed in the past (Fig. 2.3). In a mapping study of ten esophagectomy cases in 2007, we showed that intestinal metaplasia extended from the top of the columnar lined segment all the way into the dilated distal esophagus [17]. This contrasts with the mapping data of Paull et al. [55] where patients with long segments of columnar lined esophagus either had no intestinal metaplasia or intestinal metaplasia limited to the proximal part of the segment. The distal 3–4 cm of the segment in Paull et al. consisted of cardiac and oxyntocardiac epithelia [55].

The goal of treating reflux with acid suppressive drugs is to alkalinize gastric juice; the unintended consequence of this is that the esophagus is exposed to alkalinized material during reflux. This results in increased prevalence and extent of intestinal metaplasia in the columnar lined segment.

Carcinogenesis in Columnar Lined Esophagus

The only epithelium in the esophagus that is susceptible to carcinogenesis is intestinal epithelium [51]. Squamous, cardiac, and oxyntocardiac epithelia do not develop cancer.

Oxyntocardiac epithelium is particularly immune to cancer because it does not develop intestinal metaplasia [28]. It is therefore a stable epithelium that is highly desirable because it is resistant to acid, carcinogens, and agents in the gastric contents that induce intestinal metaplasia. Cardiac epithelium is

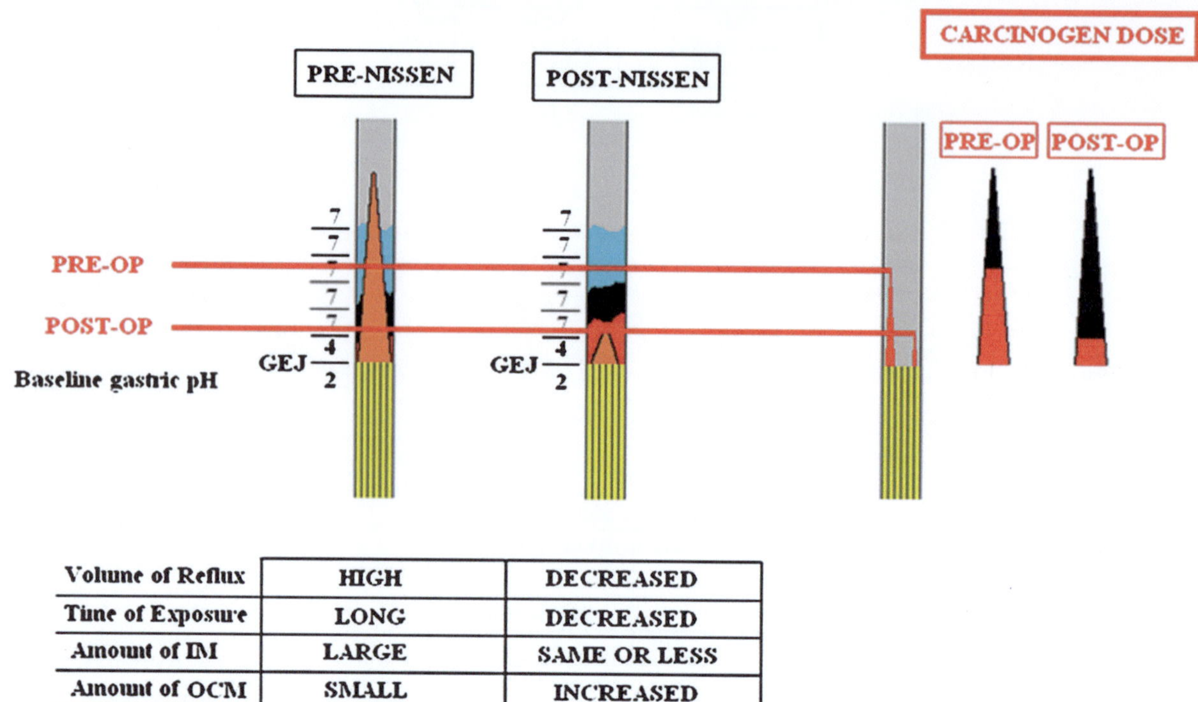

Volume of Reflux	HIGH	DECREASED
Time of Exposure	LONG	DECREASED
Amount of IM	LARGE	SAME OR LESS
Amount of OCM	SMALL	INCREASED
CANCER RISK	PRESENT	ZERO

Fig. 2.4 Similar diagram of a patient with severe reflux and a long segment of columnar lined esophagus with intestinal metaplasia limited to the proximal region. Pre-operatively, carcinogen is delivered to the intestinal metaplastic region by the severe reflux. After Nissen fundoplication, the reflux has decreased and effective carcinogen delivery is limited to the distal esophagus, never reaching the level of intestinal metaplasia. This would theoretically reduce the risk of carcinoma

also resistant to acid and carcinogens but can transform into intestinal metaplasia [28]. There is a time lag of many years between the occurrence of cardiac metaplasia and intestinal metaplasia. Children with reflux disease often develop cardiac mucosa but intestinal metaplasia only rarely develops before the third decade of life [59]. In patients who have undergone esophagectomy, cardiac mucosa commonly develops proximal to the anastomotic line. In some patients, intestinal metaplasia occurs in the cardiac mucosa, often many months to years later [60].

The carcinogen that induces oncogenic changes in esophageal intestinal metaplasia is uncertain. There is some evidence that it is a derivative of bile salts/acids that enters the stomach via duodeno-gastric reflux. Carcinogenesis is likely to be largely dependent on the concentration of carcinogen in the gastric contents. Because this cannot be measured, the risk of cancer in reflux cannot be accurately assessed. A patient who has no carcinogen will never develop cancer irrespective of any condition in the esophagus. A patient with a high carcinogen level can develop cancer only if there is intestinal metaplasia in the esophagus.

The carcinogen is delivered to the esophagus by reflux. As with all other molecules that are refluxed into the esophagus, the highest concentration of carcinogen is in the distal esophagus and progressively decreases from distal to proximal [61]. The distal esophagus is therefore at greatest risk for cancer development (Figs. 2.3 and 2.4). However, the carcinogen acts only on intestinal epithelium. This must mean that the risk of adenocarcinoma increases significantly as the distal part of the columnar lined esophagus becomes intestinalized. The role played by alkalinization of gastric contents with acid suppressive drugs in increasing the extent of intestinal metaplasia in the esophagus would therefore promote carcinogenesis in reflux (Fig. 2.3).

The most common location of reflux-induced adenocarcinoma is in the distal part of the intestinal metaplasia within the columnar lined segment near the junction of intestinal epithelium and non-intestinalized cardiac mucosa [62]. In the 1950s, adenocarcinoma was rare because intestinal metaplasia was rare and when it was present it was limited to the most proximal region of long segments of columnar lined esophagus, commonly in the mid-esophagus [37, 38]. Theoretically, carcinogen concentration in this proximal region was sufficient only if the patient had a very high carcinogen level. With increasingly effective alkalinization by drugs, the location where adenocarcinoma occurs has moved increasingly to the more distal part of the esophagus. This is the result of extension of intestinal metaplasia into lower regions of the columnar lined esophagus as a result of alkalinization of the refluxate [61].

At the present time, cancer risk is defined by the presence of intestinal metaplasia in the columnar lined esophagus. No effort is made to stratify risk in the patients with intestinal metaplasia by mapping the extent of intestinal metaplasia and the proximity of intestinal metaplasia to the distal esophagus. It can be predicted that the patients who have more reflux (i.e., a longer squamo-oxyntic gap) with its attendant higher carcinogen exposure, more intestinal metaplasia and extension of intestinal metaplasia to the more distal esophagus where carcinogen concentration is highest are at the greatest risk for cancer. If the prevalence and extent of intestinal metaplasia is promoted by alkalization of gastric juice, the use of drugs that suppress or neutralize acid may be responsible for at least some of the increased incidence of Barrett esophagus and adenocarcinoma that has been seen in the past six decades [61].

Effect of Anti-reflux Surgery on Esophageal Epithelia

Anti-reflux surgery typically consists of some type of fundoplication which artificially augments the function of the damaged lower esophageal sphincter. The most common operation is a Nissen fundoplication, which is a complete wrap of the gastric fundus around the distal esophagus, commonly with a crural repair. Partial fundoplications that produce a lesser sphincter augmentation than a Nissen are also used. Lesser procedures than surgical fundoplication are available as anti-reflux procedures. Endoscopic fundoplication has been attempted but not with sustained success. The only procedure presently being used is the transoral incisionless fundoplication which has had limited success in a small number of patients. A newer technique is LINX, a magnetic ring placed laparoscopically around the distal esophagus to augment sphincter function.

At the present time, anti-reflux surgery is recommended only to improve the quality of life in patients with GERD who fail to achieve adequate symptom control with maximum doses of acid suppressive drugs. As such, patients who undergo surgery are likely to be those with the greatest damage to their sphincter. Anti-reflux surgery is presently not recommended as a cancer-preventive surgery for patients with Barrett's esophagus.

Anti-reflux surgery differs fundamentally from medical therapy with acid suppressive drugs in that it addresses the cause of reflux. By restoring or augmenting sphincter function, surgery not only prevents acid from reaching the esophagus; it prevents reflux and sequesters the esophagus from all molecules in the gastric contents (Fig. 2.4).

At the present time, the success or failure of anti-reflux surgery is defined by:

(a) Symptom relief and improvement of quality of life: This is a low bar to achieve by anti-reflux surgery. In general, anti-reflux surgery controls symptoms in approximately 85 % of patients who have failed medical therapy. A relatively small reduction in the exposure of the esophageal epithelium to refluxate can probably achieve this objective.

(b) The ability of the patient to withdraw from proton pump inhibitor therapy: Approximately 30 % of patients require continued proton pump inhibitor therapy after anti-reflux surgery. This is commonly regarded as a failed surgery. However, it is known that many patients are placed on drug therapy without certainty that the symptoms are caused by reflux, suggesting that being on drug treatment after surgery does not equate to failure of the operation.

(c) Normalization of the 24-h pH test: Post-operative 24-h pH testing is rarely undertaken in patients after anti-reflux surgery outside academic centers and in patients where the objective of symptom control has been met. In general, normalization of the 24-h pH test is a criterion for success of surgery that is more difficult to achieve than symptom control. Nissen fundoplication has a 75-85 % probability of normalizing the 24-h pH test. Initial studies with LINX suggest that patients with early reflux disease have a high rate of success in controlling symptoms as well as normalizing the 24-h pH test. It is likely that the success of fundoplication will be greater if the operation is done earlier in the course of the disease where sphincter damage is less.

(d) Cessation of all reflux: While complete cessation of reflux with a totally flat line on a 24-h pH study is achieved in some patients after a fundoplication, this is not the stated objective for this surgery.

(e) Regression or prevention of progression of histologic changes: Anti-reflux surgery is as or more successful than the best medical therapy in reversing and preventing histologic changes in squamous epithelium caused by reflux. This is usually measured as control of heartburn and healing and prevention of erosive esophagitis. The effect of anti-reflux surgery on the histologic composition of columnar epithelium has not been studied adequately. Oberg et al. [63] reported a series of 69 patients with columnar lined esophagus without intestinal metaplasia who were treated with either long-term proton pump inhibitor therapy or anti-reflux surgery. On follow-up, 80 % of 49 patients who were treated medically developed intestinal metaplasia at 8 years, significantly higher than 40 % of 20 patients treated by anti-reflux surgery after 16 years. This suggests that anti-reflux surgery has a protective effect, at least compared with proton pump inhibitor therapy, in preventing progression of cardiac mucosa to Barrett esophagus. The significant number of patients developing Barrett esophagus after surgery indicates that the protection is incomplete but could be explained by less than complete cessation of reflux after surgery.

Anti-reflux surgery has been shown to reverse intestinal metaplasia in the columnar lined esophagus in patients with Barrett esophagus. This occurs uncommonly in patients with long segment Barrett esophagus, but was reported in 73 % of patients with intestinal metaplasia limited to a dilated distal esophagus [64, 65].

The most important question is whether anti-reflux surgery can prevent progression of reflux disease and particularly reflux disease complicated by Barrett's esophagus to adenocarcinoma. Several small individual studies with prolonged follow-up have shown that patients with non-dysplastic Barrett's esophagus were shown to remain stable without progression to high grade dysplasia and cancer after fundoplication [64, 65]. In a controlled study by Parrilla et al. [66], the protective effect of anti-reflux surgery was seen only in those patients who normalized their 24-h pH study after the surgery. In patients who did not normalize their 24-h pH test, the incidence of cancer was not significantly less than patients who were treated with acid suppressive drug therapy without surgery.

Chang et al. [67], in a meta-analysis of the literature, showed that there was a significant cancer-preventive role for anti-reflux surgery when controlled and uncontrolled studies were combined. However, when only controlled studies were included, the data supporting such a role did not reach statistical significance, possibly because the number of these studies was small.

Lagergren et al. [68] reported that the odds ratio for adenocarcinoma in patients with Barrett's esophagus who had anti-reflux surgery was 12 times the general population, and concluded that surgery did not prevent cancer. However, in a prior epidemiologic study of a similar population, Lagergren et al. [69] showed that the odds ratio for adenocarcinoma was 43.5 times the general population in the most severely symptomatic GERD patients. If one recognizes that it is likely that anti-reflux surgery is performed in the most severe GERD patients, i.e., those with Barrett's, this study actually suggests that anti-reflux surgery may play a partially protective role against cancer in severe GERD patients.

In both Chang et al. [67] and Lagergren et al. [68], there is no reporting of the success or failure of the surgery in any objective way. The available data only shows that with fundoplications being performed with the objective of symptom control and without the aim of stopping reflux completely, it possibly has a partial cancer-preventive effect in patients with severe GERD and Barrett esophagus. Lagergren et al.

[70], in fact showed that one reason for failure of anti-reflux surgery to prevent adenocarcinoma may be persistent reflux after surgery, i.e., an ailed surgery.

Theoretically, if an anti-reflux surgical procedure can be refined to completely stop reflux, and if post-operative testing proves that this has indeed happened, the likelihood is that progression of columnar epithelial changes to cancer will be prevented. This is based only on the fact that carcinogenesis in metaplastic columnar epithelium in the esophagus is the result of luminal exposure of the target epithelium to oncogenic molecules in gastric contents delivered to it by reflux. If reflux is stopped completely and the required mutations for carcinogenesis have not occurred at the time of surgery, there is a near certainty that cancer will be prevented (Fig. 2.4).

The failure of studies to show that anti-reflux surgery does not conclusively prevent cancer in patients with GERD is likely due to the fact that surgery is not designed to achieve this objective and falls short of complete or even adequate control of reflux in many cases. When this failure is at a level where symptom control is achieved but carcinogens still bombard the target epithelium in the esophagus, we declare the procedure a success. A successful surgery defined by the achievement of symptom control is not necessarily a success in terms of cancer prevention. If we are to use anti-reflux surgery to prevent adenocarcinoma in patients with GERD, we must refine surgical technique to satisfy the objective of stopping reflux almost completely while maintaining the complication rate at a level that is acceptable.

References

1. Chandrasoma PT, Wijetunge S, DeMeester SR, Hagen JA, DeMeester TR. The histologic squamo-oxyntic gap: an accurate and reproducible diagnostic marker of gastroesophageal reflux disease. Am J Surg Pathol. 2010;34:1574–81.
2. Chandrasoma P, Wijetunge S, Ma Y, Demeester S, Hagen J, Demeester T. The dilated distal esophagus: a new entity that is the pathologic basis of early gastroesophageal reflux disease. Am J Surg Pathol. 2011;35:1873–81.
3. Katz PO, Ginsberg GG, Hoyle PE, Sostek MB, Monyak JT, Silberg DG. Relationship between intragastric acid control and healing status in the treatment of moderate to severe erosive oesophagitis. Aliment Pharmacol Ther. 2007;25:617–28.
4. Yu EW, Bauer SR, Bain PA, Bauer DC. Proton pump inhibitors and risk of fractures: a meta-analysis of 11 international studies. Am J Med. 2011;124:519–26.
5. Janarthanan S, Ditah I, Adler DG, Ehrinpreis MN. *Clostridium difficile*-associated diarrhea and proton pump inhibitor therapy: a meta-analysis. Am J Gastroenterol. 2012;107:1001–10.
6. Herbella FA, Vicentine FP, Silva LC, Patti MG. Postprandial proximal gastric acid pocket and gastroesophageal reflux disease. Dis Esophagus. 2012;25:652–5.
7. Kauer WK, Burdiles P, Ireland AP, Clark GW, Peters JH, Bremner CG, DeMeester TR. Does duodenal juice reflux into the esophagus of patients with complicated GERD? Evaluation of a fiberoptic sensor for bilirubin. Am J Surg. 1995;169:98–103.

8. Tamagawa Y, Ishimura N, Uno G, Yuki T, Kazumori H, Ishihara S, Amano Y, Kinoshita Y. Notch signaling pathway and Cdx2 expression in the development of Barrett's esophagus. Lab Invest. 2012;92:896–909.

9. Jürgens S, Meyer F, Spechler SJ, Souza R. The role of bile acids in the neoplastic progression of Barrett's esophagus – a short representative overview. Z Gastroenterol. 2012;50:1028–34.

10. Csendes A, Smok G, Burdiles P, Braghetto I, Castro C, Korn O. Effect of duodenal diversion on low-grade dysplasia in patients with Barrett's esophagus: analysis of 37 patients. J Gastrointest Surg. 2002;6:645–52.

11. Miner Jr P, Katz PO, Chen Y, Sostek M. Gastric acid control with esomeprazole, lansoprazole, omeprazole, pantoprazole, and rabeprazole: a five-way crossover study. Am J Gastroenterol. 2003;98: 2616–20.

12. DeMeester TR, Peters JH, Bremner CG, Chandrasoma P. Biology of gastroesophageal reflux disease: pathophysiology relating to medical and surgical treatment. Annu Rev Med. 1999;50:469–506.

13. Theodorou D, Ayazi S, DeMeester SR, Zehetner J, Peyre CG, Grant KS, Augustin F, Oh DS, Lipham JC, Chandrasoma PT, Hagen JA, DeMeester TR. Intraluminal pH and goblet cell density in Barrett's esophagus. J Gastrointest Surg. 2012;16:469–74.

14. Karam SM. Lineage commitment and maturation of epithelial cells in the gut. Front Biosci. 1999;4:286–98.

15. McClave SA, Boyce Jr HW, Gottfried MR. Early diagnosis of columnar lined esophagus: a new endoscopic diagnostic criterion. Gastrointest Endosc. 1987;33:413–6.

16. Sharma P, McQuaid K, Dent J, Fennerty B, Sampliner R, Spechler S, Cameron A, Corley D, Falk G, Goldblum J, Hunter J, Jankowski J, Lundell L, Reid B, Shaheen N, Sonnenberg A, Wang K, Weinstein W. A critical review of the diagnosis and management of Barrett's esophagus: the AGA Chicago Workshop. Gastroenterology. 2004;127:310–30.

17. Chandrasoma P, Makarewicz K, Wickramasinghe K, Ma YL, DeMeester TR. A proposal for a new validated histologic definition of the gastroesophageal junction. Hum Pathol. 2006;37:40–7.

18. Shi L, Der R, Ma Y, Peters J, DeMeester T, Chandrasoma P. Gland ducts and multilayered epithelium in mucosal biopsies from gastroesophageal-junction region are useful in characterizing esophageal location. Dis Esophagus. 2005;18:87–92.

19. Chandrasoma PT, Der R, Ma Y, et al. Histology of the gastroesophageal junction: an autopsy study. Am J Surg Pathol. 2000;24:402–9.

20. Hayward J. The lower end of the oesophagus. Thorax 1961;16: 36–41.

21. Odze RD. Unraveling the mystery of the gastroesophageal junction: a pathologist's perspective. Am J Gastroenterol. 2005;100: 1853–67.

22. Tobey NA, Carson JL, Alkiek RA, et al. Dilated intercellular spaces: a morphological feature of acid reflux-damaged human esophageal epithelium. Gastroenterology. 1996;111:1200–5.

23. Genta RM, Spechler SJ, Kielhorn AF. The Los Angeles and Savary-Miller systems for grading esophagitis: utilization and correlation with histology. Dis Esophagus. 2011;24:10–7.

24. Rodrigo S, Abboud G, Oh D, DeMeester SR, Hagen JA, Lipham J, DeMeester TR, Chandrasoma P. High intraepithelial counts in esophageal squamous epithelium are not specific for eosinophilic esophagitis in adults. Am J Gastroenterol. 2008;103:435–42.

25. Tobey NA, Hosseini SS, Argore CM, Dobrucali AM, Awayda MS, Orlando RC. Dilated intercellular spaces and shunt permeability in non-erosive acid-damaged esophageal epithelium. Am J Gastroenterol. 2004;99:13–22.

26. Bhattacharya B, Carlsten J, Sabo E, Kethu S, Meitner P, Tavares R, Jakate S, Mangray S, Aswad B, Resnick MB. Increased expression of eotaxin-3 distinguishes between eosinophilic esophagitis and gastroesophageal reflux disease. Hum Pathol. 2007;38:1744–53.

27. Castillo D, Puig S, Iglesias M, Seoane A, de Bolós C, Munitiz V, Parrilla P, Comerma L, Poulsom R, Krishnadath KK, Grande L, Pera M. Activation of the BMP4 pathway and early expression of CDX2 characterize non-specialized columnar metaplasia in a human model of Barrett's esophagus. J Gastrointest Surg. 2012; 16:227–37.

28. Chandrasoma P. Controversies of the cardiac mucosa and Barrett's esophagus. Histopathol. 2005;46:361–73.

29. Kilgore SP, Ormsby AH, Gramlich TL, et al. The gastric cardia: fact or fiction? Am J Gastroenterol. 2000;95:921–4.

30. Chandrasoma PT, Lokuhetty DM, DeMeester TR, et al. Definition of histopathologic changes in gastroesophageal reflux disease. Am J Surg Pathol. 2000;24:344–51.

31. Chow WH, Blaser MJ, Blot WJ, et al. An inverse relation between cagA + strains of Helicobacter pylori infection and risk of esophageal and gastric cardia adenocarcinoma. Cancer Res. 1998;58: 588–90.

32. Blonski W, Vela MF, Castell DO. Comparison of reflux frequency during prolonged multichannel intraluminal impedance and pH monitoring on and off acid suppression therapy. J Clin Gastroenterol. 2009;43:816–20.

33. Tamhankar AP, Peters JH, Portale G, Hsieh C-C, Hagen JA, Bremner CG, DeMeester TR. Omeprazole does not reduce gastroesophageal reflux: new insights using multichannel intraluminal impedance technology. J Gastrointest Surg. 2004;8:890–8.

34. Agrawal A, Roberts J, Sharma N, Tutuian R, Vela M, Castell DO. Symptoms with acid and nonacid reflux may be produced by different mechanisms. Dis Esophagus. 2009;22:467–70.

35. Barrett NR. Chronic peptic ulcer of the oesophagus and 'oesophagitis'. Br J Surg. 1950;38:175–82.

36. Barrett NR. The lower esophagus lined by columnar epithelium. Surgery. 1957;41:881–94.

37. Allison PR, Johnstone AS. The oesophagus lined with gastric mucous membrane. Thorax. 1953;8:87–101.

38. Morson BC, Belcher BR. Adenocarcinoma of the oesophagus and ectopic gastric mucosa. Br J Cancer. 1952;6:127–30.

39. Rex DK, Cummings OW, Shaw M, Cumings MD, Wong RKH, Vasudeva RS, Dunne D, Rahmani EY, Helper DJ. Screening for Barrett's esophagus in colonoscopy patients with and without heartburn. Gastroenterology. 2003;125:1670–7.

40. Chandrasoma PT, Der R, Ma Y, Peters J, DeMeester T. Histologic classification of patients based on mapping biopsies of the gastroesophageal junction. Am J Surg Pathol. 2003;27:929–36.

41. Haggitt RC. Adenocarcinoma in Barrett's esophagus: a new epidemic? Hum Pathol. 1992;23:475–6.

42. Pohl H, Welch HG. The role of overdiagnosis and reclassification in the marked increase of esophageal adenocarcinoma incidence. J Natl Cancer Inst. 2005;97:142–6.

43. Chandrasoma PT, Wickramasinghe K, Ma Y, DeMeester TR. Adenocarcinomas of the distal esophagus and "gastric cardia" are predominantly esophageal adenocarcinomas. Am J Surg Pathol. 2007;31:569–75.

44. Rice TW, Blackstone EW, Rusch VW. 7th edition of the AJCC cancer staging manual: esophagus and esophagogastric junction. Ann Surg Oncol. 2010;17:1721–4.

45. Chandrasoma PT, DeMeester TR. Chapter 5: histologic definitions and diagnosis of epithelial types. In: Chandrasoma PT, DeMeester TR, editors. GERD: reflux to esophageal adenocarcinoma. San Diego: Academic; 2006. p. 89–106.

46. Chandrasoma PT, DeMeester TR. Chapter 9: the pathology of reflux disease at a cellular level: part 2 – evolution of cardiac mucosa to oxyntocardiac mucosa and intestinal metaplasia. In: Chandrasoma PT, DeMeester TR, editors. GERD: reflux to esophageal adenocarcinoma. San Diego: Academic; 2006. p. 169–200.

47. Yamanaka Y, Shiotani A, Fujimura Y, Ishii M, Fujita M, Matsumoto H, Tarumi K, Kamada T, Hata J, Haruma K. Expression of Sonic hedgehog (SHH) and CDX2 in the columnar epithelium of the lower oesophagus. Dig Liver Dis. 2011;43:54–9.

48. Feng R, Xiao C, Zavros Y. The role of Sonic Hedgehog as a regulator of gastric function and differentiation. Vitam Horm. 2012; 88:473–89.

49. Vallbohmer D, DeMeester SR, Peters JH, Oh DS, Kuramochi H, Shimizu D, Hagen JA, Danenberg KD, Danenberg PV, DeMeester TR, Chandrasoma PT. Cdx-2 expression in squamous and metaplastic columnar epithelia of the esophagus. Dis Esophagus. 2006;19:260–6.

50. Silberg DG, Swain GP, Suh ER, Traber PG. Cdx1 and Cdx2 during intestinal development. Gastroenterology. 2000;119:961–71.

51. Chandrasoma P, Wijetunge S, DeMeester S, Ma Y, Hagen J, Zamis L, DeMeester T. Columnar lined esophagus without intestinal metaplasia has no proven risk of adenocarcinoma. Am J Surg Pathol. 2012;36:1–7.

52. Vahabzadeh B, Seetharam AB, Cook MB, Wani S, Rastogi A, Bansal A, Early DS, Sharma P. Validation of the Prague C & M criteria for the endoscopic grading of Barrett's esophagus by gastroenterology trainees: a multicenter study. Gastrointest Endosc. 2012;75:236–41.

53. Oberg S, Peters JH, DeMeester TR, et al. Inflammation and specialized intestinal metaplasia of cardiac mucosa is a manifestation of gastroesophageal reflux disease. Ann Surg. 1997;226:522–32.

54. Glickman JN, Fox V, Antonioli DA, Wang HH, Odze RD. Morphology of the cardia and significance of carditis in pediatric patients. Am J Surg Pathol. 2002;26:1032–9.

55. Paull A, Trier JS, Dalton MD, Camp RC, Loeb P, Goyal RK. The histologic spectrum of Barrett's esophagus. N Engl J Med. 1976; 295:476–80.

56. Spechler SJ, Zeroogian JM, Antonioli DA, Wang HH, Goyal RK. Prevalence of metaplasia at the gastroesophageal junction. Lancet. 1994;344:1533–6.

57. Chandrasoma PT, Der R, Dalton P, Kobayashi G, Ma Y, Peters J, DeMeester T. Distribution and significance of epithelial types in columnar lined esophagus. Am J Surg Pathol. 2001;25:1188–93.

58. Barros R, Freund JN, David L, Almeida R. Gastric intestinal metaplasia revisited: function and regulation of CDX2. Trends Mol Med. 2012;18:555–63.

59. Hassall E. Columnar lined esophagus in children. Gastroenterol Clin North Am. 1997;26:533–48.

60. Dresner SM, Griffin SM, Wayman J, Bennett MK, Hayes N, Raimes SA. Human model of duodenogastro-oesophageal reflux in the development of Barrett's metaplasia. Br J Surg. 2003;90: 1120–8.

61. Chandrasoma PT, DeMeester TR. Chapter 10: the pathology of reflux disease at a cellular level: part 3 – Intestinal (Barrett) metaplasia to carcinoma. In: Chandrasoma PT, DeMeester TR, editors. GERD: reflux to esophageal adenocarcinoma. San Diego: Academic; 2006. p. 201–40.

62. Thiesen J, Stein HJ, Feith M, Kauer WK, Dittler HJ, Pirchi D, Siewert JR. Preferred location for the development of esophageal adenocarcinoma within a segment of intestinal metaplasia. Surg Endosc. 2006;20:235–8.

63. Oberg S, Johansson J, Wenner J, Johnsson F, Zilling T, von Holstein CS, Nilsson J, Walther B. Endoscopic surveillance of columnar-lined esophagus: frequency of intestinal metaplasia detection and impact of antireflux surgery. Ann Surg. 2001;234: 619–26.

64. Hofstetter WL, Peters JH, DeMeester TR, Hagen JA, DeMeester SR, Crookes PF, Tsai P, Banki F, Bremner CG. Long-term outcome of antireflux surgery in patients with Barrett's esophagus. Ann Surg. 2001;234:532–8.

65. DeMeester SR, Campos GMR, DeMeester TR, Bremner CG, Hagen JA, Peters JH, Crookes PF. The impact of antireflux procedure on intestinal metaplasia of the cardia. Ann Surg. 1998;228: 547–56.

66. Parrilla P, deHaro LFM, Ortiz A, Munitiz V, Molina J, Bermejo J, Canteras M. Long term results of a randomized prospective study comparing medical and surgical treatment of Barrett's esophagus. Ann Surg. 2003;237:291–8.

67. Chang EY, Morris CD, Seltman AK, O'Rourke RW, Chan BK, Hunter JG, Jobe BA. The effect of antireflux surgery on esophageal carcinogenesis in patients with Barrett esophagus: a systematic review. Ann Surg. 2007;246:11–21.

68. Lagergren J, Ye W, Lagergren P, Lu Y. The risk of esophageal adenocarcinoma after antireflux surgery. Gastroenterology. 2010; 138:1297–301.

69. Lagergren J, Bergstrom R, Lindgren A, Nyren O. Symptomatic gastroesophageal reflux as a risk factor for esophageal adenocarcinoma. N Engl J Med. 1999;340:825–31.

70. Lagergren J, Viklund P. Is esophageal adenocarcinoma occurring late after antireflux surgery due to persistent postoperative reflux? World J Surg. 2007;31:465–9.

Epidemiology and Socioeconomics of Reflux Disease

Vic Velanovich

Introduction

Gastroesophageal reflux disease (GERD) is a protean disease with many manifestations. The purpose of this chapter will be to review its epidemiology, emphasizing the prevalence, incidence and risk factors for GERD, and Barrett's esophagus in adult patients. The current literature on the costs of treatment, societal costs, and changing patterns of antireflux surgery will be reviewed.

Epidemiology of Gastroesophageal Reflux Disease

Prevalence

The true prevalence and incidence of GERD is difficult to determine. Much of this has to do with how the presence of GERD is determined and GERD itself is defined. Most attempts have been through surveys of the presence of symptoms, review of administrative data, or results of endoscopic evaluation. As is discussed elsewhere in this book, the symptoms of GERD are quite varied and sometimes even nonexistent. Therefore, the primary difficulty in understanding the extent of this disease is due to the variation in symptoms. Prevalence can be based on the typical symptoms, atypical symptoms, presence of erosive esophagitis, or the presence of a hiatal hernia but will never be 100 % accurate (Table 3.1).

Typical Symptoms

Studies based on surveys of general populations based on inquiring whether subjects had the "typical" symptoms of GERD, namely heartburn, show that these symptoms are experienced by a large proportion of individuals. A study synthesizing publications surveying general adult samples of Americans found 14 publications reporting GERD symptoms and five covering GERD and other dyspeptic symptoms. The pooled prevalence of GERD symptoms was 24.2 % (95 % confidence interval (CI), [18.2–30.5 %]) and for combination GERD and dyspeptic symptoms it was 35.2 % (95 % CI, [14.8–58.9 %]). The influence of covariates, that is, risk factors for GERD, evaluated as part of most multivariate analyses, is often inconsistent [1]. A survey of 2,973 people in South Australia found that about one-half experience heartburn; 21.2 % at least once a month and 12.4 % at least a few times a week. Of patients reporting symptoms, 25 % self graded the symptoms as moderate or severe and 16.9 % were taking medications for reflux symptoms [2]. However, a Canadian study found the prevalence to be much lower, that is approximately 10–20 % of the population [3]. Prevalence does seem to be affected by ethnicity. A population-based, cross-sectional survey of 1,172 American subjects showed that 50 % of Hispanics experienced heartburn at least monthly, compared to 37 % of Caucasians, 31 % of African Americans, and 20 % of Asians. Asians in the United States had higher rates of symptoms than in the Far East [4].

Another way of evaluating the prevalence of GERD has been to determine how often patients visited medical facilities for assessment and treatment. A study of 134 primary care clinics across six European countries showed that 3.4 % of all visits were for GERD-related reasons. Of these, symptom recurrence following remission was the most common (35.1 %) reason for a primary care visit, while 12.7 % were for persistence of previous symptoms, and 16.2 % had never seen a physician for GERD-related symptoms before [5]. Most primary care physicians can expect to commonly evaluate patients with GERD symptoms.

Other manifestations of GERD are atypical or extra-esophageal symptoms, which may or may not also be associated with the typical symptoms of GERD. In patients with these extra-esophageal symptoms, 81 % had abnormal acid exposure by 48 h Bravo pH monitoring. Most patients had

V. Velanovich, MD (✉)
Department of Surgery, University of South Florida,
One Tampa General Circle, F145, Tampa, FL 33606, USA
e-mail: vvelanov@health.usf.edu

L.L. Swanstrom and C.M. Dunst (eds.), *Antireflux Surgery*,
DOI 10.1007/978-1-4939-1749-5_3, © Springer New York 2015

Table 3.1 Prevalence gastroesophageal reflux disease

Prevalence				
Basis	Geographic location	Prevalence (%)	95 % CI (%)	Reference
GERD symptoms	United States	24.2	18.2–30.5	[1]
GERD/dyspeptic symptoms	United States	35.2	14.8–58.9	[1]
Any heartburn	South Australia	50		[2]
GERD symptoms	Canada	10–20		[3]
Heartburn	Hispanics	50		[4]
	Caucasians	37		
	African Americans	31		
	Asians	20		
Clinic visits for GERD	Six European countries	3.4		[5]
Non-cardiac chest pain	Various	13		
Asymptomatic	Japan, Korea, Taiwan, Sweden	26.4–45.3		[9]

only mild to moderate symptoms with a low prevalence of esophagitis (18 %) or Barrett's esophagus (0.8 %). It is well described that the degree of esophageal acid exposure, as measured by pH monitoring, cannot be predicted from the presence or absence of typical GERD symptoms [6]. In an evaluation of 18 articles of population-based studies of non-cardiac chest pain, there was an overall prevalence of 13 %, but this varied by geographic location and definition of the disease used (mere presence vs. Rome I or II criteria). There was no difference between men and women, but higher incidences in subjects reporting GERD symptoms and increased as well according to frequency of GERD symptoms [7]. In an analysis from the ProGERD cohort study of patients presenting with heartburn, 32.8 % also had extra-esophageal symptoms. Female gender, age, LA esophagitis grade C or D, duration of GERD symptoms >1 year, and smoking were significantly associated with extra-esophageal symptoms. [8]

There is a significant proportion of individuals with signs of pathologic reflux, but no overt symptoms. In this setting, the definition of "silent" GERD is the presence of esophageal mucosal injury that is typical of GERD found during upper GI endoscopy in individuals who lack the typical or atypical manifestations of GERD [9]. Population-based studies from Sweden, Japan, Taiwan, and Korea have shown that the number of patients with erosive esophagitis but who were asymptomatic varied between 26.4 and 45.3 % [10]. In a group of 594 asymptomatic patients screened with endoscopy in Taiwan, 14.5 % had findings of erosive esophagitis. Male gender (OR 2.32, 95 % CI [1.35–3.98]) and hiatal hernia (OR 4.48, 95 % CI [2.35–89.17]) were risk factors for findings of asymptomatic erosive esophagitis, while a positive CLO test for *Helicobacter pylori* was protective (OR 0.57, 95 % CI [0.34–0.95]) [11]. Therefore, it is apparent that a significant proportion of people in North American and Europe suffer from some type of GERD. It also appears that although some ethnic groups are more likely to suffer from GERD, there at least some members of all ethnic groups that do.

Incidence

As with prevalence, the determination of the incidence of GERD depends on the method and what is measured as a sign of GERD. The best data relates to progression of disease in patients already diagnosed with GERD. In a follow-up study of a Swedish general population (the Kalixandra Study), patients with initial endoscopic or histological diagnosis of GERD and nonerosive reflux disease (NERD), 9.7 % of NERD patient progressed to erosive esophagitis, and 1.8 % to Barrett's esophagus. In patients initially with erosive esophagitis, 13.3 % progress to a more severe grade and 8.9 % to Barrett's esophagus [12]. In a cohort of 3,894 patients undergoing routine care in Germany, Austria, and Switzerland (the ProGERD study), those who underwent endoscopy and found to have GERD were initially treated with esomeprazole. After 2 years, 25 % of patients who had NERD progressed to LA grade A or B esophagitis and 0.6 % to LA grade C or D esophagitis; 1.6 % of patients who had LA grade A or B esophagitis progressed to LA grade C or D and 61 % regressed to NERD; 42 % of patients with LA grade C or D esophagitis regressed to LA grade A and B, while 50 % regressed to NERD. Of the patient initially on esomeprazole, 22 % had been off medication for at least 3 months. Therefore, it seems that both progression and regression in the severity of esophagitis are common [13]. This same study published a 5-year follow-up of 2,721 patients who completed follow-up and showed only a few patients with NERD or mild/moderate erosive esophagitis progressed to severe forms of erosive esophagitis [14]. Therefore, in patients with mild acid-related mucosal damage, it is not likely that they will progress to more severe forms of mucosal injury as long as they receive appropriate treatment.

To determine the incidence of new GERD-related symptoms, our knowledge generally comes from surveys or administrative data. A survey in Canada determined the adult incidence of GERD to be 4.5–5.4 per 1,000 person–years [3]. This is similar to results from a systematic review of the General Practice Research Database in the United Kingdom, which found the incidence of new diagnoses of GERD to be 4.5 per 1,000 person–years [15]. In another systematic review of published longitudinal studies, 65 % of patients with complicated GERD and 70 % of patients with "defined" GERD had persistent disease on follow-up, whereas only 34 % with infrequent or mild symptoms had persistent symptoms. With the prevalence of GERD in the 10–20 % range and the incidence in the 4.5–19.6/1,000 person–years range, this study suggests that GERD is a disease that persists for at least 18 years [16]. A random sample of 10,000 Danish inhabitants followed for 5 years showed that 22 % had GERD symptoms at inclusion. However, over the 5 years, 43 % had symptom resolution, of which 10 % continued to receive acid reducing medication. The overall incidence of new GERD symptoms was 2.2 %/year [17]. Of course, these are new cases, as to how many individuals who had symptoms of GERD that no longer do now is unknown.

Risk Factors

Risk factors for GERD are related to patient's physiology, behavior factors, and genetic factors. Risk factors for developing gastroesophageal reflux disease include: obesity, smoking, age, parental or family history of gastroesophageal diseases, esophageal stricture, high-cholesterol diet, lung transplantation, and cystic fibrosis—all of which have been commonly associated with GERD [3].

Although age has been associated with GERD, this relationship seems to be more complex. A systematic review of nine population based studies showed no increase in GERD symptom prevalence with age, but in patients with GERD, ageing is associated with more severe patterns of acid reflux and reflux esophagitis. Despite this, symptoms associated with GERD have been shown to become less severe and more nonspecific with age. Therefore, the real prevalence of GERD may well increase with age [18]. However, it may also be that older individuals may simply have minimal or no symptoms of acid reflux, despite pathologic reflux leading even to mucosal damage. However, the evolution of hiatal hernias is clearly associated with age. A meta-analysis of 29 studies showed age >50 years was a definite risk factor for hiatal hernia (OR 2.17, 95 % confidence interval [1.35–3.51]) [19]. This study, however, did not differentiate between symptomatic and asymptomatic hiatal hernia nor for paraesophageal hernias.

The relationship between GERD and gender is also complex. In a South Australian sample of 2,973 individuals from the community and 2,152 patients presenting for antireflux surgery, females were more likely to report heartburn, and

with a higher symptom severity. Prevalence of dysphagia was similar from males and females, but dysphagia scores for solid foods were higher in females. A similar proportion of male and female took antireflux medications. Females presenting for antireflux surgery were, on average, 7 years older, had a higher BMI, and higher heartburn and dysphagia scores, while at endoscopy males were more likely to have ulcerative esophagitis and Barrett's esophagus. The authors concluded that these gender differences may reflect differences in symptom perception [20]. However, with respect to hiatal hernia, the study showed that male gender was a definite risk factor (OR 1.36, 95 % CI [1.10–1.68]) [19].

There appear to be ethnic difference associated with GERD. Evidence from both community surveys and studies of endoscopic findings report esophagitis, hiatus hernia, and Barrett's esophagus prevalences were lower among Asian and Afro-Caribbean subjects compared to Caucasians. There may also be a north–south gradient in the prevalence of GERD among western countries; that is, GERD may be more common in northern regions compared to southern regions. Studies involving other geographic regions show that GERD may be moderately common in the Middle East and less common in Asia, although the prevalence seems to be increasing in the Far East [21]. In the United States, in a study of an impoverished minority population, waist circumference and smoking were strongly associated with GERD, while overall BMI, waist/hip ratio, and diet were not [22]. Therefore, in some minority populations, the risk factors for GERD are different.

Weight is clearly associated with GERD. Being overweight, obese, or morbidly obese contributes to the development of a variety of esophageal disorders, including hiatal hernia, GERD, Barrett's esophagus, and esophageal adenocarcinoma [23]. Weight gain increases GERD symptoms and weight loss decreases symptoms [24]. A population-based study in Germany showed a pronounced dose–response relationship between BMI and heartburn occurrence in people without chronic atrophic gastritis, but this was not the case for those with chronic atrophic gastritis [25]. Comparing populations, samples of 3,633 English and 1,483 Swedish people showed that the prevalence of GERD symptoms was twice as common in the English as the Swedish, but obesity (BMI ≥ 30) was also nearly twice as likely, although tobacco smoking was similar [26]. Weight is associated with erosive esophagitis and pathologic acid-reflux related NERD, while patients with functional heartburn or a hypersensitive esophagus tended to be of normal weight. [27] Lastly, with respect to hiatal hernia, individuals with BMI's > 25 where at increased risk of having a HH (OR 1.92, 95 % CI [1.10–3.39]) [19].

Of particular interest to surgeons are the effects of other disorders on GERD. In a study of Japanese workers with GERD, 6 % of patients were found to have functional

Table 3.2 Risk factors for GERD-associated disorders

Risk factor		Pathologic acid reflux	Hiatal hernia	Esophagitis	GERD-perceived symptoms	
					Typical	Atypical
Increasing age		↑	↑	↑	↓	↑
Gender	Female				↑	↑
	Male		↑	↑		
Ethnicity	Caucasian		↑	↑	↑	
	Asian/Afro-Caribbean		↓	↓	↓	
Increasing weight		↑	↑	↑	↑	
Associated conditions	Functional GI disorders				↑	
	Depression				↑	
	Kyphosis/lordosis		↑		↑	
	H. pylori/Atrophic gastritis	↓		↓	↓	
Smoking			↑	↑	↑	↑

dyspepsia or irritable bowel syndrome. Female gender and smoking increased the risk of overlapping GERD with both functional dyspepsia and irritable bowel syndrome [28]. The severity and duration of daytime heartburn and regurgitation were independent risk factors for nocturnal GERD [29]. A diagnosis of depression is also associated with an increased risk of subsequent GERD. The incidence of GERD was 14.2/1,000 person–years in a cohort of patients with depression as compared to 8.3/1,000 person–years in a control group. The use of tricyclic antidepressants increased the risk of GERD (OR 1.71, 95 % CI [1.34–2.20]), while selective serotonin reuptake inhibitors did not [30]. Spinal issues have been recently associated with GERD. A multivariate analysis demonstrated that kyphosis, lumbar lordosis angle, sagittal balance, number of oral drugs taken per day, and back muscle strength had significant effects on the presence of GERD [31]. As these spinal conditions are more common in older individuals, this may, at least partially, explain the increase incidence of GERD with age.

The effects of lifestyle (beyond obesity) and other environmental factors have been shown to have some influence on the occurrence of GERD. Some suggest that smoking, alcohol, dietary fat, or drugs play only a minor role in shaping the epidemiologic patterns of GERD. On a population level, a high prevalence of *H. pylori* infection is likely to reduce levels of acid secretion and protect against reflux [24]. Obese/overweight people with chronic atrophic gastric actually had a much lower risk of heartburn (OR 0.31, [0.24–0.40]) [25]. On the other hand, in a South Korean population, eradication of *H. pylori* did not affect the development of reflux esophagitis or GERD symptoms [32].

Stress has been shown to affect GERD as well. The terrorist attacks of September 11, 2001 have resulted in several unique health issues, one of which is GERD. Among individuals exposed to the terrorists attacks at the World Trade Center, the cumulative incidence of GERD symptoms was 20 %, and occurred more often in individuals suffering from post-traumatic stress disorder (24 %), asthma (13 %), or both (36 %), compared with neither (8 %). The authors concluded that GERD symptoms may be accentuated in the presence of asthma or PTSD [33]. This event and its aftermath may help shed light on the relation of patient-perceived symptoms and concomitant psychoemotional disorders in GERD [34].

Risk factors for GERD-related disorders need to be organized into those which truly increase the risk of pathologic acid reflux, those which increase the risk of hiatal hernia, those which increase the risk of erosive esophagitis, and those with increase the perception of GERD-like symptoms. The later can be further divided into the typical and atypical (extra-esophageal) symptoms of GERD. Table 3.2 summarizes the previously discussed risks factors in this manner.

Economics of Gastroesophageal Reflux

Gastroesophageal reflux disease has wide-ranging economic implications. These include economic loss to the patient, health care system, and society. In addition, GERD is big business, with pharmaceutical and device companies vigorously competing for sales in drugs and surgical instrumentation. This later controversial topic will not be addressed in this review.

Personal Cost to Patients

Patients economically suffer from GERD due to both personal direct medical costs and loss of income due to missed work. Data from the 2010 National Health and Wellness Survey comparing non-GERD controls to GERD patients with diurnal, nocturnal, and both diurnal and nocturnal symptoms showed that GERD patients had an estimated burden of illness direct costs of $1,435 and a lost productivity costs of $3,134 [35]. Depending on employee benefits, loss of work can directly lead to loss of income. The true amount of this income loss is unknown.

Effects on Work and Productivity

The effects of GERD on the work place are two-fold. One is absenteeism due to missing work from GERD-related problems. The other is "presenteeism," which is reduction in the worker's effectiveness and productivity while at work due to a medical condition. The Retrospective Analysis of Gastroesophageal Reflux Disease (RANGE) study of 134 primary care clinics in Germany, Greece, Norway, Spain, Sweden, and the UK analyzed a random sample of 2,678 patients with GERD. Average absenteeism due to GERD was highest in Germany (3.2 h/week) and lowest in the UK (0.4 h/week). In Norway, an average of 6.7 h/week was lost to presenteeism. The average monetary impact of GERD-related work absenteeism and presenteeism ranged from 55 euros/week per employed patient in the UK to 273 euros/week per employed patient in Sweden. One should keep in mind that this monetary impact affects both employers and society as a whole. Reductions in productivity in daily life activities of up to 26 % were observed in this study [36]. Another study of US respondents to the Internet-based 2004 National Health and Wellness Survey who had self-reported GERD showed increased absenteeism (Median time lost: 0.9 h/week), reduced percentage productivity at work (Median percent lost: 7.5 %), and increased healthcare utilization. All tested variables deteriorated with increasing symptom severity [37]. A post hoc analysis of the 2007 National Health and Wellness Survey including respondents from France, Germany, the United Kingdom, and the United States showed that PPI-compliant respondents with persistent and intense symptoms also reported lower work productivity, greater activity impairment, and more hours missed from work due to health problems [38]. Another study showed, the total costs for absenteeism and presenteeism for employers were 10 and 1 million euros for Germany, Italy, and Spain, respectively [39]. In a Canadian survey, of 173 patients employed, 6.7 h of work time was lost each week due to GERD symptoms (16 % lost work time and activity impairment also affected as much as 21 % of nonwork-related activities [3].

Costs to Healthcare Systems

In addition to being a burden on patients, GERD burdens healthcare systems. In Germany, Italy, and Spain, the size of the population with poorly treated GERD and with Barrett's esophagus was estimated to be 29,678 in Spain, 19,327 in Germany, and 10,079 in Italy. Costs to each healthcare system were estimated to be 18, 12, and 7 million euros [39]. In 2004 and 2005, the Canadian health care system spent a mean of $6,915 per patient who had a primary diagnosis benign esophageal diseases and associated complications.

Canadian cost estimates for a 28-day supply of proton pump inhibitor therapy ranged from $40 to 70 [3]. This is much harder to estimate in the United States as what is charged for medications varies across insurance plans. In a study of commercial insurer enrollees, GERD-associated complications were classified as stage A (GERD diagnosis, no other symptoms), stage B (GERD + extra-esophageal symptoms), stage C (GERD + Barrett's esophagus), stage D (GERD + esophageal stricture), and stage E (GERD + iron deficiency anemia or acute upper gastrointestinal hemorrhage). Of 174,597 patients, 6-month costs ranged from $615/patient (stage A) to $1,714/patient (stage D); all costs ranged from $615/patient (stage A) to $11,340/patient (stage E) [40]. In a retrospective cohort study of 600 GERD patients, with age, gender, prescription pharmaceutical benefits, and insurance status matched to non-GERD controls, the mean annual direct medical costs of the GERD group was $4,906 compared to $2,054 for the non-GERD group. Among the costs of services, the GERD group had 2.00-fold higher cost associated with outpatient services, 1.70-fold higher cost associated with inpatient services, and a 2.70-fold higher cost associated with pharmacy [41].

Part of this burden has to do with hospitalizations and doctor visits. In the United Kingdom and the United States, respondents with persistent and intense symptoms reported more visits to both primary care and specialty physicians than respondents with a low symptom burden; and the United States respondents with persistent and intense symptoms reported significantly more emergency room visits [38]. During the period from 2003 to 2006, approximately 500,000 patients with a primary and 14.5 million patients with a secondary GERD-related diagnosis became hospitalized in the United States [42].

On the other hand, effective treatment can reduce this utilization. In a study of more than 25 million managed care lives from January, 2000 to February, 2005 using the National Managed Care Benchmarks database of compliant and non-compliant proton pump inhibitor users showed that of 41,837 proton pump inhibitor users, 68 % were compliant. On an annual, per-patient basis, proton pump inhibitor compliance resulted in 0.47 fewer outpatient visits, 0.03 fewer inpatient visits, and 0.47 fewer hospital days compared to pre-proton pump inhibitor use and compared to noncompliance. Proton pump inhibitor therapy increased pharmacy costs in both groups, but the total annual costs were reduced. Compliant patients experienced a greater decline in total costs from the pre-proton pump inhibitor compared to non-compliant patients ($3,261 vs. $2.406 per patient per year) [43]. Better understanding of who would actually benefit from therapy would probably lead to less medication costs. In a cost-benefit analysis of patients in an integrated health network, a break-even analysis showed that Bravo testing with esophagogastroduodenoscopy (EGD) to identify those patients who could be taken off PPI therapy, paid for itself in 33 months.

Bravo+EGD+manometry testing performed to screen for other possible pathologies paid for itself in 38 months. Bravo+barium swallow+EGD testing to screen patients for cancer paid for itself in 42 months. Early testing can realize cost savings by identifying patients that are taking double-dose PPI's unnecessarily based on a presumptive diagnosis of GERD [44]. This cost-effectiveness of therapy extends to antireflux surgery as well. A Markov analysis from data based on the REFLUX trial showed that on a base-case model, surgery is likely to be considered cost effective on average with an incremental cost-effectiveness ration of 2,648 lb sterling ($4,385) per quality adjusted life year and that the probability that surgery is cost effective is 0.94 at a threshold incremental cost-effectiveness ratio of 20,000 lb sterling. The results were sensitive to some of the assumptions within the extrapolation model such as the length of the treatment effect of surgery, if patients who return to medical management have poor health related quality of life, or if PPI's were cheaper [45].

Therefore, GERD is a significant burden to patients and the healthcare system. Successful treatment can certainly reduce costs and improve the population's quality of life.

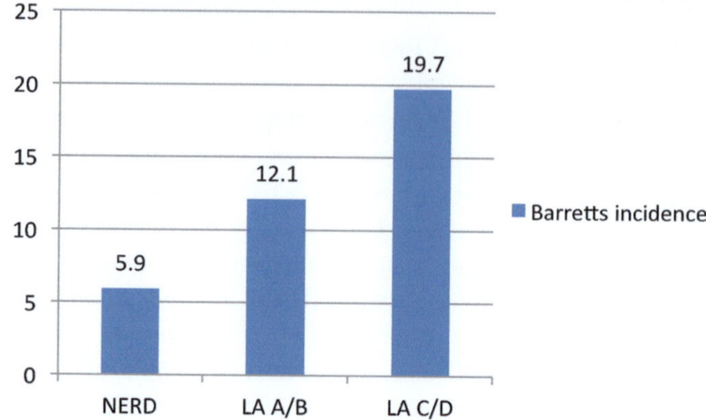

Fig. 3.1 Barrett's incidence

Epidemiology of Barrett's Esophagus

Prevalence

It is difficult to truly know the overall prevalence and incidence of Barrett's esophagus. This is due to the fact that many individuals with Barrett's metaplasia are asymptomatic and, therefore, will never be evaluated for the presence of Barrett's esophagus. Also, different populations are at risk and, therefore, prevalence may vary from location to location. The best estimate of population prevalence of Barrett's esophagus is 1.6 % of the general population [46]. In parallel, the frequency of esophageal adenocarcinoma in men has quadrupled in the past few years. The cause is unknown, but it is probably linked to an increase in incidence of gastro-esophageal reflux, and with its association with Barrett's esophagus [47]. A population-based study conducted in Sweden with the objective of validating the Gastrointestinal Symptom Rating Scale, performed endoscopy on a random selection of 1,000 individuals [48]. Patients with symptoms of reflux had an overall prevalence of Barrett esophagus of 2.3 %, whereas the prevalence in asymptomatic individuals was 1.4 %. Patients with symptoms seem to have a higher incidence of Barrett's esophagus, with one study identifying 13.2 % of symptomatic patients having Barrett's metaplasia [49]. Paradoxically, patients with short-segment Barrett esophagus had more frequent and intense symptoms than did those with long-segment Barrett's esophagus [50]. Among patients undergoing endoscopy for any reason, Barrett's esophagus was rare in children and tended to become more prevalent with increasing age [51]. Nevertheless, in a series of patients from a tertiary care clinic, about 25 % of patients with Barrett's esophagus were younger than 50 years [52]. Men and Caucasians appear to have a higher prevalence of Barrett's esophagus than other groups [51]. The "typical" patient with Barrett's esophagus is the middle-age, white male with several year history of GERD-related symptoms.

Incidence

As with prevalence, incidence of Barrett's esophagus is also difficult to determine. Most studies are based on follow-up endoscopies of defined populations. In another longitudinal study of a Swedish general population (the Kalixandra Study), looking at patients with initial endoscopic or histological evidence of GERD and NERD, the overall incidence of Barrett's esophagus was 9.9/1,000 person–years. In patients with NERD, 9.7 % progressed to erosive esophagitis, and 1.8 % to Barrett's esophagus. In patients initially presenting with erosive esophagitis, 13.3 % progress to a more severe grade of esophagitis and 8.9 % to Barrett's esophagus. Erosive esophagitis was independently associated with progression to Barrett's esophagus (Relative Risk Ratio (RRR) 5.2; 95 % CI 1.2–22.9) [12]. Patients with LA C/D esophagitis were at greatest risk for developing Barrett's esophagus at 2 years, 5.8 % vs. 1.4 % for LA A/B compared to 0.5 % for NERD [13]. A 5-year follow-up of the ProGERD study showed 5.9 % of NERD patients, 12.1 % of LA A/B patients, and 19.7 % of LA C/D patients progressed to Barrett's esophagus [14] (Fig. 3.1).

Risk Factors

In general, the risk factors for Barrett's esophagus are similar to GERD. The main risk factor is GERD with pathologic exposure of the esophagus to acid and bile refluxate. Analysis of five case–control studies from the Barrett's and Esophageal Adenocarcinoma Consortium showed that subjects with Barrett's esophagus were significantly more likely to have ever smoked cigarettes compared to population-based controls or patients with GERD. Increasing pack-years of smoking increase risk for Barrett's esophagus. There was evidence of synergy between ever-smoking and heartburn or regurgitation [53]. In a case–control study of the Kaiser Permanente Northern California population higher intake of omega-3 fatty acids (OR 0.46, 95 % CI [0.22–0.97]), polyunsaturated fat, total fiber (OR 0.34, 95 % CI [0.15–0.76]), and fiber from fruits and vegetables (OR 0.47, 95 % CI [0.25–0.88]) was associated with lower risks of Barrett's esophagus. Higher meat intakes were also associated with a lower risk of long-segment Barrett's esophagus (OR 0.25, 95 % CI [0.09–0.72]). Conversely, higher trans-fat (often found in processed foods) intakes were associated with increased risk of Barrett's esophagus (OR 1.11, 95 % CI [1.03–1.21]). Total fat intake, barbecued foods, and fiber intake from sources other than fruits and vegetables were not associated with Barrett's esophagus [54]. Interestingly, Barrett's esophagus and adenocarcinoma tend to occur slightly more often in subjects with higher income [24].

Conclusion

GERD and Barrett's esophagus are relatively common problems that nearly all physician will encounter. The incidence of both is dramatically increasing and is becoming a increasing public concern. Understanding the epidemiology of both conditions will help surgeons counsel patients more appropriately. Understanding the cost burden to patients and the healthcare system will help surgeons be better stewards of medical resources.

References

1. Sobieraj DM, Coleman SM, Coleman CI. US prevalence of upper gastrointestinal symptoms: A systematic review. Am J Mang Care. 2011;17:e449–45.
2. Watson DI, Lally CJ. Prevalence of symptoms and use of medication for gastroesophageal reflux disease in an Australian community. World J Surg. 2009;33:88–94.
3. Fedorak RN, Veldhuyzen van Zanten S, Bridges R. Canadian Digestive Health Foundation Public Impact Series: gastro-esophageal reflux disease in Canada: incidence, prevalence, and direct and indirect economic impact. Can J Gastroenterol. 2010;24:431–4.
4. Yuen E, Romney M, Toner RW, et al. Prevalence, knowledge and care patterns for gastro-oesophageal reflux disease in United States minority populations. Aliment Pharmacol Ther. 2010;32:645–54.
5. Gisbert JP, Cooper A, Karagiannis D, et al. Consultation rates and characteristics of gastro-oesophagel reflux disease in primary care: a European observational study. Eur J Gen Pract. 2009;15:154–60.
6. Fletcher KC, Goutte M, Slaughter JC, et al. Significance and degree of reflux in patients with primary extraesophageal symptoms. Laryngoscope. 2011;121:2561–5.
7. Ford AC, Suares NC, Talley NJ. Meta-analysis: the epidemiology of noncardiac chest pain in the community. Aliment Pharmacol Ther. 2011;34:172–80.
8. Jaspersen D, Kulig M, Labenz J, et al. Prevalence of extra-oesophageal manifestations in gastro-oesophageal reflux disease: an analysis based on the ProGERD study. Aliment Pharmacol Ther. 2003;17:1515–20.
9. Fass R, Dickman R. Clinical consequences of silent gastroesophageal reflux disease. Curr Gastroenterol Rep. 2006;8:195–201.
10. Goh K-L, Shiaw-Hooi H. Silent gastroesophageal disease: clinical implications of an unknown disease. J Gastroenterol Hepatol. 2011;26:941–2.
11. Wang PC, Hsu CS, Tseng TC, et al. Male sex, hiatus hernia, and Helicobacter pylori infection associated with asymptomatic erosive esophagitis. J Gastroenterol Hepatol. 2012;27:586–91.
12. Ronkainen J, Talley NJ, Storskrubb T, et al. Erosive esophagitis is a risk factor for Barrett's esophagus: a community-based endoscopic follow-up study. Am J Gastroenterol. 2011;106:1946–52.
13. Labenz J, Nocon M, Lind T, et al. Prospective follow-up data from the ProGERD study suggest that GERD is not a categorical disease. Am J Gastroenterol. 2006;101:2457–62.
14. Malfertheiner P, Nocon M, Vieth M, et al. Evolution of gastro-oesophageal reflux disease over 5 years under routine medical care—the ProGERD study. Aliment Pharmacol Ther. 2012; 35:154–64.
15. El-Serag H, Hill C, Jones R. Systematic review: the epidemiology of gastro-oesophageal reflux disease in primary care, using the UK General Practice Research Database. Aliment Pharmacol Ther. 2009;29:470–80.
16. Armstrong D. Systematic review: persistence and severity in gastro-oesophageal reflux disease. Aliment Pharmacol Ther. 2008;28:841–53.
17. Hansen JM, Wildner-Christensen M, Schaffalizky de Muckadell OB. Gastroesophageal reflux symptoms in a Danish population: a prospective follow-up analysis of symptoms, quality of life, and health-care use. Am J Gastroenterol. 2009;104:2394–403.
18. Ageing reference
19. Menon S, Trudgill N. Risk factors in the aetiology of hiatus hernia: a meta-analysis. Eur J Gastroenterol Hepatol. 2011;23:133–8.
20. Chen Z, Thompson SK, Jamieson GG, et al. Effect of sex on symptoms associated with gastroesophageal reflux. Arch Surg. 2011; 146:1164–9.
21. Kang JY. Systematic review: geographical and ethnic differences in gastro-oesophageal reflux disease. Aliment Pharmacol Ther. 2004;20:705–17.
22. Friedenberg FK, Rai J, Vanar V, et al. Prevalence and risk factors for gastroesophageal reflux disease in an impoverished minority population. Obes Res Clin Pract. 2010;4:e261–369.
23. Lagergren J. Influence of obesity on the risk of esophageal disorders. Nat Rev Gastroenterol Hepatol. 2011;8:340–7.
24. Sonnenberg A. Effects of environment and lifestyle on gastroesophageal reflux disease. Dig Dis. 2011;29:229–34.
25. Gao L, Weck MN, Rothenbacher D, Brenner H. Body mass index, chronic atrophic gastritis and heartburn: a population-based study among 8936 older adults from Germany. Aliment Pharmacol Ther. 2010;32:296–302.
26. Lofdahl HE, Lane A, Lu Y, et al. Increased population prevalence of reflux and obesity in the United Kingdom compare with Sweden: a potential explanation for the difference in incidence of esophageal adenocarcinoma. Eur J Gastroenterol Hepatol. 2011;23:128–32.
27. Savarino E, Zentilin P, Marabotto E, et al. Overweight is a risk factor for both erosive and non-erosive reflux disease. Dig Liver Dis. 2011;43:940–5.
28. Fujiwara Y, Kubo M, Kohata Y, et al. Cigarette smoking and its association with overlapping gastroesophageal reflux disease, functional dyspepsia or irritable bowel syndrome. Intern Med. 2011; 50:2443–7.

29. Gaddam S, Maddur H, Wani S, et al. Risk factors for nocturnal reflux in a large GERD cohort. J Clin Gastroenterol. 2011; 45:764–8.

30. Martin-Merino E, Ruigomez A, Garcia-Rodriguez LA, et al. Depression and treatment with antidepressants are associated with the development of gastro-oesophageal reflux disease. Aliment Pharmacol Ther. 2010;31:1132–40.

31. Imagama S, Hasegawa Y, Wakao N, et al. Influence of lumbar kyphosis and back muscle strength on the symptoms of gastro-esophageal reflux disease in middle-aged and elderly people. Eur Spine J. 2012; Feb 28 [Epub ahead of print]

32. Kim N, Lee SW, Baik GH, et al. Effect of Helicobacter pylori eradication on the development of reflux esophagitis and gastroesophageal reflux symptoms: a nationwide multi-center prospective study. Gut Liver. 2011;5:437–46.

33. Li J, Brackbill RM, Stellman SD, et al. Gastroesophageal reflux symptoms and comorbid asthma and posttraumatic stress disorder following the 9/11 terrorist attacks on World Trade Center in New York City. Am J Gastroenterol. 2011;106:1933–41.

34. Velanovich V. The effects of chronic pain syndromes and psycho-emotional disorders on symptomatic and quality of life outcomes of antireflux surgery. J Gastrointest Surg. 2003;7:53–8.

35. Wagner JS, DiBonaventura MD, Balu S, Buchner D. The burden of diurnal and nocturnal gastroesophageal reflux disease symptoms. Expert Rev Pharmacoecon Outcomes Res. 2011;11:739–49.

36. Gisbert JP, Cooper A, Karagiannis D, et al. Impact of gastroesophageal reflux disease on work absenteeism, presenteeism and productivity in daily life: a European observational study. Health Qual Life Outcomes. 2009;7:90.

37. Wahlqvist P, Karlsson M, Johnson D, et al. Relationship between symptom load of gastro-oesophageal reflux disease and health-related quality of life, work productivity, resource utilization and concomitant diseases: survey of a US cohort. Aliment Pharmacol Ther. 2008;27:960–70.

38. Toghanian S, Johnson DA, Stalhammar NO, Zerbib F. Burdent of gastro-oesophageal reflux disease in patients with persistent and intense symptoms despite proton pump inhibitor therapy: a post hoc analysis of the 2007 National Health and Wellness Survey. Clin Drug Investig. 2011;31:703–15.

39. Darba J, Kaskens L, Plans P, et al. Epidemiology and societal costs of gastroesophageal reflux disease and Barrett's syndrome in Germany, Italy and Spain. Expert Rev Pharmacoecon Outcomes Res. 2011;11:225–32.

40. Gerson L, McLaughlin T, Balu S, et al. Variation of health-care resource utilization according to GERD-associated complications. Dis Esophagus 2012; Jan 31 [Epub ahead of print]

41. Jayadevappa R, Chhatre S, Weiner M. Gastro-oesophageal acid-related disease, co-morbidity and medical care cost. Chronic Illn. 2008;4:209–18.

42. Thukkani N, Sonnenberg A. The influence of environmental risk factors in hospitalization for gastro-oesophageal reflux disease-related diagnoses in the United States. Aliment Pharmacol Ther. 2010;31:852–61.

43. Gosselin A, Luo R, Lohouses H, et al. The impact of proton pump inhibitor compliance on health-care resource utilization and costs in patients with gastroesophageal reflux disease. Value Health. 2009;12:34–9.

44. Raman A, Sternbach J, Babajide A, et al. When does testing for GERD become cost effective in an integrated health network? Surg Endosc. 2010;24:1245–9.

45. Epstein D, Bojke L, Sculpher MJ, The REFLUX trial group. Laparoscopic fundoplication compared with medical management for gastro-oesophageal reflux disease: cost effectiveness study. BMJ. 2009;339:b2576.

46. Wang KK, Sampliner RE, Practice Parameters Committee of the American College of Gastroenterology. Updated guidelines 2008 for the diagnosis, surveillance and therapy of Barrett's esophagus. Am J Gastroenterol. 2008;103:788–97.

47. Spechler SJ. Clinical practice. Barrett's esophagus. N Engl J Med. 2002;346:836–42.

48. Ronkainen J, Aro P, Storskrubb T, et al. Prevalence of Barrett's esophagus in the general population: an endoscopic study. Gastroenterology. 2005;129:1825–31.

49. Westhoff B, Brotze S, Weston A, et al. The frequency of Barrett's esophagus in high-risk patients with chronic GERD. Gastrointest Endosc. 2005;61:226–31.

50. Dickman R, Kim JL, Camargo L, et al. Correlation of gastroesophageal reflux disease symptom characteristics with long-segment Barrett's esophagus. Dis Esophagus. 2006;19:360–5.

51. Cameron AJ. Epidemiology of Barrett's esophagus and adenocarcinoma. Dis Esophagus. 2002;15:106–8.

52. Guardino JM, Khandwala F, Lopez R, et al. Barrett's esophagus at a tertiary care center: association of age on incidence and prevalence of dysplasia and adenocarcinoma. Am J Gastroenterol. 2006;101:2187–93.

53. Cook MB, Shaheen NJ, Anderson LA, et al. Cigarette smoking increases risk of Barrett's esophagus: An analysis of the Barrett's and Esophageal Adenocarcinoma Consortium. Gastroenterology 2012; Jan 11 [Epub ahead of print]

54. Kubo A, Block G, Queensberry Jr CP, et al. Effects of dietary fiber, fats, and meat intakes on the risk of Barrett's esophagus. Nutr Cancer. 2009;61:607–16.

Philip O. Katz and Jorge R. Uribe

Lifestyle Modifications

Numerous dietary and lifestyle modifications continue to be advocated as important in therapy of GERD. (Table 4.1) The physiologic basis for elimination of certain foods, change in body positions, tobacco, alcohol, and body mass index are certainly sound. Some drugs have been shown to decrease lower esophageal sphincter pressure and have the potential to exacerbate reflux. These drugs include aspirin, non-steroidal anti-inflammatory drugs, some antibiotics, potassium chloride tablets, ferrous sulfate tablets, alendronate, and other bisphosphonates. They may cause direct esophageal injury and have been shown to exacerbate reflux symptoms. On the other hand, most patients have already attempted their own lifestyle changes before seeing a specialist, often based on their own evidence of which dietary indiscretions and lifestyle issues exacerbate their symptoms.

Encouraging patients to go to bed on an empty stomach is the most logical suggestion. Proximal acid migration is greatest during sleep and sleep also delays esophageal acid clearance. As the majority of reflux is in the first 4 h of sleep, eating within 1–2 h of sleep is much more likely to cause nocturnal reflux [1].

Elevation of the head of the bed 6–8 inches is worth considering. This is based on studies using prolonged pH monitoring that have shown an acceleration of esophageal clearance when the head of the bed is elevated compared to sleeping flat [2–4]. In addition, reflux frequency as well as total time that esophageal pH was <4 is decreased in the left side down position, compared to right side down, prone, and supine [5–9]. Sleep medications increase night time reflux and should be used with care in GERD [10].

Acidic liquids (colas and teas) and citrus products are direct esophageal irritants and may exacerbate symptoms [11–16]. A high-fat meal is known to increase reflux frequency [17, 18]. Fat delays gastric emptying, so may increase the risk of reflux through this mechanism. Chocolate also decreases LESP [19], increases esophageal acid exposure [20], and is on the list of foods to potentially avoid.

Symptomatic GERD and body weight are clearly related. Weight gain is associated with an increased risk of having symptoms of GERD and weight loss associated with a decrease in incidence [21, 22]. Increase in BMI is a risk for the development of adenocarcinoma as well in patients with Barrett's esophagus [23] and a BMI of >30 may be a risk for failure of antireflux surgery [24] further suggesting that there is some link between obesity and GERD. Overall waist circumference is emerging as a bigger issue rather than BMI itself.

Overall, lifestyle changes are still reasonable adjuncts to treatment, even if they have a minimal impact [25]. Educating patients about the potential values of going to bed on an empty stomach and the overall potential of lifestyle modifications to reduce symptoms takes little time and ultimately might help. It is, however, difficult to push these interventions on patients who choose not to implement them as "hard data" are lacking.

Pharmacologic Therapy

Proton pump inhibitors (PPIs) are the agents of choice for anti-secretory therapy in GERD. Today's clinician needs, however, to be familiar with the still widely used antacids, H_2 receptor antagonists, sucralfate, and prokinetic agents to understand their synergistic potential in GERD management.

P.O. Katz, MD (✉)
Division of Gastroenterology, Department of Medicine,
Einstein Medical Center, 5401 Old York Road, Klein Professional
Building, Suite 363, Philadelphia, PA 19141, USA
e-mail: philipokatz@gmail.com

J.R. Uribe, MD
Department of Medicine, Einstein Medical Center,
5401 Old York Road, Klein Professional Building,
Suite 363, Philadelphia, PA 19141, USA
e-mail: uribejor@einstein.edu

L.L. Swanstrom and C.M. Dunst (eds.), *Antireflux Surgery*,
DOI 10.1007/978-1-4939-1749-5_4, © Springer New York 2015

Table 4.1 Lifestyle modifications and GERD

Lifestyle modification	Evidence of strength	Reasonable to recommend?
Sleep with head elevated	Equivocal	Not generally
Avoid fatty meals	Equivocal	Not generally
Avoid carbonated beverages	Moderate	Yes
Select decaffeinated beverages	Equivocal	Not generally
Avoid citrus	Weak	Not generally
Eat smaller meals	Weak	Yes
Lose weight	Equivocal	Yes[a]
Avoid alcoholic beverages	Weak	Not generally
Stop smoking	Weak	Yes (in symptomatic persons)
Avoid excessive exercise	Weak	Yes[a]
Sleep on left side	Unequivocal	Yes

[a]Obesity and smoking appear to be risk factors for cancer of the distal esophagus

Antacids

Antacids are effective only for symptom relief. It is rare that they are sufficient to adequately help a patient with other than occasional heartburn. Efficacy of antacids should be evaluated between equivalent doses, whether tablet or liquid. Alginic acid combined with antacid has a slightly different mechanism of action but is likely similar to other antacids in efficacy. Side effects of antacids are minimal when they are used intermittently. Chronic use of magnesium-containing antacids may cause diarrhea, and should be avoided in the patient with heart failure, renal insufficiency, and in late trimester pregnancy. Aluminum-containing antacids may cause constipation [26–28]. Popular over-the-counter antacids, such as Maalox® and Mylanta®, contain both magnesium and aluminum. Gaviscon® also has alginic acid and is often described as more effective for nocturnal reflux.

Barrier Agent

Sucralfate binds to inflamed tissue and may inhibit the erosive action of pepsin and bile [29]. Healing of erosive esophagitis compared to H$_2$RAs is similar [31, 32]. Constipation is seen in 2 % of patients with this sucraflate. Little systemic absorption of the agent has been demonstrated making it quite safe. Because of the need to give the drug four times a day, there is little value in GERD except perhaps in pregnant women [30]. Otherwise, this compound has little to no place in modern medical therapy for GERD.

Prokinetics

A promotility, or "motility altering" agent, theoretically may represent the ideal agent to treat GERD. Improving the strength and competence of the LES, augmenting esophageal clearance to shorten the time the esophageal mucosa is exposed to a pH < 4 and to improve gastric emptying with its potential for "overflow reflux," might constitute the ideal therapy. Unfortunately, the remaining agent available in the United States—metoclopramide—is limited in efficacy and has an unfavorable side effect profile. Usefulness is thus limited in GERD patients.

Metoclopramide is a dopamine antagonist that likely sensitizes tissues to the action of acetylcholine, increases the amplitude of gastric and esophageal contractions, transiently increases LES pressure (LESP), and predominantly accelerates gastric emptying. It produces clinically important central nervous system side effects such as drowsiness and confusion [33]. Equivalent efficacy of metoclopramide compared to Histamine receptor antagonists (H$_2$RA) in relieving heartburn and other GERD symptoms has been documented. When compared to placebo, 10 mg of metoclopramide three times daily showed little symptom improvement. When the dose was increased to 10 mg four times daily, it is more effective than placebo in improving symptoms [34–38]. Because of its centrally acting effects; antidopaminergic side effects are observed in 20–30 % of patients. Anxiety, agitation, confusion, motor restlessness, hallucinations, and drowsiness are common side effects; depression and potentially irreversible tardive dyskinesia are the most serious complications of the drug. Side effects are likely dose related and may be higher in children and the elderly. There is currently a black box warning for side effects and informed, written consent is recommended if prescribed for long-term use. In a patient with clear evidence of gastroparesis and GERD symptoms refractory to antisecretory therapy, metoclopramide may be of additional benefit. Unfortunately, it is not effective in treating patients with esophageal motility abnormalities.

Domperidone is a peripheral dopamine antagonist that stimulates esophageal peristalsis, increases LESP, and accelerates gastric emptying. It is not FDA approved in the United

States [39]. It does not have the central dopaminergic side effects of metoclopramide. There are few GERD studies with this drug, and nothing to suggest it is superior to an H_2RA. It should not be administered with antisecretory agents or antacids, as reduced gastric acidity impairs its absorption [40, 41]. Hyperprolactinemia, nipple tenderness, galactorrhea, and amenorrhea are the most common side effects. This is not a GERD drug.

Bethanechol is a cholinergic drug that has been used to treat reflux and bladder spasm since the 1970s [42]. It has been demonstrated to increase the resting tone of the clasp and sling fibers of the gastroesophageal junction which are typically defective in patients with GERD [43]. Side effects relate to the relative increase in parasympathetic tone including abdominal cramps, diarrhea, bradycardia, sweating, salivation, and flushing. Its use is mostly related to pharmacologic theory and there exists no definitive clinical data to support its use over other standard therapies.

Baclofen can be helpful for patients with mild reflux, particularly with meals. Baclofen is an agonist of GABA, the major inhibitory neurotransmitter in the central nervous system. GABA receptors are also found in the enteric nervous system where it has been shown to decrease reflux through inhibition of transient LES relaxations and elevation of LES resting pressure. In a study of 20 volunteers, a single dose of baclofen reduced acid reflux events and TLESRs by about 40 % but interestingly has no effect on overall acid exposure during the 3 h study period [44]. Baclofen is associated with only mild side effects including somnolence, dizziness, and nausea and has no adverse effects on other aspects of esophageal function [45]. Baclofen is therefore considered a fairly safe option for most patients with very mild symptoms.

Antisecretory Agents

Acid control remains the medical approach of choice to treat patient with GERD. Two classes of drugs are available, H_2RAs and PPIs. Both inhibit gastric secretion and raise intragastric pH though to varying degrees. Intragastric pH control is an indirect measure of efficacy of symptom relief, correlates with healing of erosive esophagitis, and is important in understanding the overall efficacy data of these agents. If gastric pH is <4, pepsinogen is activated to pepsin, which exacerbates the esophageal mucosal damage caused by contact with gastric acid during reflux events. There is a relationship between the duration of time (calculated over 24 h) that the intragastric pH is >4 and healing [46, 47].

H_2RAs have been available as over-the-counter agents since 1995. There are four H_2 receptor antagonists currently available—cimetidine, ranitidine, famotidine, and nizatidine. The mechanism of action for H_2RAs is via competitive inhibition of the acid stimulating histamine receptors on the gastric parietal cells. As a class, H_2RAs are relatively weak inhibitors of meal-stimulated acid secretion, reducing acid secretion by 60–70 % [48]. Antisecretory effects of H_2RAs are best at night, with duration of acid inhibition longer when the drug is taken in the evening or before bedtime. Equally potent doses of the various H_2RAs equally inhibit acid secretion.

Maintenance of symptom relief and healing with H_2RAs is variable. An illustrative study [55] examined symptom relapse over four weeks in 423 patients with GERD symptoms, randomized to either a placebo or 150 mg ranitidine twice or four times daily. At the end of 24 weeks, 52 % with baseline nonerosive disease and 67 % with erosive disease experienced symptomatic relapse [31]. In an another study [56] comparing cisapride, ranitidine, and omeprazole, ranitidine 150 mg tid maintained remission in only 49 % at 1 year. Objective healing rates are somewhat better than symptom control with H2 blockers, Twelve-week healing rates as high as 70 % are seen with ranitidine at 150 mg up to four times daily [51–53] eight-week healing rates of up to 77 % at 800 mg of cimetidine twice daily [52], and famotidine 40 mg twice daily. High healing rates are unusual in clinical practice, especially with higher grades of erosive esophagitis [53, 54]. Because these results are sufficiently lower for H_2RAs than for PPIs, H_2RAs are rarely used as a primary prescribed GERD treatment [49, 50].

H_2RAs are extremely safe. Minor GI side effects include nausea, abdominal pain, and bloating. There have been concerns about drug interactions with these agents, particularly interactions with agents affecting the cytochrome P450 system and, in particular, with cimetidine. Serum concentrations of phenytoin, procainamide, theophylline, and warfarin have been altered after administration of cimetidine, and to a lesser degree ranitidine; these effects are not seen with famotidine and/or nizatidine [57, 58]. H_2RAs may not inhibit the effect of clopidogrel. The clinical consequences of these interactions are minimal and rarely result in a clinically important interaction. Awareness of these potential complications needs to be considered if H_2RAs are prescribed.

PPIs provide superior control of intragastric pH over a 24-h period compared to H2RAs and effect greater symptom relief and healing (Fig. 4.1). They do so by inhibiting the hydrogen potassium ATPase in the parietal cell, the final common pathway of acid secretion [59]. Currently, there are seven PPIs available for use. Traditional delayed release PPIs are omeprazole, lansoprazole, rabeprazole, pantoprazole, and esomeprazole. Two newer formulations of PPIs have recently been added—omeprazole immediate release-sodium bicarbonate (a combination of non-enteric-coated omeprazole granules with sodium bicarbonate (OME-IR) [60] and dexlansoprazole, the R-enantiomer of lansoprazole). The latter differs from traditional delayed release PPIs by utilizing a dual delayed release technology, with two types of enteric-coated granules soluble at different pHs. It is designed such that part will dissolve in

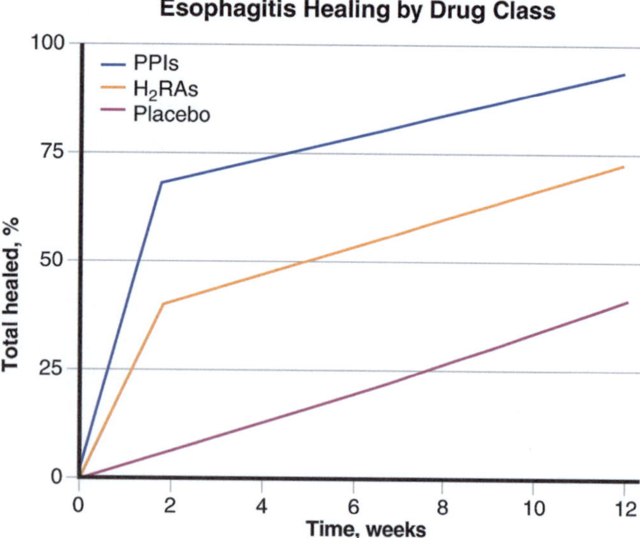

Esophagitis Healing by Drug Class

Fig. 4.1 Relative ability of the different classes of antisecretory medications to heal esophagitis

the duodenum, like the traditional delayed release PPI, and part in the distal small intestine [61].

PPIs are all weak bases that concentrate in the secretory canaliculi at pH <4. PPIs bind covalently and irreversibly to proton pumps; therefore, the degree of inhibition is related to AUC, not plasma concentration. PPIs block 70–80 % of active pumps; therefore, for acid secretion to resume, new hydrogen potassium ATPase molecules must be synthesized, a process that takes 36–96 h. Although the agents have different binding capacities, delayed release PPIs provide maximal efficacy in control of intragastric pH when taken immediately or a short time before a meal, as the drugs bind to actively secreting pumps.

Approach to the Patient

Administering PPIs before the first meal of the day, or when a second dose is needed, before the evening meal, optimizes acid control and therefore symptom relief Acid inhibition is not "complete" because of continued synthesis of new pumps [62]. When delayed release PPIs are administered twice daily, more active pumps are exposed to the drug, the steady-state inhibition of gastric acid is more rapidly achieved and more complete. Two exceptions to before meal dosing should be considered. The sodium bicarbonate in OME-IR protects the PPI granules from acid degradation and may in and of itself stimulate proton pumps. This may allow OME-IR to be effective when given at bedtime or perhaps when administered in the fasting state during the day. Dexlansoprazole uses a dual delayed release technology that results in a first peak in absorption at about 90 min after ingestion and a second 4–5 h after ingestion. The FDA label allows this drug to be given without regard to food so precise meal timing may not be required for optimal efficacy. In the vast majority of circum-

stances taking a PPI before the first meal of the day (usually breakfast) is still the preferred dosing regimen. Compliance seems better without a general compromise in efficacy [63].

A once daily dose should result in healing of erosive esophagitis in the vast majority (85–95 %) with minimal differences between PPIs and between studies. About 65 % will achieve "complete symptom resolution" defined as seven days without heartburn. There are patients who require an increase in dosage due to incomplete symptom relief, the presence of extra-esophageal symptoms (e.g., asthma, cough, laryngitis, and chest pain), and perhaps Barrett's esophagus. The second dose is given before the evening meal as this provides superior intragastric pH control, particularly at night, when compared to a double dose given once daily. No data are available assessing intragastric pH control on dexlansoprazole given twice daily.

Switching PPIs when they cease to work, infrequently but occasionally, offers dramatic change in symptom relief. Observations from intragastric pH studies find wide intersubject variability in intragastric pH control despite similar dosing regimens, which may account [64] for the occasional patient who responds to a switch from one PPI to another after one seemingly fails. Switching PPIs more than once is rarely indicated in actual practice.

Nocturnal GERD

Reflux that occurs while the patient is asleep (nocturnal reflux) whether or not it produces symptoms has the potential to be more damaging to the esophageal mucosa, as esophageal clearance is delayed during sleep.

If patients have reflux symptoms during the sleeping period on a standard once daily morning dose PPI there are several options. The single dose can be given before the dinner (evening) meal, consideration can be given to using OME-IR at bedtime, adding an H₂RA at bedtime, increasing the PPI to twice daily (before breakfast and dinner or OME-IR before breakfast and bedtime), or in some cases twice daily PPI plus H₂RA at bedtime. The use of OME-IR at bedtime is based on a study comparing overnight intragastric pH control in GERD patients with nocturnal symptoms treated with OME-IR 40 mg at bedtime, compared with esomeprazole 40 mg and lansoprazole 30 mg given at a similar time [65]. The former showed more rapid onset of pH control and improved overnight pH control in the vulnerable period (first 4 h of sleep) compared to the other PPIs. It is important to be aware, however, that 24-h pH control with this dosing regimen of OME-IR was not as effective as esomeprazole 40 mg given at bedtime [65].

Another potential means of controlling nocturnal reflux is to add an H₂RA at bedtime to a PPI given once or twice daily to control overnight gastric pH. Once popular, this practice has diminished primarily based on studies [66, 67] that evaluated longer-term use of nocturnal H₂RAs on control of

Table 4.2 Hierarchy of intragastric pH control

PPI once a day
PPI plus H₂RA (OTC probably acceptable)[a]
PPI bid[a] (OME-IR at bedtime)
PPI bid plus H₂RA[a]

[a]These regimens have never been tested head to head in clinical trials. I use OME-IR in selected patients but this has not been compared head to head with PPI BID plus H₂RA

intragastric pH. A clinically important number of patients will lose the initial overnight pH control (tachyphylaxis) suggesting a limit to long-term efficacy of H₂RAs at bedtime. The findings of tachyphylaxis and the availability of OME-IR have limited the use of H₂RAs at bedtime. In practice, an on demand H₂RA at bedtime is reasonable in those situations in which night time reflux is likely to occur. Some patients experience good results with H₂RAs long-term.

These studies underscore the importance of prolonged ambulatory reflux monitoring as a means of documenting the need for aggressive acid control regimen, and the need to individualize antisecretory therapy in difficult-to-treat patients. A hierarchy of intragastric pH control is outlined in Table 4.2.

Unexplained Chest Pain (Non-cardiac Chest Pain)

Many patients with unexplained chest pain will have GERD as the proximate cause of their symptoms. The key to managing patients with chest pain is to rule out cardiac disease prior to treatment with PPI.

A trial of antireflux therapy with a PPI is often recommended as initial therapy for suspected GERD in patients with chest pain. This so-called "PPI test" was studied in a randomized, double-blind, placebo-controlled crossover trial that evaluated one week of high-dose omeprazole as a diagnostic test for GERD in patients with non-cardiac chest pain [68]. All patients had chest pain at least three times a week. Endoscopy and 24-h ambulatory esophageal pH monitoring were performed in all. GERD was based on the presence of erosive esophagitis or abnormal 24-h pH monitoring.

The so-called "omeprazole test" (the PPI test) was diagnostic of GERD if chest pain scores improved after treatment. Seventy-eight percent of GERD-positive patients and 14 % of GERD-negative patients had positive test results, (sensitivity 78.3 % (95 % CI [confidence interval], 61.4–95.1) and specificity of 85.7 % (95 % CI, 67.4–100)), compared with endoscopy and ambulatory pH monitoring for the diagnosis of GERD. Economic analysis has estimated that this approach is cost effective.

A more recent systematic review found that PPI response compared to placebo could be predicted by endoscopy and pH studies. Incremental response to PPI over placebo is only seen in patients with an abnormal objective study [69]. This latter review suggests an early workup is perhaps the best way to avoid unneeded treatment for patients without GERD.

Extra-Esophageal Disease

There are many patients who present with a symptom other than heartburn or regurgitation that is felt to be caused by GERD. Clinical trials of treatment involving patients with extra-esophageal manifestations of GERD, specifically asthma, cough, and voice changes are few, small and in many instances uncontrolled. Early uncontrolled observations have led to the clinical impression that these patients require higher doses of PPIs (usually twice daily) for longer periods of time (up to 3–6 months) than patients with the typical symptoms of heartburn and regurgitation. Performing clinical trials in these patients is more difficult than patients with erosive esophagitis as the "gold standard" for diagnosis of GERD with extra-esophageal symptoms is not clear. As such, few randomized trials have been performed. The best of these trials offer several important generalizations:

- A once daily PPI is more likely to be ineffective.
- Response to symptoms is slower.
- A poor response to PPI twice daily suggests a poor response to surgery.

The optimal treatment for patients with unexplained chest pain and other extra-esophageal manifestations of GERD is not clear. Until better diagnostic tests are developed, the most efficient approach is to begin empirical therapy with twice daily PPI before breakfast and dinner for two to three months (note again that dexlansoprazole has not been studied twice daily). If patients do not respond to a trial of antireflux therapy, an evaluation with prolonged ambulatory reflux monitoring with impedance/pH testing while continuing therapy may be the procedure of choice [70]. This allows assessment of both pH control and symptom correlation. In the event that pH control is incomplete—especially when overnight [71] esophageal acid exposure continues [72], and/or symptoms continue in association with continued reflux—adjustment in antisecretory therapy or addition of a reflux inhibitor may be indicated [71, 73]. Baclofen, a skeletal muscle relaxant [73], can be considered if non-acid reflux is present and associated with symptoms though the latter is not approved by the FDA. Patients successfully treated with acid suppression should be considered for long-term maintenance with PPI therapy, although no study has specifically addressed this issue (Fig. 4.2). Patients with incomplete control or onerous medical regimes may be better off with referral for antireflux surgery.

Side Effects of PPIS

As a class, PPIs have been amongst the safest in the treatment of reflux disease [74, 75]. Potential side effects associated with PPI therapy include headache, diarrhea, and dyspepsia in less than 2 % of users. Switching to another PPI

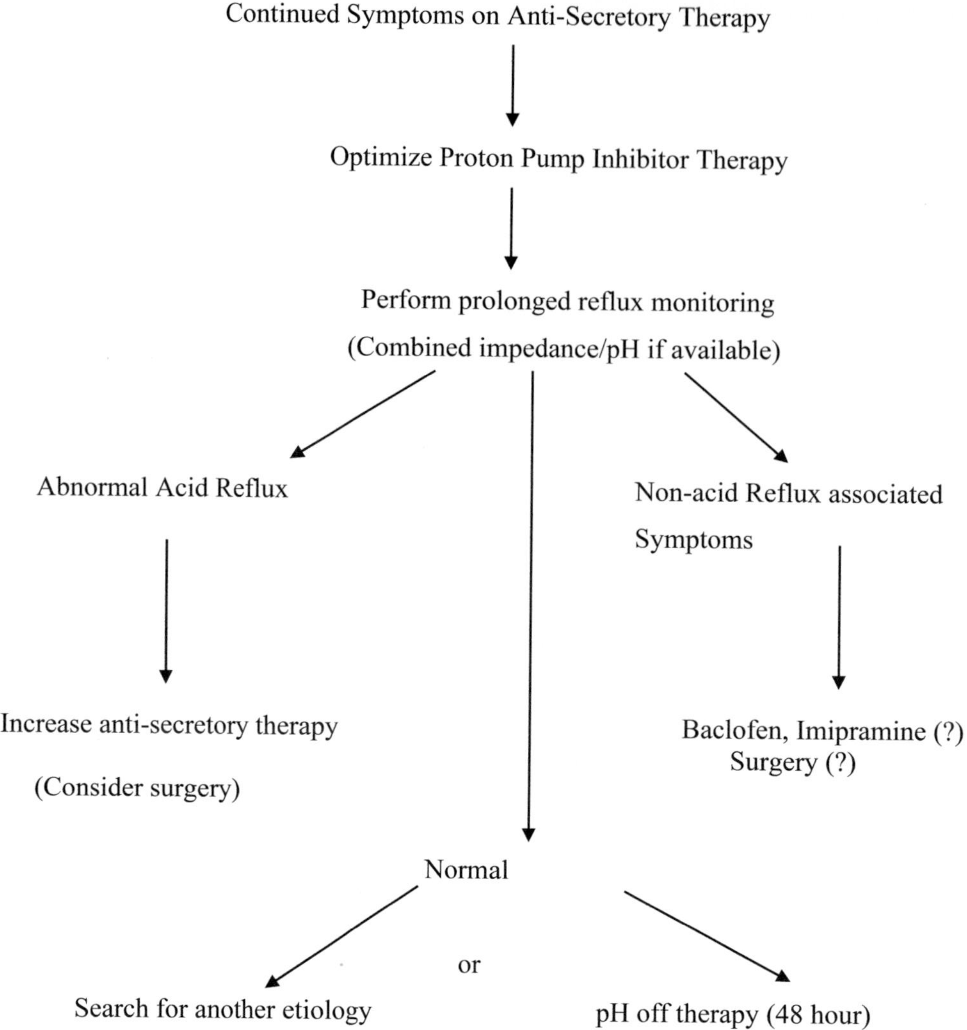

Fig. 4.2 Suggested approach to a patient with symptoms suspected due to gastroesophageal reflux who is symptomatic despite antisecretory therapy. This approach is designed to establish whether continued symptoms are due to continued reflux

can be considered in these patients. Other much discussed associations are vitamin and mineral deficiencies, infections such as pneumonia and *Clostridium difficile*, long bone fractures, and cardiovascular events in patients using concomitant clopidogrel therapy. The FDA issued warnings regarding the potential for wrist, hip, and spine fractures among PPI users in 2010 and warnings regarding potential for adverse cardiovascular events among clopidogrel users taking PPI therapy in 2009.

Two recent reviews demonstrated evidence that PPI therapy reduces the absorption of protein-bound vitamin B12, but not enough clinical evidence to document B12 deficiency or the need to check B12 levels in chronic PPI users. Recent studies have suggested that in elderly, institutionalized long-term PPI users, B12 deficiency is more likely to develop and should be considered.

Gastric acid is needed to allow absorption of non-heme iron and also enhances iron salt dissociation from ingested food. Iron deficiency anemia has been reported in patients with atrophic gastritis, gastric resection, or vagotomy. To date, no data are available demonstrating the development of iron deficiency anemia in normal subjects on PPI therapy without mucosal injury.

By their effects in increasing gastric pH levels, PPIs may encourage growth of gut microflora and increase susceptibility to organisms including *Salmonella*, *Campylobacter jejuni*, *Escherichia coli*, *Clostridium difficile*, *Vibrio cholerae*, and *Listeria*. An increased susceptibility in PPI users for *Salmonella* infections, *Campylobacter*, and *C. difficile* infections was found in a systematic review [76]. Current recommendations are to carefully evaluate the need for PPI therapy in hospitalized patients who need intravenous antibiotics.

An increased risk for community-acquired pneumonia is difficult to demonstrate in association with PPI therapy but has been suggested. A meta-analysis showed that the overall risk of pneumonia was higher among people using PPIs. If only randomized controlled trial data was analyzed, H_2RAs were associated with an elevated risk of hospital-acquired pneumonia not PPIs. A more recent meta-analysis did find an increased risk of pneumonia associated with PPI usage, but the results were confounded by methodologic issues. Paradoxically, short duration of use was associated with an increase in the odds of community-acquired pneumonia but chronic use was not. No definite recommendation can be given [77, 78].

Clinical studies in patients taking PPI therapy have shown mixed results regarding bony fracture [79–81]. The study with the longest clinical follow-up matched cases with abnormal bone mineral density (osteoporosis) at the hip or lumbar vertebrae (T-score< or +=−2.5) to controls with normal bone mineral density (T-score> or −1.0). PPI use was not associated with having osteoporosis either the hip or the lumbar spine for PPI use >1,500 doses over the previous 5 years. In the longitudinal study no significant decrease was observed in bone mineral density at either site attributable to PPI use. This suggests the association between PPI use and hip fracture was probably related to factors independent of osteoporosis.

In a recent meta-analysis, the pooled odds ratio (OR) for fracture was 1.29 (95 % confidence interval [CI], 1.18–1.41) with PPIs and 1.10 (95 % CI, 0.99–1.23) with H_2RA use compared to non-users. Another study showed that the hip fracture risk among PPI users was seen only in persons with at least one other fracture risk factor. A meta-analysis covering 1,521,062 patients showed significant risk for spine fractures (OR 1.50, 95 % CI 1.32–1.72, $p<0.001$). For hip fractures, there was an increased risk of fractures with PPIs (OR 1.23, 95 % CI 1.11–1.36, $p<0.001$) [78]. Overall an OR of 1.20 is seen for PPIs, and OR of 1.08 (95 % CI 1.00–1.18, $p=0.06$) for H_2RAs. Again, even short durations of PPI use may be associated with increased risk of developing hip fracture (OR=1.24; 95 % CI=1.19–1.28), however, this is not as clear in long-term PPI users (OR=1.30; 95 % CI=0.98–1.70).

In 2009, the FDA issued a warning regarding potential for increased adverse cardiovascular events in concomitant users of PPI and clopidogrel therapy, particularly among users of omeprazole, lansoprazole, and esomeprazole. The concern arises from the fact that the antiplatelet activity of clopidogrel requires activation by CYP 2C19, the same pathway required for metabolism of some PPIs. In vitro studies have been conflicting. The newest data suggests that dexlansoprazole does not inhibit platelets in vitro to the same degree as the three former PPIs. Pantoprazole appears to have less inhibition as well. A recent meta-analysis [83] (27 studies) focused on primary (myocardial infarction, stroke, stent occlusion, or death) and secondary outcomes (re-hospitalization for cardiac symptoms or revascularization procedures). Outcomes from the two randomized controlled trials did not show an increased risk for adverse outcomes. Meta-analysis of primary and secondary outcomes showed an increased risk difference for all studies. Essentially, the risk of adverse cardiac outcomes was 0 % based on data from well-controlled randomized trials [84]. Data from retrospective studies and the addition of probable vascular events slightly but significantly increased the risk estimates, likely due to lack of adjustment for potential confounders.

References

1. Hila A, Castell DO. Nighttime reflux is primarily an early event. J Clin Gastroenterol. 2005;39(7):579–83.
2. Johnson LF, DeMeester TR. Evaluation of the head of the bed, bethanechol, and antacid foam tablets on gastroesophageal reflux. Dig Dis Sci. 1981;26:673–80.
3. Hamilton JW, Boisen RJ, Yamamoto DT, et al. Sleeping on a wedge diminishes exposure of the esophagus to refluxed acid. Dig Dis Sci. 1988;33(5):518–22.
4. Pollman. Z Gastroenterol. 1996.
5. Khoury RM, Camacho-Lobato LC, Katz PO, et al. Influence of spontaneous sleep positions on nighttime recumbent reflux in patients with gastroesophageal reflux disease. Am J Gastroenterol. 1999;94:2069–73.
6. Kapur KC, Trudgill NJ, Riley SA. Mechanism of gastroesophageal reflux in the lateral decubitus position. Neurogastroenterol Motil. 1998;10:517–22.
7. Katz LC, Just R, Castell DO. Body position affects recumbent postprandial reflux. J Clin Gastroenterol. 1994;18:280–3.
8. VanHerwaarden M, Katzka D, Smout AJPM, et al. Effect of different recumbent positions on postprandial reflex in normal subjects. Am J Gastroenterol. 2000;95:2731–6.
9. Dickman R, Parthasarathy S, Malagon IB, et al. Comparisons of the distribution of oesophageal acid exposure throughout the sleep period among the different gastro-oesophageal reflux disease groups. Aliment Pharmacol Ther. 2007;26(1):41–8.
10. Gagliardi GS, Shah AP, Goldstein M, et al. Effect of zolpidem on the sleep arousal response to nocturnal esophageal acid exposure. Clin Gastroenterol Hepatol. 2009;7(9):948–52.
11. McArthur K, Hogan D, Isenberg JI. Relative stimulatory effects of commonly ingested beverages on gastric acid secretion in humans. Gastroenterology. 1982;83:199–203.
12. Babka JC, Castell DO. On the genesis of heartburn: the effects of specific foods on the lower esophagus sphincter. Dig Dis. 1973;18:391–7.
13. Castell DO. Diet and the lower esophageal sphincter. Am J Clin Nutr. 1975;28:1296–8.
14. Vakily M, Lee RD, Wu J, et al. Drug interaction studies with dexlansoprazole modified release (TAK-390MR), a proton pump inhibitor with a dual delayed-release formulation: results of four randomized, double-blind, crossover, placebo-controlled, single centre studies. Clin Drug Investig. 2009;29:35–50.
15. Nebel OT, Castell DO. Lower esophageal sphincter pressure changes after food ingestion. Gastroenterology. 1972;63:778.
16. Pehl C, Pfeiffer A, Wendl B, et al. The effect of decaffeination of coffee on gastro-esophageal reflux in patients with reflux disease. Aliment Pharmacol Ther. 1997;11:483.
17. Becker DJ, Sinclair J, Castell DO, et al. A comparison of high and low fat meals on postprandial esophageal acid exposure. Am J Gastroenterol. 1989;84:782.
18. Nebel OT, Castell DO. Lower esophageal sphincter pressure changes after food ingestion. Gastroenterology. 1972;63:778–83.

19. Wright LE, Castell DO. Adverse effect of chocolate on lower esophageal sphincter pressure. Dig Dis Sci. 1975;20:703–7.

20. Murphy DW, Castell DO. Chocolate and heartburn: evidence of increased esophageal acid exposure after chocolate ingestion. Am J Gastroenterol. 1988;83:633–6.

21. Kjellin A, Ramel S, Rossner S, et al. Gastroesophageal reflux in obese patients is not reduced by weight reduction. Scand J Gastroenterol. 1996;31:1047–51.

22. Jacobson BC, Somers SC, Fuchs CS, et al. Body-mass index and symptoms of gastroesophageal reflux in women. N Engl J Med. 2006;354(22):2340–8.

23. Chow WH, Blot WJ, Vaughan TL, et al. Body mass index and risk of adenocarcinoma of the esophagus and gastric, cardia. J Natl Cancer Inst. 1998;90:150–5.

24. Perez AR, Moncure AC, Rattner DW. Obesity adversely affects the outcome of antireflux operations. Surg Endosc. 2001;15:986–9.

25. DeVault KR, Castell DO. Updated guidelines for the diagnosis and treatment of gastroesophageal reflux disease. Am J Gastroenterol. 2005;100(1):190–200.

26. Tytgat GNJ, Nio CY. The medical therapy of reflux oesophagitis. Bailleres Clin Gastroenterol. 1987;1:791–807.

27. Klinkenberg-Knol EC, Festen HPM, et al. Pharmacologic management of gastro-oesophageal reflux disease. Drugs. 1995;49:695–710.

28. Furman D, Mensh R, Winan G, et al. A double-blind trial comparing high dose liquid antacid to placebo and cimetidine in improving symptoms and objective parameters in gastroesophageal reflux. Gastroenterology. 1992;82:A1062.

29. Eslborg L, Beck B, Stubgaard M. Effect of sucralfate on gastroesophageal reflux in esophagitis. Hepatogastroenterology. 1985; 32:181–4.

30. Katz PO, Castell DO. Gastroesophageal reflux disease during pregnancy. Gastroenterol Clin. 1998;27:153–67.

31. Simon B, Mueller P. Comparison of the effect of sucralfate and ranitidine in reflux esophagitis. Am J Med. 1987;83:43–7.

32. Hameeteman W, van de Boomgaard DM, Dekker W, et al. Sucralfate versus cimetidine in reflux esophagitis: single blind multicenter study. J Clin Gastroenterol. 1987;9:390–4.

33. Barone JA, Jessen LM, Colaizzi JL, et al. Cisapride: a gastrointestinal prokinetic drug. Ann Pharmacother. 1994;28:488–500.

34. McCallum RW, Ippoliti AF, Cooney C, et al. A controlled trial of metoclopramide in symptomatic gastroesophageal reflux. N Engl J Med. 1977;296:354–7.

35. Bright-Asare P, El-Bassoussi M. Cimetidine, metoclopramide or placebo in the treatment of symptomatic gastroesophageal reflux. J Clin Gastroenterol. 1980;2:149–56.

36. Temple JG, Bradby GVH, O'Connor F, et al. Cimetidine and metoclopramide in esophageal reflux disease. BMJ. 1983;286:1863–5.

37. Paull A, Kerr A, Grant AK. A controlled trial of metoclopramide in reflux esophagitis. Med J Aust. 1974;2:627–9.

38. Venables CW, Bell D, Eccleston D. A double-blind study of metoclopramide in symptomatic peptic esophagitis. Postgrad Med J. 1973;49 suppl 4:73–7.

39. Ramirez B, Richter JE. Review article: promotility drugs in the treatment of gastro-oesophageal reflux disease. Aliment Pharmacol Ther. 1993;7:5–20.

40. Blackwell JN, Heading RC, Fettes MR. Effects of domperidone on lower oesophageal sphincter pressure and gastro-oesophageal reflux in patients with peptic esophagitis. Progress with domperidone. In: International congress and symposium series, vol 36. London: Royal Society of Medicine Press; 1981. p. 57.

41. Richter JE, Sabesin SM, Kogut DG, et al. Omeprazole versus ranitidine or ranitidine/metoclopramide in poorly responsive symptomatic gastroesophageal reflux disease. Am J Gastroenterol. 1996;91:1766–72.

42. Miller WN, Ganeshappa KP, Dodds WJ, Hogan WJ, Barreras RF, Arndorfer RC. Effect of bethanechol on gastroesophageal reflux. Am J Dig Dis. 1977;22(3):230–4.

43. Miller L, Dai Q, Vegesna A, Korimilli A, Ulerich R, Schiffner B, Brassuer J. A missing sphincteric component of the gastro-esophageal junction in patients with GERD. Neurogastroenterol Motil. 2009;21(8):813–e52.

44. Zhang Q, Lehmann A, Rigda R, Dent J, Holloway RH. Control of transient lower oesophageal sphincter relaxations and reflux by the GABAB agonist baclofen in patients with gastro-oesophageal reflux disease. Gut. 2002;50(1):19–24.

45. Sidhu AS, Triadafilopoulos G. Neuro-regulation of lower esophageal sphincter function as treatment for gastroesophageal reflux disease. World J Gastroenterol. 2008;14(7):985–90.

46. Bell NJV, Burget DL, Howden CW, et al. Appropriate acid suppression for the management of gastro-esophageal reflux disease. Digestion. 1992;51 suppl 1:59–67.

47. Katz PO, Ginsberg GG, Hoyle PE, et al. Relationship between intragastric acid control and healing status in the treatment of moderate to severe erosive esophagitis. Aliment Pharmacol Ther. 2007;25(5):617–28.

48. Jones DB, Howden CW, Burget DW, et al. Acid suppression in duodenal ulcer: a meta-analysis to define optimal dosing with antisecretory drugs. Gut. 1987;28:1120–7.

49. DeVault KR, Castell DO. Guidelines for the diagnosis and treatment of gastroesophageal reflux disease. Arch Intern Med. 1995; 155:2165–73.

50. Bell NJV, Hunt RH. Role of gastric acid suppression in the treatment of gastro-oesophageal reflux disease. Gut. 1992;33:118–24.

51. Cloud ML, Offen WW. Nizatidine versus placebo in gastroesophageal reflux disease: a six-week, multicenter, randomized, double-blind comparison. Dig Dis Sci. 1992;37:865–74.

52. McCarty-Dawson D, Sue S, Morrill B, et al. Ranitidine versus cimetidine in the healing of erosive esophagitis. Clin Ther. 1996; 18:1150–60.

53. Wesdorp ICE, Dekker W, Festen HPM. Efficacy of famotidine 20 mg twice a day versus 40 mg twice a day in the treatment of erosive or ulcerative reflux esophagitis. Dig Dis Sci. 1993;38:2287–93.

54. Euler AR, Murdock Jr RH, Wilson TH, et al. Ranitidine is effective therapy for erosive esophagitis. Am J Gastroenterol. 1993;88: 520–4.

55. Hallerback B, Glise H, Johansson B, et al. Gastroesophageal reflux symptoms: clinical findings and effect of ranitidine treatment. Eur J Surg Suppl. 1998;583:6–13.

56. Vignieri S, Termini R, Leandor G, et al. A comparison of five maintenance therapies for reflux esophagitis. N Engl J Med. 1995; 333:1106–10.

57. Feldman M, Burton ME. Histamine2-receptor antagonists: standard therapy for acid-peptic diseases. N Engl J Med. 1990; 323:1672–80.

58. Lipsy RJ, Fennerty B, Fagan TC. Clinical review of histamine2 receptor antagonists. Arch Intern Med. 1990;150:745–51.

59. Robinson M. Review article: current perspectives on hypergastrinemia and enterochromaffin-like-cell hyperplasia. Aliment Pharmacol Ther. 1999;13 suppl 5:5–10.

60. Castell D. Review of immediate-release omeprazole for the treatment of gastric acid-related disorders. Expert Opin Pharmacother. 2005;6(14):2501–10.

61. Metz D, Vakily M, Dixit T, Mumford D. Review article: dual delayed release formulation of dexlansoprazole MR, a novel approach to overcome the limitations of conventional single release proton pump inhibitor therapy. Aliment Pharmacol Ther. 2009; 29(9):928–37.

62. Wolfe MM, Sachs G. Acid suppression: optimizing therapy for gastroduodenal ulcer healing, gastroesophageal reflux disease, and stress-related erosive syndrome. Gastroenterology. 2000;118(suppl):9–31.

63. Hatlebakk JG, Katz PO, Castell DO. Proton pump inhibitors: better acid suppression when taken before a meal than without a meal. Aliment Pharmacol Ther. 2000;14:1267–72.

64. Katz PO, Hatlebakk JG, Castell DO. Gastric acidity and acid break-through with twice daily omeprazole or lansoprazole. Aliment Pharmacol Ther. 2000;14:709–14.

65. Katz PO, Koch FK, Ballard ED, et al. Comparison of the effects of immediate-release omeprazole oral suspension, delayed-release lansoprazole capsules and delayed-release esomeprazole capsules on nocturnal gastric acidity after bedtime dosing in patients with night-time GERD symptoms. Aliment Pharmacol Ther. 2007; 25(2):197–205.

66. Fackler WK, Tm O, Vaezi MF, et al. Long-term effect of H_2RA therapy on nocturnal gastric acid breakthrough. Gastroenterology. 2002;122:625–32.

67. Katz PO, Xue S, Castell DO. Control of intragastric pH with omeprazole 20 mg, omeprazole 40 mg and lansoprazole 30 mg. Aliment Pharmacol Ther. 2001;15:647–52.

68. Fass R, Fennerty MB, Ofman JJ, et al. The clinical and economic value of a short course of omeprazole in patients with non-cardiac chest pain. Gastroenterology. 1998;1(15):42–9.

69. New reference

70. Klinkenberg-Knol E, Meuwissen S. Combined gastric and oesoph-ageal 24 hour monitoring in patients with reflux disease resistant to treatment with omeprazole. Aliment Pharmacol Ther. 1990; 4:485–95.

71. Peghini PL, Katz PO, Bracy NA, et al. Nocturnal recovery of gas-tric acid secretion with twice-day dosing of proton pump inhibitors. Am J Gastroenterol. 1998;93:763–7.

72. Katz PO, Anderson C, Khoury R, et al. Gastro-oesophageal reflux associated with nocturnal gastric acid breakthrough on proton pump inhibitors. Aliment Pharmacol Ther. 1998;12:1231–4.

73. Peghini PL, Katz PO, Castell DO. Ranitidine controls nocturnal gastric acid breakthrough on omeprazole: a controlled study in normal subjects. Gastroenterology. 1998;115:1335–9.

74. Lodato F, Azzaroli F, Turco L, et al. Adverse effects of proton pump inhibitors. Best Pract Res Clin Gastroenterol. 2010;24:193–201.

75. Aseeri M, Schroeder T, Kramer J, Zackula R. Gastric acid suppres-sion by proton pump inhibitors as a risk factor for clostridium-difficile-associated diarrhea in hospitalized patients. Am J Gastroenterol. 2008;103:2308–13.

76. Bavishi C, Dupont HL. Systematic review: the use of proton pump inhibitors and increased susceptibility to enteric infection. Aliment Pharmacol Ther. 2011;34:1269–81.

77. Eom CS, Jeon CY, Lim JW, et al. Use of acid-suppressive drugs and risk of pneumonia: a systematic review and meta-analysis. CMAJ. 2011;183:310–9.

78. Johnstone J, Nerenberg K, Loeb M. Meta-analysis: proton pump inhibitor use and the risk of community-acquired pneumonia. Aliment Pharmacol Ther. 2010;31:1165–77.

79. Targownik LE, Lix LM, Leung S, et al. Proton-pump inhibitor use is not associated with osteoporosis or accelerated bone mineral density loss. Gastroenterology. 2010;138:896–904.

80. Eom CS, Park SM, Myung SK, et al. Use of acid-suppressive drugs and risk of fracture: a meta-analysis of observational studies. Ann Fam Med. 2011;9:257–67.

81. Corley DA, Kubo A, Zhao W, et al. Proton pump inhibitors and histamine-2 receptor antagonists are associated with hip fractures among at-risk patients. Gastroenterology. 2010;139:93–101.

82. Ngamruengphong S, Leontiadis GI, Radhi S, et al. Proton pump inhibitors and risk of fracture: a systematic review and meta-analysis of observational studies. Am J Gastroenterol. 2011;106: 1209–18. quiz 1219.

83. Gerson LB, McMahon D, Olkin I, et al. Lack of significant interac-tions between clopidogrel and proton pump inhibitor therapy: meta-analysis of existing literature. Dig Dis Sci. 2012;57: 1304–13.

84. Kwok CS, Jeevanantham V, Dawn B, et al. No consistent evidence of differential cardiovascular risk amongst proton-pump inhibitors when used with clopidogrel: meta analysis. Int J Cardiol. 2013;167:965–74.

Indications for Antireflux Surgery

Renato A. Luna, Nathan W. Bronson, and John G. Hunter

Introduction

In the United States 45 % of the adult population experienced at least one symptom related to the upper gastrointestinal tract in a 3-month period, with 27–38 % reporting heartburn and regurgitation [1, 2]. Disruptive gastroesophageal reflux disease (GERD) symptoms, defined as those occurring at least 2 days per week, at night, or requiring medication at least 2 times per week, are estimated to be present in 44 % of the US population. GERD patients are higher utilizers of health care resources, have higher absenteeism from work, and demonstrate reduced productivity in daily activities. In total, it is estimated that patients with frequent GERD symptoms cost the healthcare system 95 % more than non-GERD patients, with an incremental health benefit cost estimated at $23 billion annually [3].

The spectrum of the disease is wide and ranges from mildly symptomatic to more complicated disease manifested as peptic stricture, esophageal ulceration, or Barrett's esophagus. Two populations can be clearly defined by the burden of GERD symptoms: patients with sporadic symptoms, and those with frequent or constant symptoms. Patients with frequent symptoms or complications of the disease are candidates for surgical treatment. The objective of this chapter is to review the indications for surgical treatment in this patient population.

R.A. Luna, MD, MS
Servidores do Estado do Rio de Janeiro Hospital,
R. Sacadura Cabral, 178, Rio de Janeiro, Brazil
e-mail: luna_renato@hotmail.com

N.W. Bronson, MD
Department of Surgery, Oregon Health and Science University,
3181 SW Sam Jackson Park Road, Mail Code L223,
Portland, OR 97239, USA
e-mail: bronsonn@ohsu.edu

J.G. Hunter, MD (✉)
Department of Surgery, L223A, Oregon Health & Science University,
3181 Sam Jackson Park Rd., Portland, OR 97239-3098, USA
e-mail: hunterj@ohsu.edu

Clinical Presentation

Patients with GERD can be classified into two groups according to whether they experience typical or atypical symptoms. Typical symptoms are heartburn and regurgitation, while atypical symptoms are defined by extra gastrointestinal manifestations of GERD such as cough, asthma, laryngitis, chest pain, or hoarseness. Surgical outcomes differ significantly between these groups so patients must be carefully selected. Furthermore, GERD symptoms do not confirm or disprove the existence of acid reflux. It is well known that some patients with classic reflux symptoms do not have gastroesophageal reflux and likewise, some patients may present with complications of the disease and no symptoms of GERD at all.

To optimize patient selection, objective evidence of reflux is required before surgical treatment. This usually includes esophageal pH study (considered the golden standard), upper gastrointestinal endoscopy, and a barium swallow. High-resolution esophageal manometry is usually performed to exclude esophageal motility disorders, to assess esophageal body contractility, and to place the pH catheter. Patients with significant gas bloating, nausea/vomiting, or early satiety may benefit from gastric scintigraphy as well.

Pre-operative Predictors of Surgical Outcomes

Many pre-operative predictors of good surgical outcomes have been identified, and they form the basis for surgical patient selection.

Clinical Variables

Patients with GERD who respond to antireflux medications have better long-term surgical outcomes than those who do not [4, 5]. A trial of medical treatment is therefore advised for every patient considering surgical treatment.

L.L. Swanstrom and C.M. Dunst (eds.), *Antireflux Surgery*,
DOI 10.1007/978-1-4939-1749-5_5, © Springer New York 2015

Patients who complain of pre-operative dysphagia are more likely to report post-operative dysphagia after laparoscopic antireflux surgery (LARS) than those without this complaint. However, the severity of their dysphagia will likely be reduced. Seventy eight to 87 % of patients who reported post-operative dysphagia had a lower score when their dysphagia was quantified [6, 7]. Patients with delayed esophageal transit at barium swallow are more likely to present with persistent dysphagia post operatively [6].

Obesity is related to an increased incidence of GERD and has been implicated as a risk factor for poor post-operative outcomes [4, 8], but the literature is mixed, with some authors reporting similar symptomatic results between normal weight and obese patients [9–11]. The only prospective data available compared 70 morbidly obese patients to 70 non-obese patients with subjective and objective outcomes measured 6 months after surgery. The post-operative symptomatic reflux score in the obese group was significantly higher than in the non-obese group. However, esophageal pH studies failed to show an objective difference between groups and both groups showed similar improvement in post-operative symptom scores. In long-term follow-up, the incidence of recurrent symptoms and reoperations were similar in both groups [12]. Although reports are mixed, it is clear that LARS is at least more demanding in obese patients, with longer operative times, occasional need for extra port insertion, and longer hospital length of stays [8, 9, 12]. Surgeons serving this subgroup of patients must keep in mind that morbidly obese patients may benefit from a bariatric procedure, and should be offered referral to a bariatric surgeon prior to undergoing LARS. However, symptomatic obese patients who do not fulfill the criteria for a bariatric procedure should not be denied an antireflux operation based only on BMI.

Typical and Atypical Symptoms

It is well established that patients with typical symptoms have better surgical outcomes than those with atypical symptoms [13, 14, 6, 5]. This seems to be true at both short and long-term follow-up. At 1-year follow-up 99 % of patients with typical symptoms demonstrated improvement, as compared to 93 % of patients with atypical symptoms. Complete resolution is seen in 87 % of patients with typical symptoms, as compared to only 43 % of those patients with atypical symptoms [15]. At 10-year follow-up of the same group, 85 % of patients with typical symptoms had a successful outcome compared with 41 % of patients with atypical symptoms [4]. Similar results were demonstrated in a recent published prospective cohort. This is likely due to the indirect nature of many extraesophageal symptoms, the fact that many of these problems have multiple possible etiologies

and the possibility of irreparable damage from years of uncontrolled reflux. Interestingly, hypomotile patterns as measured by high-resolution manometry (HRM) correlated with less marked improvement in atypical symptoms when compared to normal or spastic motility [16].

GERD and asthma are common conditions that frequently coexist, but the relation between them is not entirely clear and difficult to prove. Many mechanisms have been proposed, including micro-aspiration, vagally mediated esophagobronchial reflex, direct neuronal connection between the esophagus and lung, and neurogenic inflammation. Patient reported symptoms and objective evidence alone are sometimes inconsistent in asthmatic patients. Approximately 25 % of asthmatic patients will complain of typical GERD symptoms without any objective evidence of GERD, and about 10 % will have objective evidence of GERD by pH study, but no typical symptoms [17]. The results of GERD treatment for asthmatic patients have traditionally been mixed. A Cochrane systematic review failed to establish any clear benefit of GERD treatment in unselected asthmatic patients, but it remains possible that GERD therapy may improve asthma in a subgroup of patients in whom GERD precipitates asthma [18]. A small randomized trial that compared LARS with ranitidine in asthmatic patients demonstrated better asthma symptom control and improvement in overall clinical status in the surgical group [19]. However, because few published trials have been specifically designed to address the effectiveness of antireflux surgery in controlling the symptoms of asthmatic patients, insight must be extrapolated from a combination of the medical literature and secondary outcomes of surgical papers. A randomized trial of asthmatic patients with a pathological pH study reported that 16 weeks of omeprazole and domperidone provided greater improvement in asthma symptom scores and less use of asthma rescue medication than placebo regardless of whether they had GERD symptoms [20]. Conversely, a randomized trial of poorly controlled asthmatic patients with asymptomatic GERD diagnosed by pH study did not demonstrate any benefit in the use of esomeprazole in this subgroup [21]. Likewise, poorly controlled asthmatic patients with pathologic esophageal pH study but without typical GERD symptoms may not benefit from antireflux surgery, and caution must be used when assessing these patients.

Patients with laryngeal symptoms have the best outcomes when their complaints are associated with typical GERD symptoms and typically have a good response to PPIs [13, 22]. In this subset of patients the improvement or resolution of symptoms was nearly twice as likely as patients who had only throat symptoms [23]. Also, abnormalities seen on direct laryngoscopy of the inter-arytenoid mucosa and true vocal cords are associated with a favorable response to antireflux treatment [24].

GERD has been strongly associated with end stage lung disease (ESLD), and remains highly prevalent after lung transplant (LTx). It afflicts 87 % of patients with idiopathic pulmonary fibrosis, and 75 % of LTx patients will have an abnormal pH study. GERD has also been implicated as one possible cause for bronchiolitis obliterans syndrome (BOS), the major cause of lung transplant failure. The refluxate may drive the evolution of BOS, and antireflux surgery is thought to slow this progression [25]. After LARS, nearly all measurements of lung function improve, with 91 % of LTx patients and 85 % of ESLD patients demonstrating an improvement in FEV1. The incidence of pneumonia and acute rejection after LTx are significantly reduced by antireflux surgery. In this subset of patients proximal reflux is more prevalent and laryngopharyngeal reflux as measured by impedance pH testing seems to correlate with more frequent episodes of acute rejection. Additionally, declining FEV1 is more likely to be reversed after antireflux surgery [26, 27]. The 30-day morbidity and mortality in LTx patients who later undergo LARS seems to be similar to patients without a history of LTx [26].

Non-cardiac chest pain is defined as retrosternal pain without evidence of cardiac ischemia. Its prevalence is around 30 % of the western population, and is usually related to GERD in up to 60 % of these patients [28]. The diagnosis is usually established after cardiac ischemic disease has been ruled out, and the 24 h esophageal pH study is the most sensitive and definitive test. Another important tool in establishing this diagnosis is the PPI empiric test, which has a sensitivity of 69–92 % and specificity of 67–91 %, depending on the type and dose of the PPI used [28]. The strongest predictors of good response to therapy are an acid exposure time (AET) greater than 4 % in the distal esophagus and a positive symptom association probability index (SAP). When both AET and SAP are positive, the chance of definite and sustained response to PPI therapy is around 88 % [29]. Although no specific surgical study has addressed this issue, it is reasonable to extrapolate these findings to surgical practice. Patients with both non-cardiac chest pain and paraesophageal hernia usually benefit from LARS, with good response to surgical treatment in long-term follow-up [30].

Non-erosive and Erosive Reflux Disease

A patient with GERD symptoms usually undergoes upper gastrointestinal endoscopy to evaluate the extent and severity of the disease. Two broad groups are readily defined by these findings: those with erosive findings (ERD-erosive reflux disease) and those without erosive findings (NERD-non-erosive reflux disease). Patients with either ERD or NERD, and a pathological pH study, benefit equally from LARS [31–33].

The spectrum of erosive reflux disease ranges from mild esophagitis, to esophageal ulcers, strictures, and Barrett's esophagus. Although these groups may differ clinically, they demonstrate equivalent resolution of typical symptoms [32]. One prospective trial reported better symptom control and better resolution of esophagitis at 2 years of follow-up with surgery as compared to medical therapy. This trial included only patients with esophageal ulcers, stricture, erosive esophagitis, or Barrett's esophagus [34]. The long-term follow-up of the same trial reported frequent antireflux medication use in the surgical group, and no benefit of surgery in preventing cancer or better controlling strictures [35]. Although this is a frequently cited paper, it is underpowered for any definitive conclusions. In 2003 another trial addressed the impact of antireflux surgery in the evolution of Barrett's esophagus to adenocarcinoma, and found that acid and bile reflux are better controlled by surgery than medication, but again, they could not demonstrate a difference in cancer incidence between the two groups. Interestingly, when surgical patients who did not normalize their pH study (15 %) were excluded, the surgical group showed a significant decrease in the progression of Barrett's esophagus (BE) to esophageal cancer. Because this subgroup was not compared to patients in whom medical therapy alone normalized the esophageal pH study, this analysis is biased [36]. The LOTUS trial reported that in patients with Barrett's esophagus, the esophageal pH was better controlled by surgery than by esomeprazole although the symptom questionnaire and quality of life scores did not differ between them. Unfortunately no conclusions about the evolution from intestinal metaplasia to cancer could be made [37]. In a recent observational study, symptomatic outcomes were similar in surgically and medically treated patients with BE. However, patients with short segment BE had complete regression of the BE more frequently when treated surgically than when treated by PPI (42 vs. 16 %, respectively). No patient with long segment BE had regression. Patients with short segment BE treated surgically also had a decrease in Cdx2 expression more frequently than the medically treated group, suggesting that in this subgroup surgery might have a role in preventing the progression of BE to cancer [38].

The incidence of peptic esophageal stricture has decreased with the widespread use of PPI and is currently a rare condition. There are no trials specifically designed to address this issue and most data are retrospective. It has been suggested that after antireflux surgery, patients with refractory strictures have good symptom control, minimal complications, and up to 87 % of patients need no further dilations after surgery [39, 40].

Special attention must be given to patients with severe disease for the presence of the "short esophagus." Patients with esophageal peptic stricture, hiatal hernia bigger than 5 cm, type III paraesophageal hiatal hernia, recurrent hiatal

Table 5.1 The relative strengths of different presentations for recommending antireflux surgery [0=avoid, + weak recommendation, ++ moderate recommendation, +++ very strong recommendation, ++++ absolute indication]

Presenting problem	24 h pH +	24 h pH −
GERD symptoms		
Regurgitation	++++	+++
Heartburn	+++	+
Regurg and HB	++++	+++
Esophagitis	+++	++
Dysphagia	++	+
Barretts	+/−	0
Supraesophageal sx		
Cough	+++	+
Hoarseness	++	0
Sore throat	++	0
Pulmonary fibrosis	++++	0

hernia, and Barrett's esophagus are especially at risk [41]. The presence of a short esophagus demands a change in surgical technique. A more detailed discussion of this issue is beyond the scope of this chapter and is covered in Chap. 19. Table 5.1 summarizes the strengths of different indications for recommending ARS.

Esophageal pH Study

The esophageal pH study was first described in 1974 [42] and is considered the gold standard for the diagnosis of GERD. Three different patterns of reflux can be identified based on esophageal pH study: supine, upright, and bipositional. Although once thought that different patterns would have different surgical outcomes, [43] the most recent literature indicates an equivalent surgical result irrespective of these pH study patterns [44, 45].

Symptomatic patients with a positive pH study generally do better than patients with symptoms and a negative pH study [46]. The symptom association probability index (SAP), which associates reflux episodes with patient reported symptoms, is an important instrument for surgical patient selection, and is especially valuable in the selection of patients with atypical symptoms for surgical treatment [47, 29]. Unfortunately, only half of patients with abnormal esophageal acid exposure have a positive SAP [48]. In a well-controlled trial, patients with an abnormal pH study and typical symptoms were randomized according to the SAP. The surgical outcomes were similar between patients with positive and negative SAP when measured objectively and subjectively at 3 months and 5 years, as were the number of reoperations within 6 years (12.8 and 14 %, respectively) [49]. The same group reported that the response to surgery is similar in reflux proven patients (abnormal pH study)

irrespective of the presence or absence of esophagitis [33]. Esophageal acid hypersensitivity is defined by a technically normal physiologic 24 h pH study and positive SAP correlation. Although caution must be exercised in this population, there are reports of good surgical results in patients with esophageal acid hypersensitivity [50]. The 48 h-wireless pH study and impedance pH study increase the sensitivity and SAP compared to traditional 24 h pH study. This can be of value in patients with initially negative 24 h pH study, and in patients with atypical symptoms [51–54]. Older methods such as the Bernstein test are rarely performed today.

Medical and Surgical Treatment for GERD: Randomized Trials

After reviewing the main predictors of good surgical outcomes and consequently how to select patients for surgical treatment of GERD, the final decision is whether surgery or medical treatment would be best for the patient.

In 2011 two randomized trials published results comparing medical and surgical GERD treatment. Anvari et al. [55] demonstrated that at 3-year follow-up surgery provided better symptomatic control and quality of life than the PPI alone, but there was no difference in GERD symptom scale or pH study results. Treatment failures were similar in both groups, being 11.8 % for surgery and 16 % for medical therapy. The LOTUS trial reported that at 5 years patients who underwent surgery had better control of regurgitation, but similar heartburn control, and an increased frequency of dysphagia and gas bloat. Treatment failure, the main outcome of the report, occurred in 15 % of surgical patients and 6 % of PPI therapy patients, a statistically significant difference [56]. It is important to highlight that both studies included only patients with typical symptoms responsive to PPI prior to randomization, and the surgical technique and medical treatment were standardized.

A meta-analysis of four randomized trials reported before 2010, which included 1,232 patients, reported an improvement in quality of life at 1 year after surgery when compared to medical therapy. It also suggested that heartburn and regurgitation are better controlled by surgery, but persistent dysphagia is more common after surgical procedure. Unfortunately, these conclusions are only valid for short and medium term follow-up [57].

Cost effectiveness analysis has been applied to compare the results of medical and surgical therapy for GERD. Two reports, one from the REFLUX Trial Group and another for Anvari et al., suggested that surgery might be cost effective in the treatment of patients who need long-term control of GERD [58, 59], Figure 5.1 (graph from Anvari Study). Although both studies suggested that surgery is more cost effective, the results are dependent on which measure was

Table 4 – Mean costs, quality-adjusted life years (QALYs) and cost-effectiveness of laparoscopic Nissen fundoplication (LNF) compared to proton pump inhibitor (PPI) treatment.

	LNF (n = 52)	PPI (n = 52)	LNF-PPI
Total costs	$15,948 (11,281)	$12,743 (12,488)	$3,205 (16,828)
Change in QALYs from baseline (based on HUI3)	0.276 (0.517)	0.167 (0.589)	0.109 (0.784)
ICUR			$29,404/QALY gained

Values are mean (SD).
ICUR, incremental cost-utility ratio; HUI3, Health Utilities Index version 3.

Fig. 5.1 Relative cost effectiveness of Nissen vs. medical treatment of GERD (from Goeree et al. [59])

used for the analysis, the cost of the PPI, and the long-term effectiveness of the surgical repair. The long-term results of surgical therapy are specifically discussed in the literature, and a recent report of 15-year follow-up of 86 patients after LARS and open fundoplication demonstrated that 76.7 % of patients were asymptomatic, with only 10.5 % of patients complaining of heartburn and regurgitation that affects their everyday life. Of those, nearly half had no objective evidence of GERD. Dysphagia was observed in 3.5 % of the series, with two cases related to previous strictures and one secondary to the fundoplication. Gas bloat was by far the most common adverse event, being reported in 43 % of the patients. In the laparoscopic group 91 % of the patients were satisfied with the surgical results. Fifteen percent ($n = 13$) of the patients were using PPI on a daily basis, but only six of them had objective endoscopic signs related to recurrent reflux [60].

Conclusion

In summary, antireflux surgery can be used to treat GERD with symptomatic long-terms results at least similar to the best medical therapy. As assessed by pH study, surgically treated patients have better objective control of reflux than medically treated patients.

For optimal outcomes patient selection is of pivotal importance. Patients who respond to PPI therapy, at least partially, and have objective evidence of GERD demonstrated on upper endoscopy or pH study have better outcomes after surgery. For those patients with GERD symptoms and no objective evidence of reflux or atypical symptoms, caution must be exercised; the SAP index and more elaborate tests such as 48 h pH study or pH impedance test add valuable information for more precise patient selection. Patients with esophageal peptic stricture are better controlled with surgery, needing fewer dilations than with medical therapy, and patients with Barrett's esophagus have good symptom control and more effective pH control. For now, there is no clear evidence that antireflux surgery prevents the progression of Barrett's epithelium to dysplasia or cancer, but some reports suggest that surgery may have a preventive role in patients with short segment BE.

References

1. Camilleri M, Dubois D, Coulie B, Jones M, Kahrilas PJ, Rentz AM, et al. Prevalence and socioeconomic impact of upper gastrointestinal disorders in the United States: results of the US Upper Gastrointestinal Study. Clin Gastroenterol Hepatol. 2005;3(6):543–52.
2. Toghanian S, Wahlqvist P, Johnson DA, Bolge SC, Liljas B. The burden of disrupting gastro-oesophageal reflux disease: a database study in US and European cohorts. Clin Drug Investig. 2010;30(3): 167–78.
3. Brook RA, Wahlqvist P, Kleinman NL, Wallander MA, Campbell SM, Smeeding JE. Cost of gastro-oesophageal reflux disease to the employer: a perspective from the United States. Aliment Pharmacol Ther. 2007;26(6):889–98.
4. Morgenthal CB, Lin E, Shane MD, Hunter JG, Smith CD. Who will fail laparoscopic Nissen fundoplication? Preoperative prediction of long-term outcomes. Surg Endosc. 2007;21(11):1978–84.
5. Hamdy E. Long-term outcomes of laparoscopic antireflux surgery. Hepatogastroenterology. 2011;58(105):56–63.
6. Oelschlager BK, Quiroga E, Parra JD, Cahill M, Polissar N, Pellegrini CA. Long-term outcomes after laparoscopic antireflux surgery. Am J Gastroenterol. 2008;103(2):280–7. quiz 288.
7. Tsuboi K, Lee TH, Legner A, Yano F, Dworak T, Mittal SK. Identification of risk factors for postoperative dysphagia after primary anti-reflux surgery. Surg Endosc. 2011;25(3):923–9.
8. Tekin K, Toydemir T, Yerdel MA. Is laparoscopic antireflux surgery safe and effective in obese patients? Surg Endosc. 2012;26(1): 86–95.
9. Chisholm JA, Jamieson GG, Lally CJ, Devitt PG, Game PA, Watson DI. The effect of obesity on the outcome of laparoscopic antireflux surgery. J Gastrointest Surg. 2009;13(6):1064–70.
10. D'Alessio MJ, Arnaoutakis D, Giarelli N, Villadolid DV, Rosemurgy AS. Obesity is not a contraindication to laparoscopic Nissen fundoplication. J Gastrointest Surg. 2005;9(7):949–54.
11. Winslow ER, Frisella MM, Soper NJ, Klingensmith ME. Obesity does not adversely affect the outcome of laparoscopic antireflux surgery (LARS). Surg Endosc. 2003;17(12):2003–11.
12. Anvari M, Bamehriz F. Outcome of laparoscopic Nissen fundoplication in patients with body mass index > or = 35. Surg Endosc. 2006;20(2):230–4.
13. So JB, Zeitels SM, Rattner DW. Outcomes of atypical symptoms attributed to gastroesophageal reflux treated by laparoscopic fundoplication. Surgery. 1998;124(1):28–32.

14. Morgenthal CB, Shane MD, Stival A, Gletsu N, Milam G, Swafford V, et al. The durability of laparoscopic Nissen fundoplication: 11-year outcomes. J Gastrointest Surg. 2007;11(6):693–700.

15. Farrell TM, Richardson WS, Trus TL, Smith CD, Hunter JG. Response of atypical symptoms of gastro-oesophageal reflux to antireflux surgery. Br J Surg. 2001;88(12):1649–52.

16. Brown SR, Gyawali CP, Melman L, Jenkins ED, Bader J, Frisella MM, et al. Clinical outcomes of atypical extra-esophageal reflux symptoms following laparoscopic antireflux surgery. Surg Endosc. 2011;25(12):3852–8.

17. Kiljander TO, Laitinen JO. The prevalence of gastroesophageal reflux disease in adult asthmatics. Chest. 2004;126(5):1490–4.

18. Gibson PG, Henry RL, Coughlan JL. Gastro-oesophageal reflux treatment for asthma in adults and children. Cochrane Database Syst Rev. 2003;2, CD001496.

19. Sontag SJ, O'Connell S, Khandelwal S, Greenlee H, Schnell T, Nemchausky B, et al. Asthmatics with gastroesophageal reflux: long term results of a randomized trial of medical and surgical antireflux therapies. Am J Gastroenterol. 2003;98(5):987–99.

20. Sharma B, Sharma M, Daga MK, Sachdev GK, Bondi E. Effect of omeprazole and domperidone on adult asthmatics with gastroesophageal reflux. World J Gastroenterol. 2007;13(11):1706–10.

21. American Lung Association Asthma Clinical Research Centers, Mastronarde JG, Anthonisen NR, Castro M, Holbrook JT, Leone FT, et al. Efficacy of esomeprazole for treatment of poorly controlled asthma. N Engl J Med. 2009;360(15):1487–99.

22. Allen CJ, Anvari M. Preoperative symptom evaluation and esophageal acid infusion predict response to laparoscopic Nissen fundoplication in gastroesophageal reflux patients who present with cough. Surg Endosc. 2002;16(7):1037–41.

23. Ratnasingam D, Irvine T, Thompson SK, Watson DI. Laparoscopic antireflux surgery in patients with throat symptoms: a word of caution. World J Surg. 2011;35(2):342–8.

24. Park W, Hicks DM, Khandwala F, Richter JE, Abelson TI, Milstein C, et al. Laryngopharyngeal reflux: prospective cohort study evaluating optimal dose of proton-pump inhibitor therapy and pretherapy predictors of response. Laryngoscope. 2005;115(7):1230–8.

25. Fisichella PM, Davis CS, Lundberg PW, Lowery E, Burnham EL, Alex CG, et al. The protective role of laparoscopic antireflux surgery against aspiration of pepsin after lung transplantation. Surgery. 2011;150(4):598–606.

26. Fisichella PM, Davis CS, Gagermeier J, Dilling D, Alex CG, Dorfmeister JA, et al. Laparoscopic antireflux surgery for gastroesophageal reflux disease after lung transplantation. J Surg Res. 2011;170(2):e279–86.

27. Hoppo T, Jarido V, Pennathur A, Morrell M, Crespo M, Shigemura N, et al. Antireflux surgery preserves lung function in patients with gastroesophageal reflux disease and end-stage lung disease before and after lung transplantation. Arch Surg. 2011;146(9):1041–7.

28. Wang WH, Huang JQ, Zheng GF, Wong WM, Lam SK, Karlberg J, et al. Is proton pump inhibitor testing an effective approach to diagnose gastroesophageal reflux disease in patients with noncardiac chest pain?: a meta-analysis. Arch Intern Med. 2005;165(11):1222–8.

29. Kushnir VM, Sayuk GS, Gyawali CP. Abnormal GERD parameters on ambulatory pH monitoring predict therapeutic success in noncardiac chest pain. Am J Gastroenterol. 2010;105(5):1032–8.

30. Oelschlager BK, Petersen RP, Brunt LM, Soper NJ, Sheppard BC, Mitsumori L, et al. Laparoscopic paraesophageal hernia repair: defining long-term clinical and anatomic outcomes. J Gastrointest Surg. 2012;16(3):453–9.

31. Kamolz T, Granderath FA, Schweiger UM, Pointner R. Laparoscopic Nissen fundoplication in patients with nonerosive reflux disease. Long-term quality-of-life assessment and surgical outcome. Surg Endosc. 2005;19(4):494–500.

32. Lord RV, DeMeester SR, Peters JH, Hagen JA, Elyssnia D, Sheth CT, et al. Hiatal hernia, lower esophageal sphincter incompetence, and effectiveness of Nissen fundoplication in the spectrum of gastroesophageal reflux disease. J Gastrointest Surg. 2009;13(4):602–10.

33. Broeders JA, Draaisma WA, Bredenoord AJ, Smout AJ, Broeders IA, Gooszen HG. Long-term outcome of Nissen fundoplication in non-erosive and erosive gastro-oesophageal reflux disease. Br J Surg. 2010;97(6):845–52.

34. Spechler SJ. Comparison of medical and surgical therapy for complicated gastroesophageal reflux disease in veterans. The Department of Veterans Affairs Gastroesophageal Reflux Disease Study Group. N Engl J Med. 1992;326(12):786–92.

35. Spechler SJ, Lee E, Ahnen D, Goyal RK, Hirano I, Ramirez F, et al. Long-term outcome of medical and surgical therapies for gastroesophageal reflux disease: follow-up of a randomized controlled trial. JAMA. 2001;285(18):2331–8.

36. Parrilla P, Martinez de Haro LF, Ortiz A, Munitiz V, Molina J, Bermejo J, et al. Long-term results of a randomized prospective study comparing medical and surgical treatment of Barrett's esophagus. Ann Surg. 2003;237(3):291–8.

37. Attwood SE, Lundell L, Hatlebakk JG, Eklund S, Junghard O, Galmiche JP, et al. Medical or surgical management of GERD patients with Barrett's esophagus: the LOTUS trial 3-year experience. J Gastrointest Surg. 2008;12(10):1646–54. discussion 1654-5.

38. Zaninotto G, Parente P, Salvador R, Farinati F, Tieppo C, Passuello N, et al. Long-term follow-up of Barrett's epithelium: medical versus antireflux surgical therapy. J Gastrointest Surg. 2012;16(1):7–14. discussion 14-5.

39. Klingler PJ, Hinder RA, Cina RA, DeVault KR, Floch NR, Branton SA, et al. Laparoscopic antireflux surgery for the treatment of esophageal strictures refractory to medical therapy. Am J Gastroenterol. 1999;94(3):632–6.

40. Spivak H, Farrell TM, Trus TL, Branum GD, Warring JP, Hunter JG. Laparoscopic fundoplication for dysphagia and peptic esophageal stricture. J Gastrointest Surg. 1998;2(6):555–60.

41. Urbach DR, Khajanchee YS, Glasgow RE, Hansen PD, Swanstrom LL. Preoperative determinants of an esophageal lengthening procedure in laparoscopic antireflux surgery. Surg Endosc. 2001;15(12):1408–12.

42. Johnson LF, Demeester TR. Twenty-four-hour pH monitoring of the distal esophagus. A quantitative measure of gastroesophageal reflux. Am J Gastroenterol. 1974;62(4):325–32.

43. Winslow ER, Frisella MM, Soper NJ, Clouse RE, Klingensmith ME. Patients with upright reflux have less favorable postoperative outcomes after laparoscopic antireflux surgery than those with supine reflux. J Gastrointest Surg. 2002;6(6):819–29. discussion 829–30.

44. Hong D, Swanstrom LL, Khajanchee YS, Pereira N, Hansen PD. Postoperative objective outcomes for upright, supine, and bipositional reflux disease following laparoscopic Nissen fundoplication. Arch Surg. 2004;139(8):848–52. discussion 852–4.

45. Meneghetti AT, Tedesco P, Galvani C, Gorodner MV, Patti MG. Outcomes after laparoscopic Nissen fundoplication are not influenced by the pattern of reflux. Dis Esophagus. 2008;21(2):165–9.

46. Khajanchee YS, Hong D, Hansen PD, Swanstrom LL. Outcomes of antireflux surgery in patients with normal preoperative 24-hour pH test results. Am J Surg. 2004;187(5):599–603.

47. Hersh MJ, Sayuk GS, Gyawali CP. Long-term therapeutic outcome of patients undergoing ambulatory pH monitoring for chronic unexplained cough. J Clin Gastroenterol. 2010;44(4):254–60.

48. Zerbib F, Roman S, Ropert A, des Varannes SB, Pouderoux P, Chaput U, et al. Esophageal pH-impedance monitoring and symptom analysis in GERD: a study in patients off and on therapy. Am J Gastroenterol. 2006;101(9):1956–63.

49. Broeders JA, Draaisma WA, Bredenoord AJ, Smout AJ, Broeders IA, Gooszen HG. Impact of symptom-reflux association analysis on long-term outcome after Nissen fundoplication. Br J Surg. 2011;98(2):247–54.

50. Broeders JA, Draaisma WA, Bredenoord AJ, de Vries DR, Rijnhart-de Jong HG, Smout AJ, et al. Oesophageal acid hypersensitivity is not a contraindication to Nissen fundoplication. Br J Surg. 2009;96(9):1023–30.

51. Sweis R, Fox M, Anggiansah A, Wong T. Prolonged, wireless pH-studies have a high diagnostic yield in patients with reflux symptoms and negative 24-h catheter-based pH-studies. Neurogastroenterol Motil. 2011;23(5):419–26.

52. Gruebel C, Linke G, Tutuian R, Hebbard G, Zerz A, Meyenberger C, et al. Prospective study examining the impact of multichannel intraluminal impedance on antireflux surgery. Surg Endosc. 2008;22(5):1241–7.

53. Gillies RS, Stratford JM, Booth MI, Dehn TC. Oesophageal pH monitoring using the Bravo catheter-free radio capsule. Eur J Gastroenterol Hepatol. 2007;19(1):57–63.

54. del Genio G, Tolone S, del Genio F, Aggarwal R, d'Alessandro A, Allaria A, et al. Prospective assessment of patient selection for antireflux surgery by combined multichannel intraluminal impedance pH monitoring. J Gastrointest Surg. 2008;12(9):1491–6.

55. Anvari M, Allen C, Marshall J, Armstrong D, Goeree R, Ungar W, et al. A randomized controlled trial of laparoscopic Nissen fundoplication versus proton pump inhibitors for the treatment of patients with chronic gastroesophageal reflux disease (GERD): 3-year outcomes. Surg Endosc. 2011;25(8):2547–54.

56. Galmiche JP, Hatlebakk J, Attwood S, Ell C, Fiocca R, Eklund S, et al. Laparoscopic antireflux surgery vs esomeprazole treatment for chronic GERD: the LOTUS randomized clinical trial. JAMA. 2011;305(19):1969–77.

57. Wileman SM, McCann S, Grant AM, Krukowski ZH, Bruce J. Medical versus surgical management for gastro-oesophageal reflux disease (GORD) in adults. Cochrane Database Syst Rev. 2010;3, CD003243.

58. Epstein D, Bojke L, Sculpher MJ, REFLUX Trial Group. Laparoscopic fundoplication compared with medical management for gastro-oesophageal reflux disease: cost effectiveness study. BMJ. 2009;339:b2576.

59. Goeree R, Hopkins R, Marshall JK, Armstrong D, Ungar WJ, Goldsmith C, et al. Cost-utility of laparoscopic Nissen fundoplication versus proton pump inhibitors for chronic and controlled gastroesophageal reflux disease: a 3-year prospective randomized controlled trial and economic evaluation. Value Health. 2011;14(2):263–73.

60. Salminen P, Hurme S, Ovaska J. Fifteen-year outcome of laparoscopic and open Nissen fundoplication: a randomized clinical trial. Ann Thorac Surg. 2012;93(1):228–33.

The Relation of Hiatal Hernia to Gastroesophageal Reflux Disease

Dustin A. Carlson and John E. Pandolfino

Abbreviations

LES   Lower esophageal sphincter
CD   Crural diaphragm
GEJ   Gastroesophageal junction
GER (D) Gastroesophageal reflux (disease)
HH   Hiatal hernia
TLESR   Transient lower esophageal sphincter relaxation
EndoFLIP Endoscopic functional luminal imaging probe

Introduction

The anti-reflux barrier is a complex anatomical region that is dependent upon numerous factors: intra-luminal pressure generated by the smooth muscle of the lower esophageal sphincter (LES), extra-luminal compression generated by the crural diaphragm (CD), compliance of the gastroesophageal junction (GEJ), integrity of the phrenoesophageal ligaments (which anchor the lower esophagus to the diaphragmatic hiatus), and the gastroesophageal "flap-valve," a conformational change associated with maintenance of the angle of His and an intra-abdominal LES (the acute angle formed between the esophagus and the greater curvature of the stomach) [1]. Gastroesophageal reflux (GER) can occur when the gastroesophageal pressure gradient overcomes the anti-reflux barrier and favors the proximal flow of gastric contents. Gastroesophageal reflux disease (GERD) is defined as a condition that occurs when refluxed

stomach contents cause troublesome symptoms and/or complications [2]. The propensity for reflux is dependent on perturbations in the various components of the anti-reflux barrier and severity of GER will increase as the number of components affected increases. The proximal displacement of the GEJ in relation to the diaphragmatic hiatus that occurs with a "type I" or "sliding" hiatal hernia (HH) contributes to or is associated with disturbances in numerous anti-reflux mechanisms, thus it is no surprise that the prevalence of GERD, as well as the severity of symptoms and erosive esophagitis, is increased in patients with HH compared to those without [3–10].

Clinical Significance of Hiatal Hernia

As mentioned, HH is seen more frequently in patients with GERD than in patients without GERD; prevalence estimates range from 50 to 90 % of patients with GERD having HH, whereas HH is seen in significantly lower percentages of patients without signs or symptoms of GERD. However, prevalence data does need to be taken with a grain of salt as diagnostic methods (endoscopic, radiographic, and manometric) and diagnostic criteria (distance of GEJ-CD separation, > 2 cm often used) for HH, as well as definition of GERD (e.g., symptoms, esophagitis, abnormal pH study) vary between studies. While small axial disruptions in the GEJ may be grouped with normal controls or non-HH patients in some studies, the impact of these small axial hernias should not be ignored. A study examining small HH (0.5–2 cm) demonstrated the importance of those small disruptions in the GEJ, as erosive esophagitis and Barrett's esophagus were still observed to be more common in patients with small HH than normal controls [8].

The presence of a HH appears to have an effect on the pattern of GERD symptoms, as patients with HH are observed to more commonly have GER-associated extraesophageal and pulmonary symptoms (e.g., cough or hoarseness) and may be more prone to nocturnal symptoms [11]. HH also appears to have an effect on response to GERD treatment as

D.A. Carlson, MD
Department of Medicine, Northwestern Memorial Hospital, 676 North St. Clair Street, Suite 1400, Chicago, IL 60611, USA
e-mail: dustin-carlson@fsm.northwestern.edu

J.E. Pandolfino, MD, MSCI (✉)
Department of Medicine, Northwestern Memorial Hospital, 676 North St. Clair Street, Suite 1409, Chicago, IL 60611, USA
e-mail: j-pandolfino@northwestern.edu

L.L. Swanstrom and C.M. Dunst (eds.), *Antireflux Surgery*,
DOI 10.1007/978-1-4939-1749-5_6, © Springer New York 2015

patients with HH may be more likely to continue to have symptoms and abnormal esophageal acid exposure while on once daily acid-suppressive therapy than GERD patients without HH [12–14].

In addition, the presence, as well as increased size, of HH is also a risk factor for development of Barrett's esophagus and esophageal adenocarcinoma [9, 15, 16]. Furthermore, progression from Barrett's to high grade dysplasia or adenocarcinoma is associated with the size of HH [17]. HH also has been associated with an increased risk of lack of regression of Barrett's after treatment with medical acid-suppressive therapy or radio-frequency ablation [18, 19].

Mechanisms of Reflux

Reflux occurs when the trans-gastroesophageal pressure gradient is sufficient to overcome the anti-reflux barrier of the GEJ to permit flow. Transient lower esophageal sphincter relaxation (TLESR) is the predominant mechanism for reflux events in normal controls, accounting for nearly 100 % of reflux episodes, and the most common mechanism in patients with GERD, accounting for 65–82 % of reflux episodes [20–22]. Reflux events associated with swallow-induced LES relaxation and abdominal strain and/or deep breaths make up smaller percentages of reflux events [20–22]. TLESRs have been demonstrated to occur more frequently in response to gastric distension in GERD patients with HH than GERD patients without HH and normal controls—a finding that was also directly correlated with the size of the HH [23].

However, in patients with HH, other mechanisms of reflux play a more prominent role as well. A study by van Herwaarden et al. [24] demonstrated that GERD patients with and without HH had a similar number of reflux episodes associated with TLESRs (and also swallow-associated prolonged LES relaxation) during 24 h of ambulatory esophageal pH and manometric monitoring. However, GERD patients with HH demonstrated more reflux episodes associated with swallow-associated normal LES relaxation, and low LES pressure (with and without abdominal straining and/or deep inspiration) than GERD patients without HH. In addition, the HH patients demonstrated more overall reflux episodes and greater esophageal acid exposure—a difference likely accounted for by the increase in reflux episodes caused by non-TLESR mechanisms.

The increased number of reflux events and overall esophageal acid exposure in patients with HH can be related to the amount of time that the anti-reflux barrier is permissive of gastroesophageal flow, which can be better understood with examination of the components that make up the anti-reflux barrier and are disrupted with hiatal hernia.

The Role of the Crural Diaphragm in Reflux

Maintaining Closure of the GEJ

The "two-sphincter" hypothesis proposes that the CD provides a second sphincteric component by applying external pressure to the GEJ. Manometric examinations of patients with HH demonstrate dual high-pressure zones that are accounted for by independent contributions of the LES and the CD. Numerous studies support that the LES pressure is reduced in patients with HH compared with normal controls and GERD patients without HH [10, 25–29]. However, simulated reduction of the hiatal hernia (i.e., additive overlap of the LES and CD high-pressure zones) has been demonstrated to produce LES pressure similar to normal control [29]. Thus, the normal "distal esophageal high-pressure zone" is composed of direct contributions from both the CD and the LES.

The striated muscle of the CD is rapidly activated during respiration and abdominal strain, which adds closure pressure to the GEJ during these activities that can predispose people to reflux due to generation of increased intra-abdominal pressure [30, 31]. A study utilizing concurrent manometry and fluoroscopy demonstrated that there was an indirect interaction between HH size and LES pressure that made patients more susceptible to GERD induced by maneuvers that increased abdominal pressure (e.g., Valsalva) [28]. In other words, the axial displacement of the GEJ into the negative pressure environment of the thoracic cavity decreases its effectiveness as a reflux barrier to the positive pressure environment of the abdomen. Another study which utilized high-resolution manometry to examine the role of the CD in GERD showed that, while lower LES pressure, the length of CD-LES separation, and reduced GEJ inspiratory augmentation were all associated with GERD, it was reduced GEJ inspiratory augmentation that displayed the strongest relationship and was the only independent predictor of GERD based on additional logistic regression analysis [27]. In addition, the correlation between CD-LES separation was weak, which may imply the importance of other factors involved in the CD's role in the anti-reflux barrier, such as primary CD dysfunction (e.g., reduced thickness), and/or changes in the radial dimensions or compliance of the hiatal canal.

Not only does the CD act as a second esophageal sphincter, it also helps maintain the acute angle of His. In this respect, the crural diaphragm plays a similar role in preventing GER as does the puborectalis muscle in maintaining fecal continence (see Fig. 6.1): The puborectalis muscle forms a sling around the lower rectum which when normally contracted, maintains the acute angle of the anorectal junction and prevents flow of stool. With defecation, relaxation of the puborectalis muscle leads to opening of the angle of the anorectal junction, reducing resistance to stool outflow

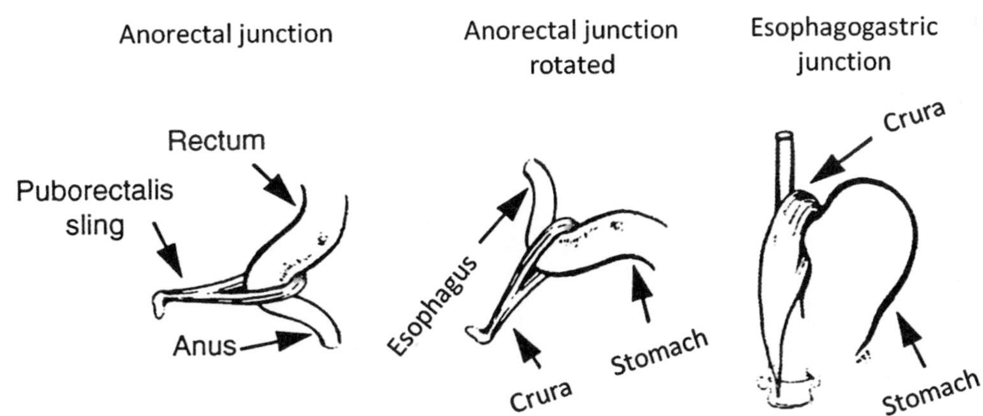

Fig. 6.1 Comparison of gastroesophageal and anorectal junctions. When the anorectal junction is graphically rotated (*middle image*), note the similarity in conformations of the rectum and the esophagus/stomach. In both instances, relaxation or contraction of the "sling" (i.e., the puborectalis and crural diaphragm) is able to facilitate or prevent flow, respectively. Modified from the original illustrations of Allison. Reprinted with permission from the Journal of the American College of Surgeons, formerly Surgery Gynecology & Obstetrics

and facilitating defecation. The crural diaphragm similarly forms a sling that wraps around the esophagus which maintains the acute angle of His that helps prevent GER. When the crural diaphragm relaxes, the angle of His can open up and create a preferential configuration for retrograde flow and allow belching, reflux, and vomiting to occur.

At the intra-luminal portion of the esophagus at the angle of His, there is a ridge of tissue that appears to act as a "flap-valve" in helping to prevent GER. Hill et al. described this "flap-valve" and supported the concept by a study in which they measured the GEJ pressure gradient required to generate gastroesophageal flow in cadavers [1]. As there is no LES or CD contraction in cadavers, the measured pressure gradient suggested that a barrier to reflux flow must be generated by a functional "flap-valve." The required pressure gradient was shown to augment with accentuation of the flap valve with sutures and also to be lower and often absent in cadavers with a HH. When a HH was present, a pressure gradient could be restored and/or increased with applying posterior fixation, which returned the GEJ to its intra-abdominal position.

Hill et al. further examined a group of GERD patients and normal controls and developed a grading system based on the endoscopic appearance of the GEJ (see Fig. 6.2). Flap-valve grades I and II were more common in normal controls and grades III and IV were more common in GERD patients. When applied prospectively, they showed that this grading scheme could accurately predict the GERD status of patients. Another study demonstrated that this flap-valve grading scheme was also associated with increased esophageal acid exposure during exercise, which causes intra-abdominal strain (flap-valve grades III and IV had greater acid exposure than grades I and II) [32]. Furthermore, these findings were shown to be independent of decreased LES pressure.

The flap-valve concept nicely demonstrates how multiple components can interact to promote the anti-reflux barrier.

Reduce Gastric Reflux Flow and Volume

Poiseuille's Law of Flow states that flow (F) is directly proportional to the pressure gradient (ΔP) multiplied by the radius (r) to the fourth power and is inversely proportional to the fluid viscosity (η) and length (L) of the system ($F \propto \Delta P r^4 / \eta \ell$). While this equation makes several assumptions of the system to which it applies, the concept remains apparent that the radius of the tube is the dominant variable of flow.

Given the relationship of opening dimensions to flow, it has been hypothesized that increased GEJ distensibility and dimensions would affect the volume of reflux in patients with GERD and HH. A series of studies using a trans-GEJ placed barostat and manometry device combined with concurrent fluoroscopy to measure the radial dimensions of the GEJ in response to low distension pressures were utilized to assess the radial dimensions of the GEJ in GERD [25, 33]. They found that patients with HH had greater relaxed GEJ distensibility, i.e., the GEJ opening occurred at lower pressures and opened wider for a given pressure, than in GER patients without HH and normal controls (Fig. 6.3). In addition, further examination using distension pressures just above and just below intragastric pressure demonstrated that only the group of patients with GER and HH (not GER without HH or normal controls) demonstrated GEJ opening at pressures below intragastric pressure [25].

An alternative method of measuring GEJ distension to the cumbersome hydrostat/fluoroscopy is an endoscopic functional luminal imaging probe (EndoFLIP; Crospon Inc. Galway, Ireland). The EndoFLIP is a device that utilizes impedance planimetry to measure intra-luminal cross-sectional area and thus when positioned across the GEJ and utilized with concurrent pressure measurements, can measure GEJ compliance. A study utilizing EndoFLIP compared the GEJ distensibility of normal controls with patients with

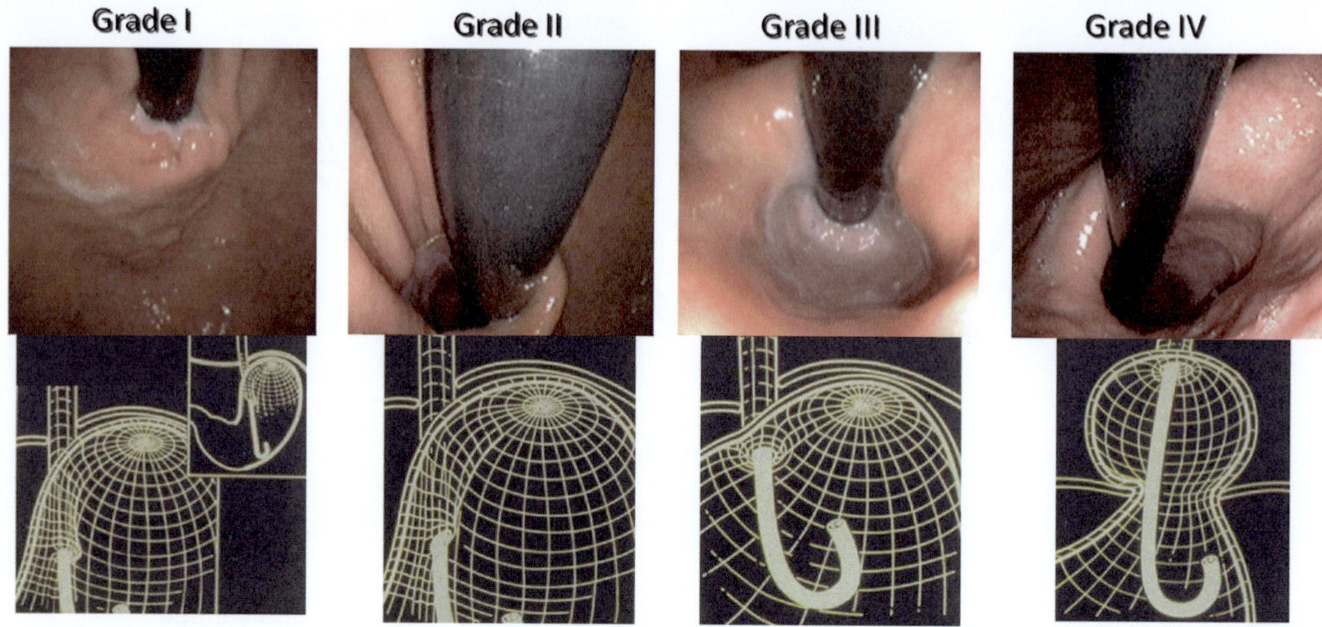

Fig. 6.2 Flap-valve grading system. Grade I—a normal, prominent ridge or fold of tissue at the lesser curvature, closely approximated to the endoscope; Grade II—fold present but with periodic opening and closing (often associated with respiration) around the endoscope; Grade III— fold not prominent and hiatus freely open, hiatal hernia may or may not be present; Grade IV—no fold, large hiatal hernia (i.e., axial displacement of the squamocolumnar junction) with open esophagus. Modified from Hill Gastrointest Endosc., 1996;**44**(5):541–7) with permission

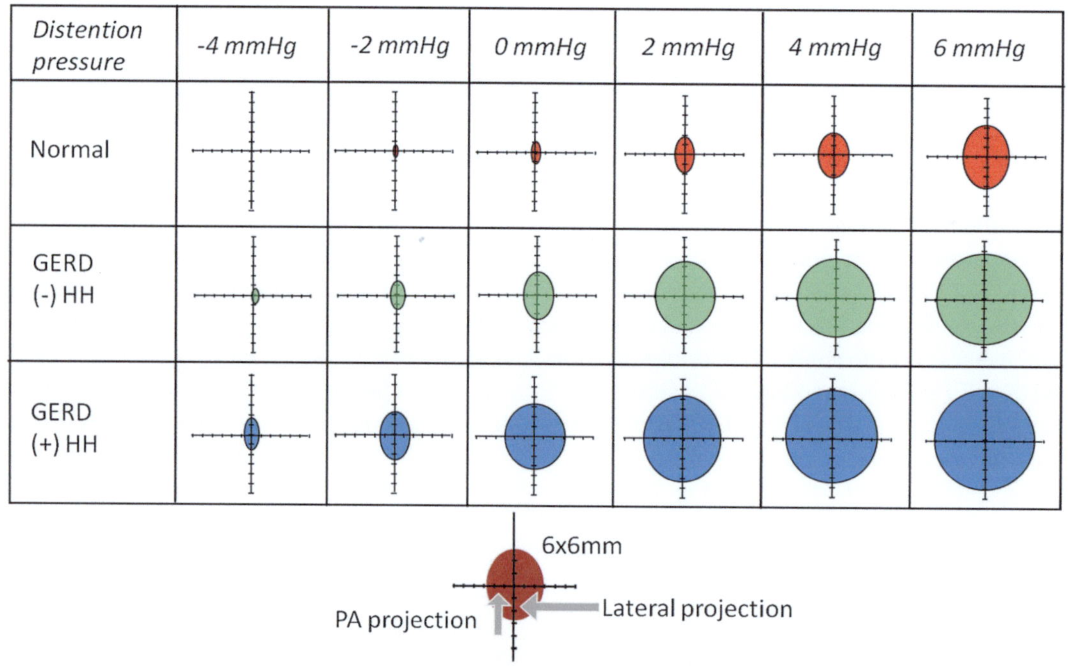

Fig. 6.3 Radial dimensions of the GEJ in response to distension pressures. Increased compliance of the GEJ in patients with GERD +/− HH is demonstrated with the plotted measurements of GEJ opening diameters made from posteroanterior (PA) and lateral fluoroscopic projections in response to intra-hydrostat bag pressures (relative to gastric pressure). While radial asymmetry was seen in all three groups, the asymmetry is most pronounced in the normal patients due to the comparably increased PA diameters seen in the GERD HH (+) and GERD HH (−) groups. Modified from Pandolfino et al. Gastroenterology 2003;**125**(4):1018–24 with permission

GERD [34]. Patients also underwent endoscopy to assess the flap-valve grade. The study demonstrated that in all patients, the diaphragmatic hiatus was the least distensible region in both controls and GERD patients, but that the GEJ distensibility was greater in GERD patients than in normal controls. Interestingly, there was poor correlation between the FLIP-measured GEJ distensibility and the flap-valve grade. This demonstrates that there is radial, as well as axial, disruption that occurs at the hiatus. Given the relationship of flow with the opening diameter, a more distensible GEJ can facilitate the presence and volume of reflux.

While radius is the dominant variable in flow, length is inversely proportional to flow to a lesser degree. The lengths of the LES, the GEJ high-pressure zone, and the intra-abdominal esophagus are observed to be shorter in patients with HH [10, 26, 28, 29, 35]. The intra-abdominal esophagus is an area of the esophagus subject to increased external pressures of the intra-abdominal compartment and is a crucial component of the flap valve, as in-vitro demonstrations have shown increased gastroesophageal pressure gradients required to generate flow through longer intra-abdominal esophageal lengths [35]. Thus, shorter lengths of LES and intra-abdominal esophagus may further add a component of incompetence to the anti-reflux barrier when a HH is present.

Impaired Esophageal Acid Clearance and Re-reflux

Esophageal acid exposure is increased in the presence of a hiatal hernia, but is due to more than just the deficiencies in *preventing* reflux as described above. Not only is more reflux and acid able to cross the GEJ, but the esophagus's ability to clear the acid is further impaired and occurs more slowly in patients with HH [36, 37]. A study utilizing concurrent video-fluoroscopy and manometry to examine esophageal emptying in normal controls and patients with HH showed that complete esophageal emptying occurred less frequently in patients with HH [37]. In addition, they showed that whether or not the hernia reduced between swallows was a factor that appeared to have an effect on esophageal emptying and the timing of reflux from the hernia sac (patients with a hernia that completely reduced between swallows had more frequent complete esophageal clearance and their reflux from the hernia sac occurred early after LES relaxation, where as patients with a non-reducing HH were observed to have late flow).

Because of incompetence at the hiatus and the potential for re-reflux from fluid retained within the hernia sac, the environment of the proximal stomach is important in determining the make-up of the refluxate. A post-prandial "acid pocket" in the proximal stomach has been described that may allow for increased esophageal acid exposure during LES relaxation [38]. Using a pH catheter pull-through method, a "pocket" of acid was demonstrated to be present at the GEJ after meals, suggesting this acid pocket may not be subjected to the buffering effects of the meal.

In an elegant study performed by Beaumont et al. [39] the post-prandial acid pocket was examined in healthy volunteers (without GERD or HH), and patients with GERD with no or small (<3 cm) HH and large (>3 cm) HH. The "acid-pocket" was visualized with nuclear medicine imaging while LES relaxation, esophageal reflux, and pH were concurrently measured with esophageal manometry, impedance, and a pull-through pH catheter (Fig. 6.4). They observed that the post-prandial acid pocket remained below the GEJ in all the healthy volunteers and most (84 %) of those with GERD and small HH. However, in GERD patients with large HH, the acid pocket extended above the diaphragm for the entire duration of the study (2 h) in half of the patients and intermittently migrated above the diaphragm in 90 % of the patients. In addition, while all three groups of patients had a similar number of TLESRs, those with HH were more likely to have *acidic* reflux (large HH more likely than small). The position of the acid pocket above the diaphragm during a TLESR was more likely to lead to acidic reflux. Thus, patients with large HH and acid pocket about the diaphragm were observed to have more esophageal acid exposure. Multivariate regression analysis indicated that presence of HH and position of the acid pocket above the diaphragm were statistically significant risk factors for acidic reflux, while distance between the acid pocket and the squamocolumnar junction was protective against acidic reflux.

While the hernia sac itself may provide a nidus for acid to re-reflux into the esophagus, it has been proposed that abnormalities in esophageal motility may also contribute to impaired esophageal acid clearance in patients with HH. Studies have shown that esophageal dysmotility is more common in patients with HH and have suggested that esophageal acid exposure may be more related to impaired esophageal motility (low distal amplitude and impaired bolus transport/ineffective esophageal contractions) than the presence or absence of HH [40, 41]. However, no significant difference was noted in the distribution of esophageal motility patterns defined by high-resolution manometry between 90 patients with large (>5 cm) HH and normal controls; normal and weak peristalsis remained the most frequent patterns seen [26]. Thus, while esophageal dysmotility may contribute to increased esophageal acid exposure, this does not appear to be a primary mechanism behind the pathophysiology of GER in patients with HH, and it remains possible that some of the findings of dysmotility in patients with HH may be related to other co-existing factors.

Summary

The GEJ is a complex region with multiple components that each plays a role in the anti-reflux barrier. The conformational change that occurs within this region when a hiatal hernia is present results in a variety of disruptions in anti-reflux protective factors which makes patients with HH more

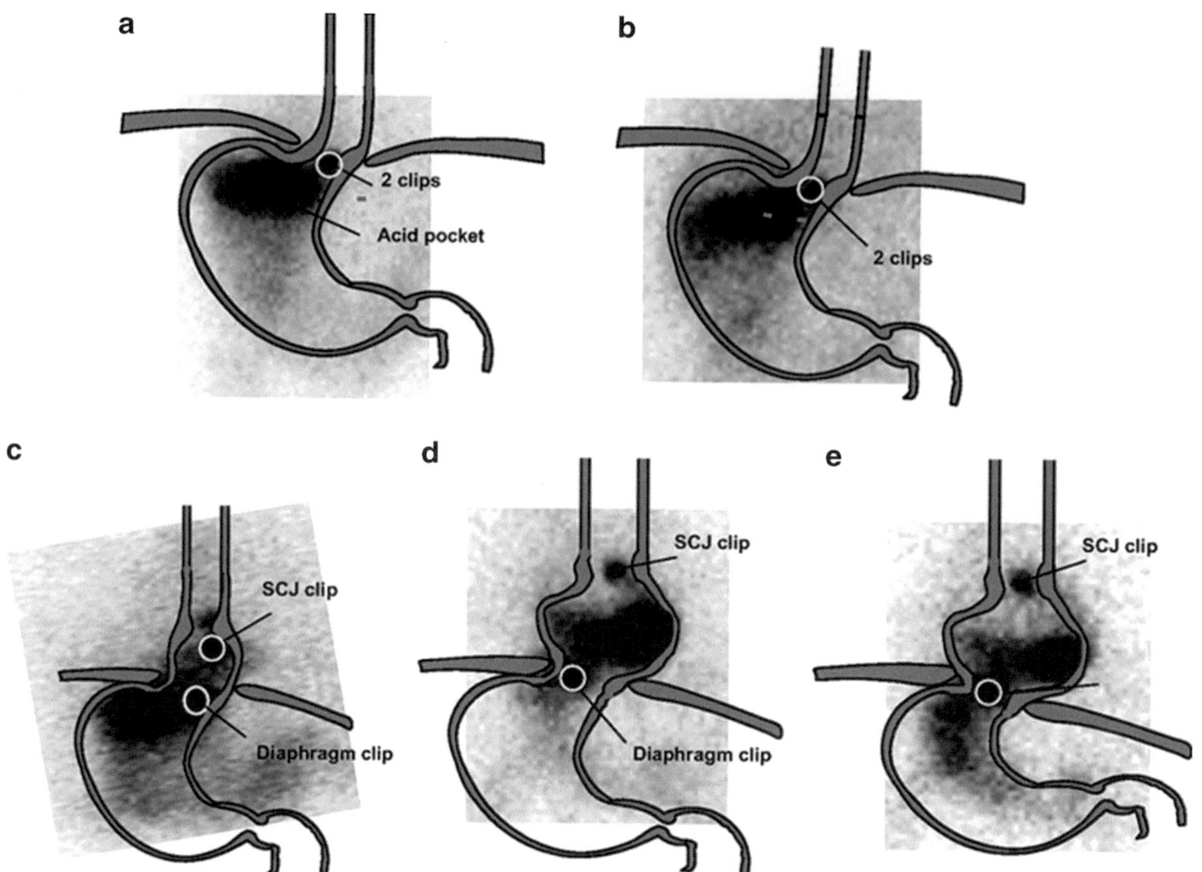

Fig. 6.4 Scintigraphic images of the post-prandial acid pocket. Nuclear-labeled acid (*black*) is visualized in relation to the squamocolumnar junction (SCJ) and diaphragmatic impression, which were marked with endoscopically placed clips. The acid pocket remained below the SCJ in normal patients (**A**) and most patients with a small HH (**B**). However, in patients with a large HH (**C–E**), the acid pocket was partially (**C, E**) or completely (**D**) located within the HH. Modified from Beaumont H, et al. Gut 2010; **59**(4): 441–51 with permission

susceptible to acid reflux and its complications. On a study population level, it is apparent that various mechanisms can account for the increased reflux and esophageal acid exposure that occurs in the presence of a HH. Future study will dictate if assessment of these components (e.g., GEJ distensibility via EndoFLIP) on an individual basis can elucidate possible targets for individually tailored mechanical corrective therapies of GERD.

References

1. Hill LD, et al. The gastroesophageal flap valve: in vitro and in vivo observations. Gastrointest Endosc. 1996;44(5):541–7.
2. Vakil N, et al. The Montreal definition and classification of gastroesophageal reflux disease: a global evidence-based consensus. Am J Gastroenterol. 2006;101(8):1900–20.
3. Petersen H, et al. Relationship between endoscopic hiatus hernia and gastroesophageal reflux symptoms. Scand J Gastroenterol. 1991;26(9):921–6.
4. Kaul B, et al. Hiatus hernia in gastroesophageal reflux disease. Scand J Gastroenterol. 1986;21(1):31–4.
5. Sontag SJ, et al. The importance of hiatal hernia in reflux esophagitis compared with lower esophageal sphincter pressure or smoking. J Clin Gastroenterol. 1991;13(6):628–43.
6. Berstad A, et al. Relationship of hiatus hernia to reflux oesophagitis. A prospective study of coincidence, using endoscopy. Scand J Gastroenterol. 1986;21(1):55–8.
7. Zagari RM, et al. Gastro-oesophageal reflux symptoms, oesophagitis and Barrett's oesophagus in the general population: the Loiano–Monghidoro study. Gut. 2008;57(10):1354–9.
8. Hyun JJ, et al. Short segment hiatal hernia: is it a clinically significant entity? J Neurogastroenterol Motil. 2010;16(1):35–9.
9. Cameron AJ. Barrett's esophagus: prevalence and size of hiatal hernia. Am J Gastroenterol. 1999;94(8):2054–9.
10. Fein M, et al. Role of the lower esophageal sphincter and hiatal hernia in the pathogenesis of gastroesophageal reflux disease. J Gastrointest Surg. 1999;3(4):405–10.
11. Patti MG, et al. Hiatal hernia size affects lower esophageal sphincter function, esophageal acid exposure, and the degree of mucosal injury. Am J Surg. 1996;171(1):182–6.
12. Loffeld SM, Dackus GM, Loffeld RJ. The long-term follow-up of patients with endoscopically diagnosed reflux oesophagitis with

specific emphasis to complaints. Eur J Gastroenterol Hepatol. 2011;23(12):1122–6.

13. Dickman R, et al. Comparison of clinical characteristics of patients with gastroesophageal reflux disease who failed proton pump inhibitor therapy versus those who fully responded. J Neurogastroenterol Motil. 2011;17(4):387–94.

14. Peng S, et al. High-dose esomeprazole is required for intraesophageal acid control in gastroesophageal reflux disease patients with hiatus hernia. J Gastroenterol Hepatol. 2012;27(5):893–8.

15. Avidan B, et al. Hiatal hernia and acid reflux frequency predict presence and length of Barrett's esophagus. Dig Dis Sci. 2002;47(2):256–64.

16. Chow WH, et al. The relation of gastroesophageal reflux disease and its treatment to adenocarcinomas of the esophagus and gastric cardia. JAMA. 1995;274(6):474–7.

17. Weston AP, Badr AS, Hassanein RS. Prospective multivariate analysis of clinical, endoscopic, and histological factors predictive of the development of Barrett's multifocal high-grade dysplasia or adenocarcinoma. Am J Gastroenterol. 1999;94(12):3413–9.

18. Weston AP, Badr AS, Hassanein RS. Prospective multivariate analysis of factors predictive of complete regression of Barrett's esophagus. Am J Gastroenterol. 1999;94(12):3420–6.

19. Krishnan K, et al. Increased risk for persistent intestinal metaplasia in patients with Barrett's esophagus and uncontrolled reflux exposure before radiofrequency ablation. Gastroenterology. 2012;143(3):576–81.

20. Dodds WJ, et al. Mechanisms of gastroesophageal reflux in patients with reflux esophagitis. N Engl J Med. 1982;307(25):1547–52.

21. Mittal RK, McCallum RW. Characteristics and frequency of transient relaxations of the lower esophageal sphincter in patients with reflux esophagitis. Gastroenterology. 1988;95(3):593–9.

22. Dent J, et al. Mechanisms of lower oesophageal sphincter incompetence in patients with symptomatic gastrooesophageal reflux. Gut. 1988;29(8):1020–8.

23. Kahrilas PJ, et al. Increased frequency of transient lower esophageal sphincter relaxation induced by gastric distention in reflux patients with hiatal hernia. Gastroenterology. 2000;118(4):688–95.

24. van Herwaarden MA, Samsom M, Smout AJ. Excess gastroesophageal reflux in patients with hiatus hernia is caused by mechanisms other than transient LES relaxations. Gastroenterology. 2000;119(6):1439–46.

25. Pandolfino JE, et al. Gastroesophageal junction opening during relaxation distinguishes nonhernia reflux patients, hernia patients, and normal subjects. Gastroenterology. 2003;125(4):1018–24.

26. Roman S, et al. Effects of large hiatal hernias on esophageal peristalsis. Arch Surg. 2012;147(4):352–7.

27. Pandolfino JE, et al. High-resolution manometry of the GEJ: an analysis of crural diaphragm function in GERD. Am J Gastroenterol. 2007;102(5):1056–63.

28. Sloan S, Rademaker AW, Kahrilas PJ. Determinants of gastroesophageal junction incompetence: hiatal hernia, lower esophageal sphincter, or both? Ann Intern Med. 1992;117(12):977–82.

29. Kahrilas PJ, et al. The effect of hiatus hernia on gastro-oesophageal junction pressure. Gut. 1999;44(4):476–82.

30. Mittal RK, Rochester DF, McCallum RW. Electrical and mechanical activity in the human lower esophageal sphincter during diaphragmatic contraction. J Clin Invest. 1988;81(4):1182–9.

31. Mittal RK, Rochester DF, McCallum RW. Sphincteric action of the diaphragm during a relaxed lower esophageal sphincter in humans. Am J Physiol. 1989;256(1 Pt 1):G139–44.

32. Pandolfino JE, et al. Gastroesophageal junction morphology predicts susceptibility to exercise-induced reflux. Am J Gastroenterol. 2004;99(8):1430–6.

33. Pandolfino JE, et al. Gastroesophageal junction distensibility: a factor contributing to sphincter incompetence. Am J Physiol Gastrointest Liver Physiol. 2002;282(6):G1052–8.

34. Kwiatek MA, et al. Gastroesophageal junction distensibility assessed with an endoscopic functional luminal imaging probe (EndoFLIP). Gastrointest Endosc. 2010;72(2):272–8.

35. DeMeester TR, et al. Clinical and in vitro analysis of determinants of gastroesophageal competence. A study of the principles of antireflux surgery. Am J Surg. 1979;137(1):39–46.

36. Mittal RK, Lange RC, McCallum RW. Identification and mechanism of delayed esophageal acid clearance in subjects with hiatus hernia. Gastroenterology. 1987;92(1):130–5.

37. Sloan S, Kahrilas PJ. Impairment of esophageal emptying with hiatal hernia. Gastroenterology. 1991;100(3):596–605.

38. Fletcher J, et al. Unbuffered highly acidic gastric juice exists at the gastroesophageal junction after a meal. Gastroenterology. 2001;121(4):775–83.

39. Beaumont H, et al. The position of the acid pocket as a major risk factor for acidic reflux in healthy subjects and patients with GORD. Gut. 2010;59(4):441–51.

40. Stacher G, et al. Esophageal acid exposure in upright and recumbent postures: roles of lower esophageal sphincter, esophageal contractile and transport function, hiatal hernia, age, sex, and body mass. Dig Dis Sci. 2006;51(11):1896–903.

41. Conrado LM, et al. Is there an association between hiatal hernia and ineffective esophageal motility in patients with gastroesophageal reflux disease? J Gastrointest Surg. 2011;15(10):1756–61.

Christina L. Greene and Steven R. DeMeester

Location, Anatomy, and Embryology of the Lower Esophageal Sphincter

The lower esophageal sphincter (LES) is an area in the distal esophagus that functions to keep gastric juice from refluxing up into the esophagus. It is formed from the primitive gut endoderm and mesoderm during the fourth week of development. As the esophagus elongates and the gastric fundus grows the angle of His and gastroesophageal junction (GEJ) appear. Extensive cadaveric dissections of the distal esophagus by Libermann–Meffert have shown that there is a 3–4 cm segment of circular muscle fibers that condense in the terminal esophagus and that may represent the LES. The "sphincter" action of the LES is believed to be due to these circular esophageal muscles and the intersecting fibers from the lesser and greater curves of the stomach at the level of the GEJ. Clasp fibers come from the lesser curve and go around the terminal esophagus toward the angle of His, while sling fibers from the greater curvature go in the direction of the lesser curvature (Fig. 7.1). Together they produce the sphincter function of the LES. The LES has no clear anatomic boundaries and is not visible endoscopically, by CT scan or by endoscopic ultrasound [1]. Instead, the location and function of the LES is identified by esophageal manometry and to some extent with the newly developed Endoflip device. The Endoflip is an imaging catheter that uses impedance planimetry to provide a real-time 3-D graphical display of luminal distensibility within the gastrointestinal tract (Fig. 7.2). On esophageal manometry the LES is defined distally as the site where there is an increase in pressure over gastric baseline that persists until there is a sudden drop to below gastric baseline, representing the negative pressure of the intra-

thoracic esophagus and the proximal extent of the LES (Fig. 7.3). Three important characteristics of the LES can be defined with motility: total LES length, intra-abdominal length, and resting pressure.

Evaluation

The classic method to evaluate the LES is with stationary manometry using a slow motorized pull-through technique. With this technique all three critical components of the LES can be evaluated. These components interact and are codependent to maintain the competency of the LES. On stationary manometry a structurally defective valve is defined as one with a resting pressure below 6 mmHg, an overall length less than 2 cm, or an intra-abdominal length less than 1 cm [2] (Table 7.1).

An abnormal value for any component can make the valve incompetent, and the likelihood of an incompetent valve increases when more than one component is abnormal [3]. Failure of these three interdependent factors to maintain an adequate resistance at the LES leads to free reflux of gastric juice into the esophagus.

Competency of the LES is a function of pressure and length. Low resting pressure is the most common abnormality reported by most laboratories. However if careful attention is paid to length, the most common abnormality of the LES is actually a short intra-abdominal length. The abdominal length of the LES is critical because studies have shown that below a minimum abdominal length of 1 cm there is essentially no pressure that will allow the LES to remain competent [4]. Using a specially designed catheter and a three-dimensional computer construct, LES resistance can be represented as a volume diagram. This is called the "Sphincter Pressure Vector Volume" (SPVV) and a calculated volume of less than the fifth percentile of normal indicates a defective LES [5] (Fig. 7.4).

High-resolution manometry has become widely accepted for the evaluation of the esophageal body and

C.L. Greene, MD • S.R. DeMeester, MD (✉)
Department of Surgery, Keck School of Medicine of the University of Southern California, 1510 San Pablo Street, Suite 514, Los Angeles, CA 90033, USA
e-mail: Christina.Greene@med.usc.edu;
Steven.DeMeester@med.usc.edu

L.L. Swanstrom and C.M. Dunst (eds.), *Antireflux Surgery*,
DOI 10.1007/978-1-4939-1749-5_7, © Springer New York 2015

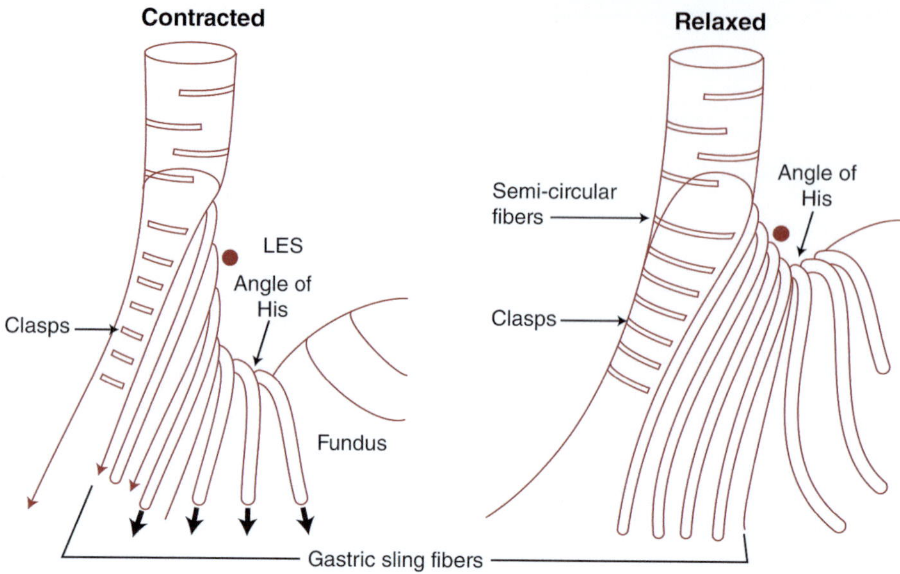

Fig. 7.1 The clasp and sling muscle fibers that make up the lower esophageal reflux barrier in the contracted and relaxed state

Fig. 7.2 The EndoFlip (Crospon, Cork, Ireland) is a physiology measuring tool that uses impedance planimetry to present a 3 dimensional "map" of the LES

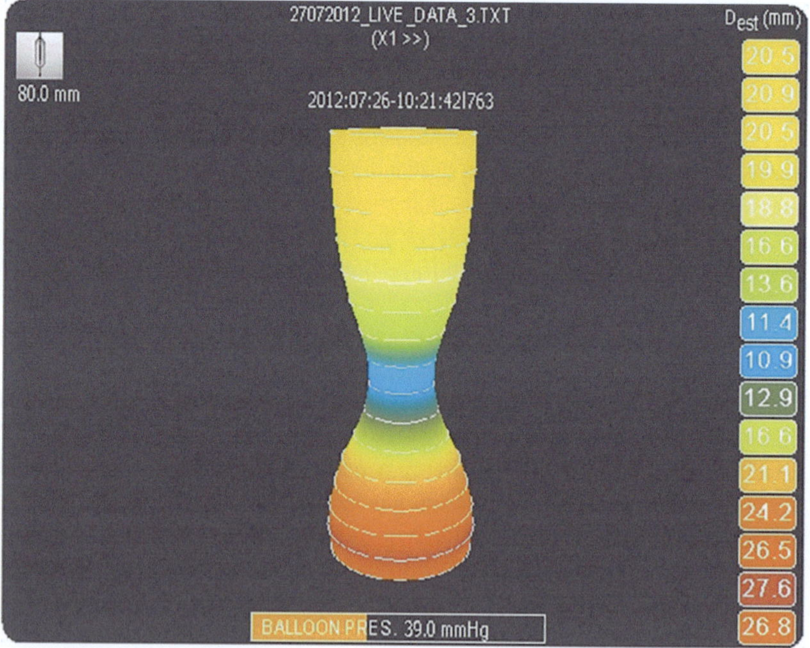

has replaced water perfusion methods. Unfortunately, while it has enhanced many aspects of esophageal manometry, it is unable to give an accurate portrayal of the length of the LES, and as such a detailed understanding of the LES is not possible. This deficit is being addressed with new technology, entitled high-definition manometry. This technology will once again allow detailed assessment of the length and vector volume of the LES. Other tests that are useful for esophageal evaluation offer limited insights into the LES, including upper endoscopy, CT scans, and barium esophagrams.

Function

The purpose of the LES is to maintain a barrier between the acid-sensitive esophageal squamous mucosa and the acid-secreting gastric mucosa. Without this barrier gastric contents would follow the natural pressure gradient from the positive pressure environment of the abdomen towards the negative pressure of the intra-thoracic esophagus. In its resting state, the LES maintains a pressure of 13–43 mmHg, and given that a portion of the sphincter is within the

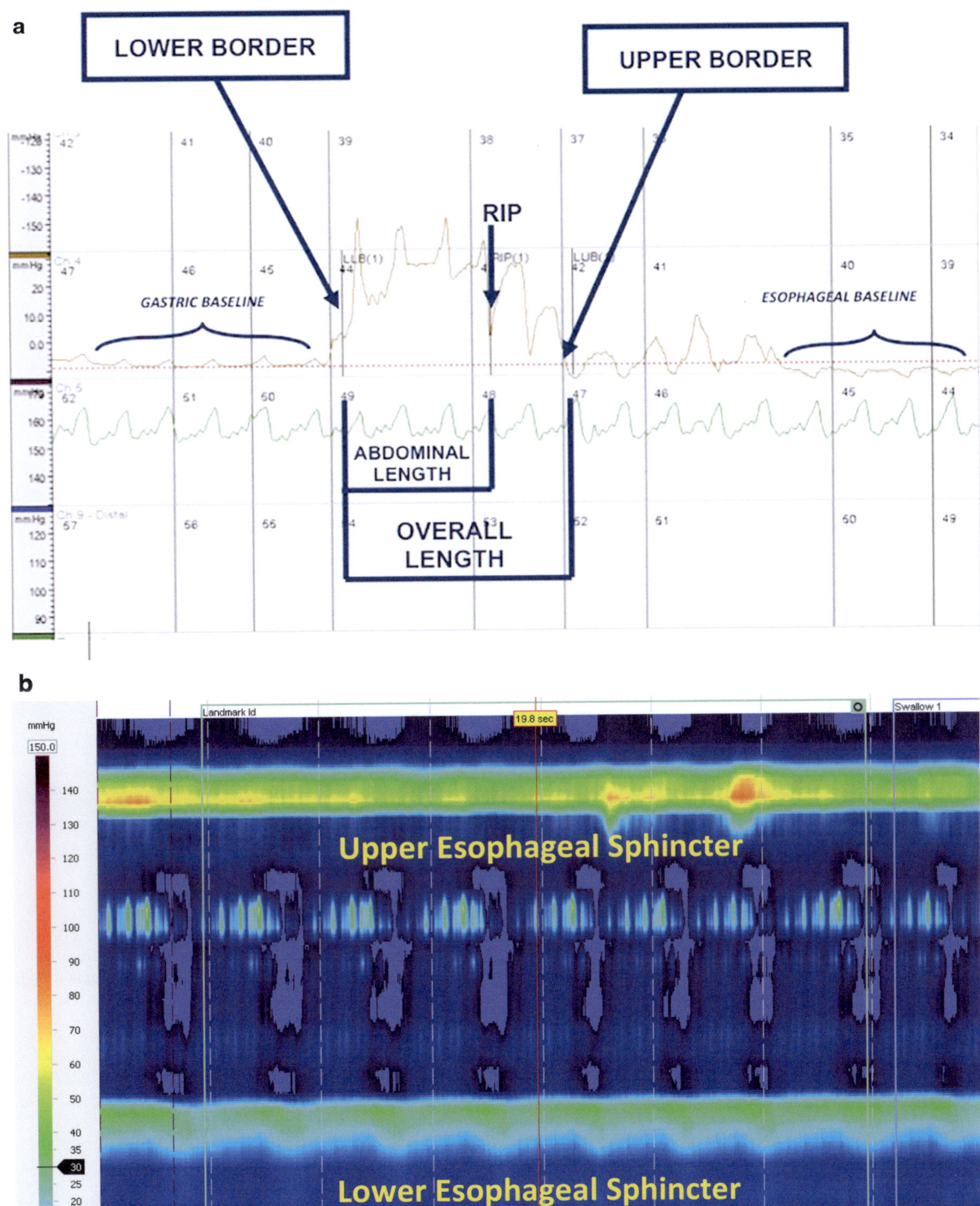

Fig. 7.3 Typical stationary (**a**) and high-resolution (**b**) manometric depictions of the LES. In the tracing from the stationary motility study (**a**) the catheter is drawn back in 1 cm increments every 15 s allowing each of the eight channels to pass through the LES. A persistent 2 mmHg rise in pressure above gastric baseline marks the distal border of the sphincter while the drop below gastric baseline marks the top of the sphincter. The LES straddles the hiatus such that the lower portion is in the abdomen and exposed to intra-abdominal pressures, while the upper portion is in the negative pressure environment of the thorax. The distinction is made on a motility study by the site of the respiratory inversion point, which is the location where the positive deflections associated with respirations become negative. Below the RIP is the abdominal length of the LES, and above represents the intra-thoracic portion of the LES. In the HRM Clouse plot (**b**) a 36-channel solid state catheter with 12 pressure sensors in each channel is inserted through the nose. The upper and lower esophageal sphincters and esophageal body peristalsis are evaluated during a swallow of 15 cc of water. Pressure is denoted by *color on the left*. In this image the esophagus is at rest. The upper esophageal sphincter is indicated by the high-pressure band on the top of the image opens while the lower band of pressure is the lower esophageal sphincter

Table 7.1 Normal manometric parameters of the LES

	Low normal	High normal
Length	2 cm	4 cm
Resting pressure	6 mmHg	35 mmHg
Relaxing nadir pressure	NA	10 mmHg
Position	<1 cm intra-abdominal length	NA

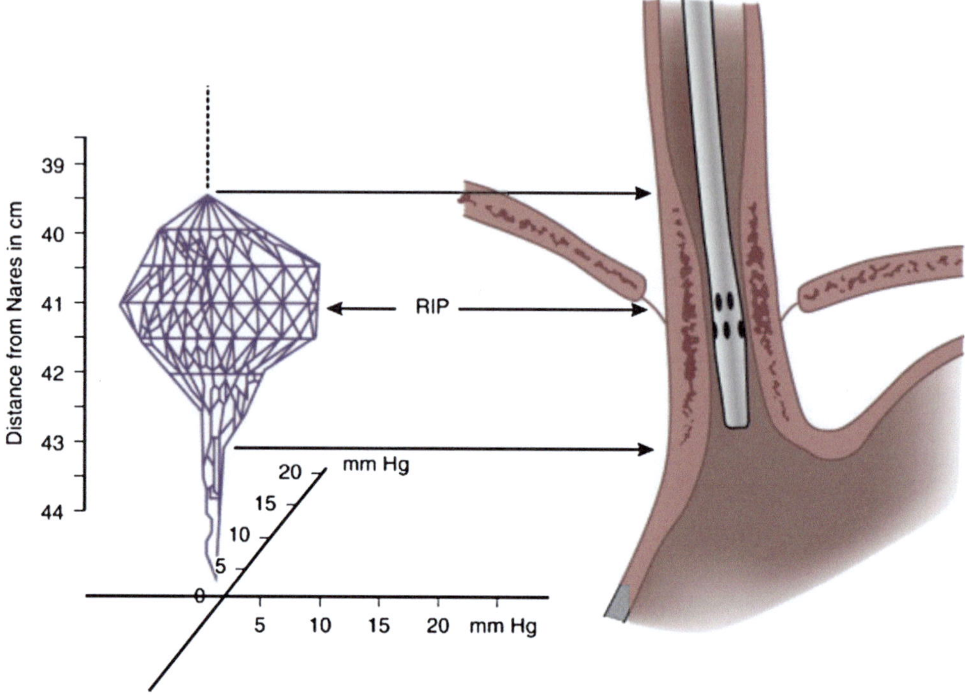

Fig. 7.4 The Sphincter Pressure Vector Volume (SPVV) is a 3-D image of the LES obtained by pulling a catheter through the gastroesophageal junction. At each level of pullback the pressure is measured radially around the catheter and plotted against the gastric baseline creating for a volume diagram of LES resistance. With permission from Stein HJ, DeMeester TR, Naspetti R, et al. Three-dimensional imaging of the lower esophageal sphincter in gastroesophageal reflux disease. Ann Surg. 1991;214:374

abdomen it can compensate for sudden increases in intra-abdominal pressure that occur with straining, coughing, or bending over. In addition to maintaining a barrier, the LES must also relax to allow a bolus of food or liquid to enter the stomach, and to allow gas and sometimes gastric contents to vent upwards as a belch or as emesis when necessary. The tonic resting pressure of the normal LES and deglutitive lower esophageal sphincter relaxation (DLESR) with a swallow is nicely seen with high-resolution esophageal manometry (Fig. 7.5). At the start of a swallow, the UES opens to allow a bolus to move from the pharynx into the cervical esophagus. Tactile stimulation of the striated muscle of the pharynx stimulates the vagus nerve, which in turn stimulates the LES to relax. Relaxation of the LES should coincide with UES opening and persist until the bolus passes through into the stomach. Once the bolus passes through the LES there is a post-relaxation contraction after which the LES returns to its basal resting pressure. From start to finish the entire LES relaxation usually lasts about 8–10 s.

In addition to relaxation initiated by a swallow, the LES can also relax to vent the stomach. The term transient LES relaxation (TLESR) was coined by Dent and Dodds in 1980. Originally believed to be a neurologic phenomenon, newer theories favor a mechanical cause. The neurologic theory states that TLESRS are the result of vagally induced relaxation, much like DLESRS. The mechanical theory proposes that gastric distention increases wall tension thus pulling and flattening the GEJ, effectively effacing the sphincter. Once the LES is effaced below a critical length it loses competence and opens.

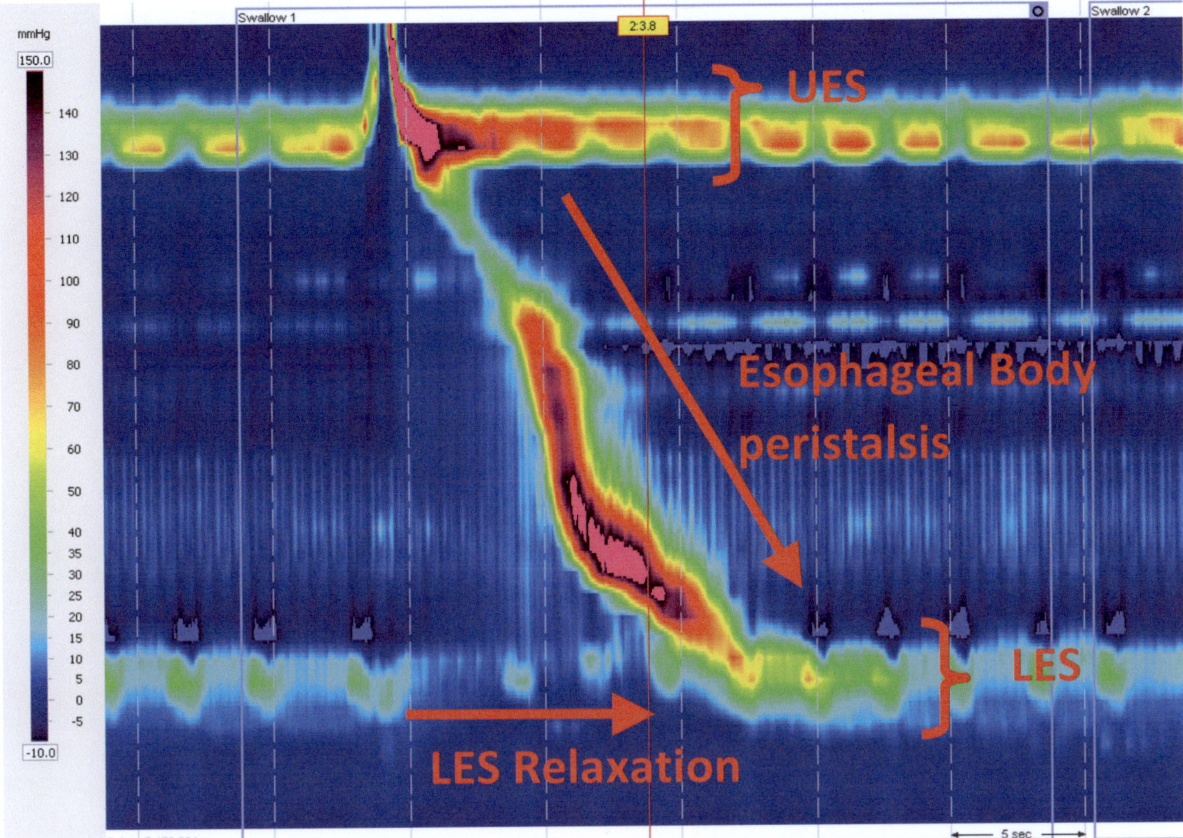

Fig. 7.5 Normal HRM swallow with appropriate relaxation is seen. Upper esophageal sphincter (UES) opening is followed by a progressive peristaltic esophageal wave with a corresponding opening of the lower esophageal sphincter (LES). The opening of the LES indicates relaxation of the sphincter and the LES returns to resting pressure after the swallow

The Role of the Diaphragmatic Crura

The diaphragmatic crura play a role in maintaining the barrier between the stomach and the esophagus. Crural augmentation of LES pressure has been shown to aid in competency of the LES. Martin et al. [6] showed in dogs that partial diaphragmatic relaxation is a necessary event for reflux to occur. During inspiration, when the chest cavity becomes most negative in pressure, the crura tighten and augment the sphincter. When a hiatal hernia is present the crura are no longer aligned with the LES and the risk of reflux is increased. During a swallow respiration is inhibited and the crura are open along with the LES, but any refluxed material is pushed into the stomach along with the bolus.

Lastly, the geometry of the angle of His also contributes to the function of the LES. In an elegant cadaver experiment Marchand showed that the pressure necessary to induce regurgitation was increased by 50 % when the left leaf of the diaphragm was removed and the fundus was allowed to bulge upwards into the left chest, thereby accentuating the angle of His. Decreasing or accentuating the angle of His made it harder for reflux to occur. In contrast, when the liver and right diaphragm were removed the angle of His was splayed out or increased and it was easier to induce reflux [7].

LES Dysfunction

Dysfunction of the LES occurs in two forms. The first and most common is loss of competence with increased esophageal exposure to refluxed gastric juice. The second less common form of dysfunction is when the LES fails to relax.

Loss of Competence

Most gastroesophageal reflux events occur in the daytime after a meal. As the stomach distends with a meal the LES is effaced and the abdominal length shortens [8]. An adequate intra-abdominal length is critical for the LES to remain competent and to accommodate to changes in intra-abdominal pressure. Gastric distension with a large meal effaces the lowermost portion of the LES, exposes this area to gastric

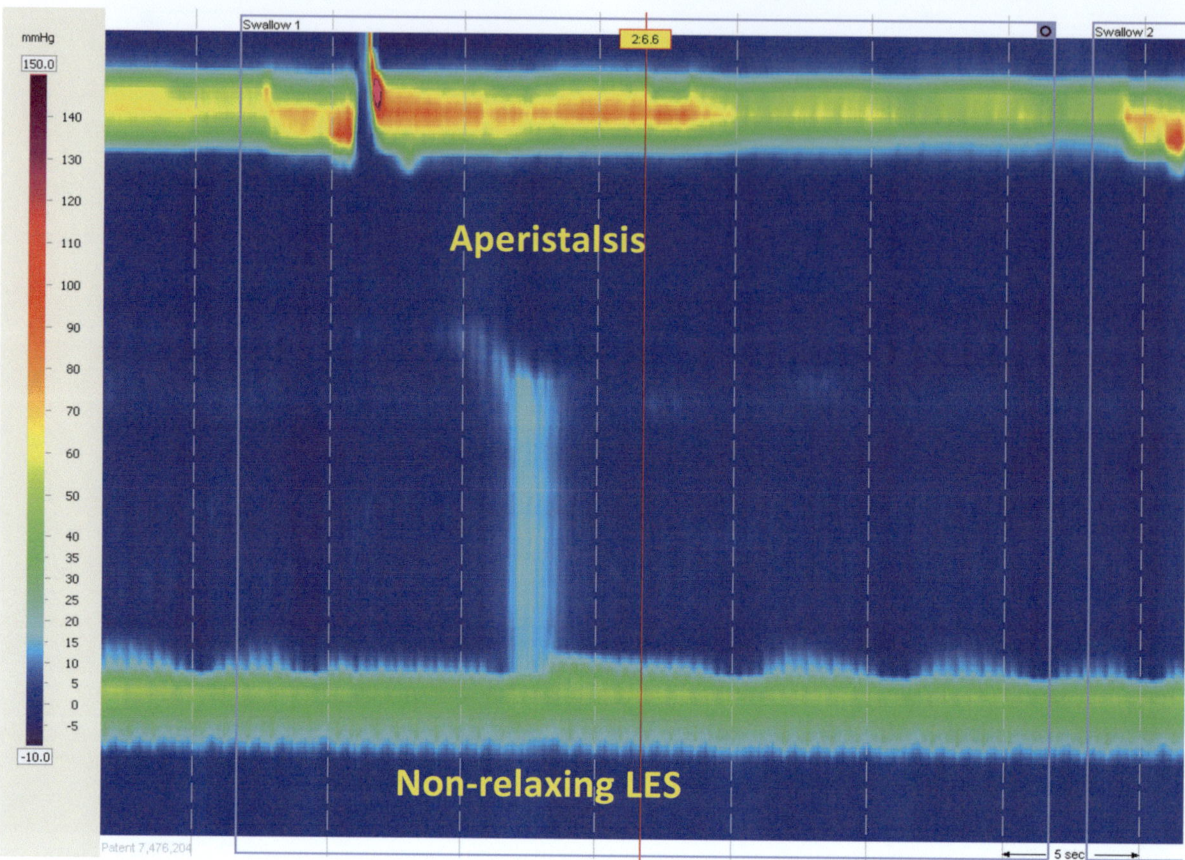

Fig. 7.6 This HRM Clouse plot is an example of classic achalasia characterized by an incompletely relaxing LES with esophageal body aperistalsis

juice, and over time leads to loss of function of this portion of the sphincter. It is likely that this gradual loss of intra-abdominal sphincter length is what ultimately leads to free gastroesophageal reflux in many patients.

In light of the fact that sphincter competence is mostly a function of length and pressure, efforts to restore competency can be aimed at pressure, length, or both. A fundoplication restores both length and pressure, while devices such as the LINX Reflux® management system (Torax®Medical Inc.) focus on restoring length and the EndoStim® (St. Louis, MO) focuses on restoring pressure [9, 10].

Failure to Relax

Dysfunction of the LES can also occur as a consequence of failure of the LES to relax. The most well described condition where this occurs is achalasia. Symptoms in these patients are related to impaired esophageal emptying rather than reflux of gastric juice back into the esophagus and include dysphagia for both solids and liquids and often regurgitation of bland material. Classically, the hallmark and necessary conventional manometric findings in achalasia

have been an incompletely relaxing LES and esophageal body aperistalsis (Fig. 7.6). With the advent of HRM, new variations of achalasia have been identified. Carlson and Pandolfino sub-classified achalasia into three types based on the function of the esophageal body. Type I Achalasia is characterized by aperistalsis and is consistent with the classic definition from stationary motility. Type II Achalasia has panesophageal pressurization in greater than 20 % of the swallows and Type III Achalasia is characterized by spastic contractions and pre-mature contractions in greater than 20 % of swallows without normal peristalsis. In each sub-class the LES fails to relax [11]. Although GERD and achalasia are opposite ends of the spectrum of LES dysfunction, the symptoms may be similar enough to lead to confusion in the diagnosis, and commonly patients with achalasia are treated with acid-suppression medications for some time before the true diagnosis is established.

Achalasia must be differentiated from pseudo-achalasia. Pseudo-achalasia shares many clinical features with achalasia, but is caused by a tumor of the gastric cardia. Another condition with some similarities to achalasia is Hypertensive LES. In this condition there is a high resting pressure in the LES with incomplete relaxation, but in contrast to achalasia

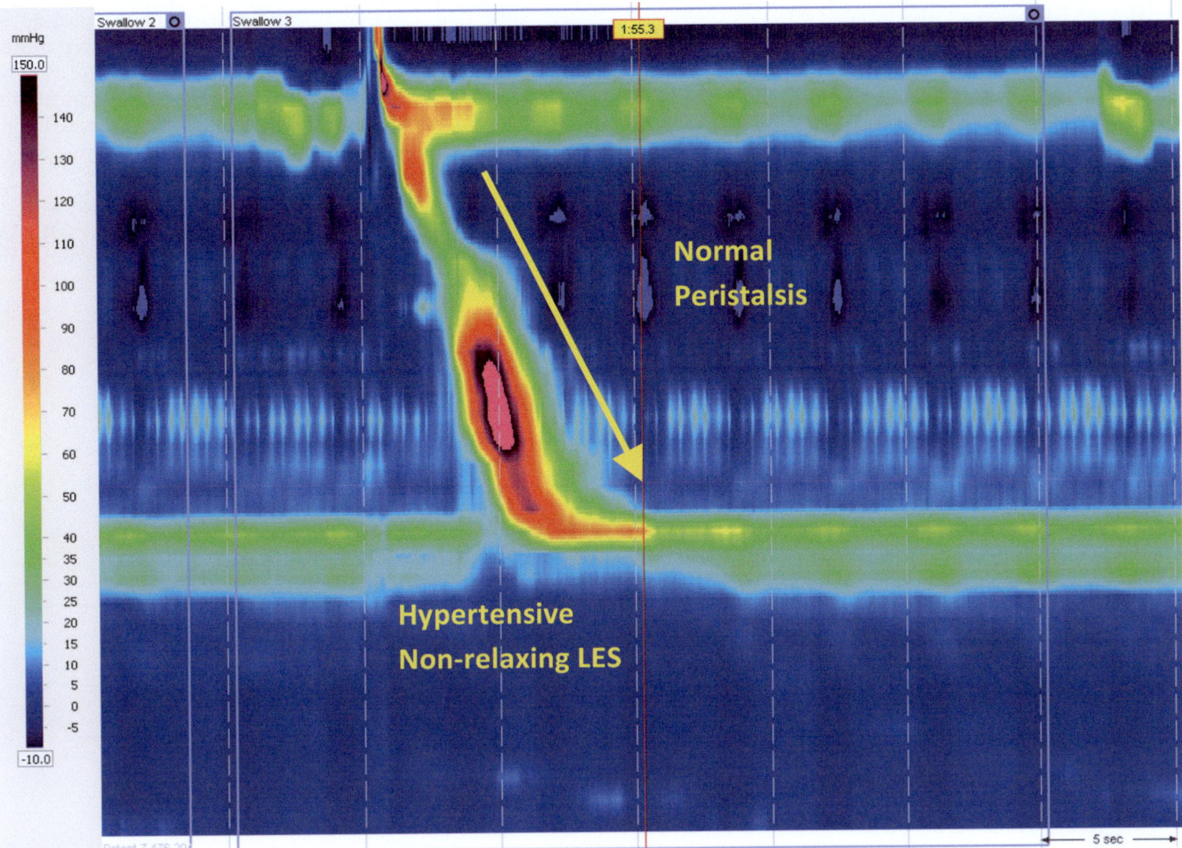

Fig. 7.7 This HRM Clouse plot shows a hypertensive non-relaxing LES with a normal peristalsis of the esophagus. After the UES opens there is no corresponding relaxation of the LES

where there is absence of peristalsis in the esophageal body, with hypertensive LES the esophageal body function is normal (Fig. 7.7). The role of manometry and careful esophageal testing to establish a firm diagnosis in patients being evaluated for esophageal symptoms cannot be over-emphasized.

In patients with impaired relaxation of the LES, treatment is aimed at improving esophageal emptying. The function of the valve cannot be restored, but by opening the LES with balloon dilatation or laparoscopic or endoscopic myotomy the symptoms of dysphagia can be dramatically improved. A drawback to opening the LES is that this can allow GERD to develop, and the efficacy of these procedures at relieving the esophageal outflow obstruction must be balanced with the long-term risk for GERD in these patients.

augmented by the crural diaphragm and the angle of His. The most common form of dysfunction is related to gastroesophageal reflux which occurs as a consequence of loss of competency of the LES, often in combination with a hiatal hernia. Competency of the LES is dependent upon the length of the valve and the resting pressure, and the most common initial change with reflux is loss of abdominal length. Failure of the LES to relax leads to impaired esophageal emptying and the symptoms of dysphagia and regurgitation of food and liquids that never reached the stomach. Treatment for GERD is augmentation of LES length, pressure, or both, while treatment for achalasia requires opening of the LES to relieve the outflow obstruction.

Conclusion

In conclusion, the LES is a remarkable physiologic structure that is designed to protect the acid-sensitive esophageal squamous mucosa from the reflux of gastric juice, yet also open to allow a swallowed bolus to enter the stomach or air to escape as a belch. The barrier function of the LES is

References

1. Libermann-Meffert D, et al. Gastroenterology. 1979;76(1):31–8.
2. Zaninotto G, et al. Am J Surg. 1988;155(1):104–11.
3. Bonavina L, Evander A, DeMeester TR, et al. Length of the distal esophageal sphincter and competency of the cardia. Am J Surg. 1986;151(1):25–34.
4. DeMeester TR, Johnson WE. Outcome of respiratory symptoms after surgical treatment of swallowing disorders. Semin Respir Crit Care Med. 1995;16:514.

5. Stein HJ, et al. Ann Surg. 1991;214(4):374–84.
6. Martin CJ, et al. Diaphragmatic contributions to the gastroesophageal competence and reflux in dogs. Am J Physiol. 1992;263 (1):G551–7.
7. Marchand P. The gastro-oesophageal 'Sphincter' and the mechanism of regurgitation. Br J Surg. 1955;42:504–13.
8. Mason RJ, et al. Nissen fundoplication prevents shortening of the sphincter during gastric distention. Arch Surg. 1997;132(7): 719–24.
9. Ganz RA, Peters JH, Horgan S, et al. Esophageal sphincter device for gastroesophageal reflux disease. N Engl J Med. 2013; 368(8):719–27.
10. Rodriguez L, Rodriguez P, Gomez B, et al. Electrical Stimulation therapy of the lower esophageal sphincter is successful in treating GERD: final results of open-label prospective trial. Surg Endosc. 2013;27(4):1084–92.
11. Carlson D, Pandolfino J. High-resolution manometry and esophageal pressure topography. Gastroenterol Clin North Am. 2013;42:1–15.

Preoperative Evaluation and Testing for GERD

Joerg Zehetner and John C. Lipham

Introduction

Symptoms alone are not a reliable indicator for the presence or persistence of troublesome reflux. A comprehensive diagnostic foregut evaluation, in addition to standard history and physical and selective cardiopulmonary evaluation, is imperative when considering surgical therapy for reflux to ensure that the patient is an appropriate candidate and to help to choose the best surgical therapy. Preoperative evaluation should focus on specific anatomic and functional details that might impact technical surgical decision making such as the presence of hiatal hernias, motility disorders, diverticulum, or esophageal mucosal problems. The key components of mandatory preoperative testing for anti-reflux surgery are discussed below.

Videoesophagram

This test is usually the first test for the preoperative evaluation of GERD. It informs the physician or surgeon about the anatomy of the esophagus, providing a roadmap for further diagnostic testing like endoscopy and pH monitoring. Further, it helps to rule out with a high sensitivity achalasia (94 %) and scleroderma (100 %) [1].

The act of swallowing as a dynamic process cannot be assessed with static images; therefore all studies should be saved as a video recording on a compact disc, DVD, or hard

J. Zehetner, MD, MMM
Department of Surgery, Keck Medical Center, Keck School of Medicine of USC, 1510 San Pablo Street, Suite 514, Los Angeles, CA 90033, USA
e-mail: joerg.zehetner@surgery.usc.edu

J.C. Lipham, MD (✉)
Division of Upper GI and General Surgery, Department of Surgery, Keck Medical Center of USC, 1510 San Pablo St., Los Angeles, CA 90033, USA
e-mail: lipham@surgery.usc.edu

drive. The overall sensitivity for detecting esophageal disorders by videoesophagram (VEG) is 55 %. A VEG is sensitive for achalasia and scleroderma, but relatively insensitive for detecting non-specific motility disorders [2].

The VEG can also show obstruction, narrowing or delay in passage of the contrast (either gastrografin or barium), bolus separation, primary and secondary peristalsis, tertiary contraction, stasis and assessment of clearance. Further, with the VEG a crico-pharyngeal bar, esophageal web, esophageal diverticula, and a hiatal hernia can be detected which may not be evident on endoscopy alone. The videoesophagram is therefore recommended as the first test in any patient who presents with dysphagia, as well as any patient with the diagnosis of GERD undergoing preoperative work-up.

Unfortunately, videoesophagram is extremely dependent on the quality and dedication of the radiology department and therefore a quality exam may be difficult to obtain in some centers. In such instances, a standard barium esophagram should be performed in all patients with atypical symptoms including chronic cough, halitosis, sore throat, and recurrent pneumonia to rule out anatomic abnormalities that can be missed with other tests such as diverticulum, proximal reflux, and aspiration. Furthermore, esophageal length and hiatal hernia reduction can still be estimated which aids in proper preoperative planning.

Analysis of the VEG

The pharynx and the upper esophageal sphincter are evaluated in the upright position, and timing and coordination of the events of pharyngeal transit are assessed: the oropharyngeal bolus transport, pharyngeal contraction, opening of the pharyngoesophageal segment, and the degree of airway protection during swallowing. Anatomical findings as earlier described can be appreciated early in the VEG. The assessment of peristalsis often adds to or complements the information obtained by esophageal manometry. Esophageal motility is best assessed with the VEG by observing 5 individual swallows of barium with the patient in both the upright and supine positions. Further, after

L.L. Swanstrom and C.M. Dunst (eds.), *Antireflux Surgery*,
DOI 10.1007/978-1-4939-1749-5_8, © Springer New York 2015

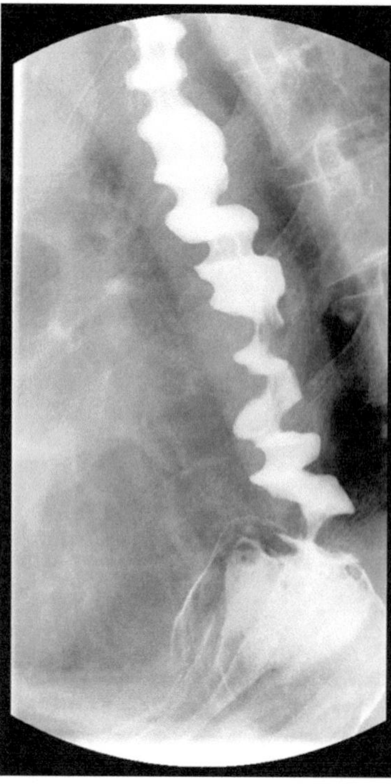

Fig. 8.1 Barium swallow radiographs can be the first indication of an esophageal motility disorder as seen here in this classic corkscrew appearance of diffuse esophageal spasm

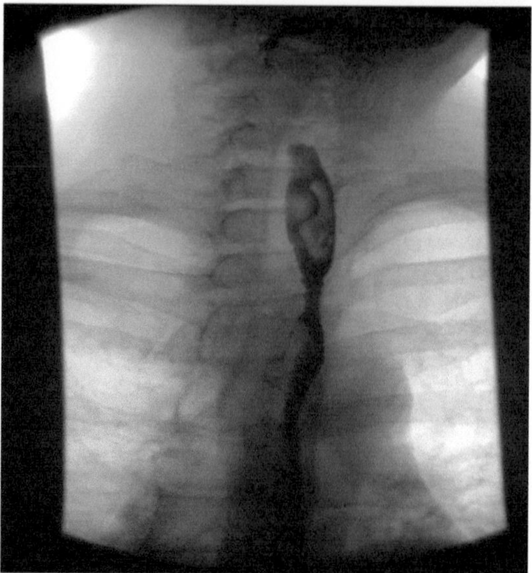

Fig. 8.2 Barium esophagram demonstrating a mod-esophageal stricture as a cause for dysphagia

testing the motility with liquid bolus material, there should be at least 2 swallows recorded and analyzed with solid bolus material like a barium hamburger. In a patient with normal swallowing, a primary peristaltic wave is generated that completely strips the bolus out of the esophagus into the stomach. Residual material rarely stimulates a secondary peristaltic wave; rather an additional pharyngeal swallow is usually required.

Normal subjects in the prone position can clear at least 3 out of 5 10 cc liquid barium boluses with 1 swallow and have only 1 episode of proximal escape or distal retention of a barium bolus with the 5 swallows. Further, normal subjects can clear a solid barium bolus with 4 or more swallows in the upright position. Motility disorders with disorganized or simultaneous esophageal contraction give a segmented appearance to the barium column (Fig. 8.1).

Hiatal or Paraesophageal Hernia

The assessment of a hiatal hernia is best done with the patient in prone position: the increased intraabdominal pressure produced in this position promotes displacement of the hernia above the diaphragm. It is a very important component of the preoperative surgical planning to understand the size and configuration of the hernia. A large hernia (>5 cm) or irreducible hiatal hernia may suggest a shortening of the esophagus, which could require an esophageal lengthening procedure (e.g., Collis gastroplasty) during the surgical

repair. Reflux is not seen easily on VEG, and only rarely in patients with classic symptoms of GERD does the radiologist observe spontaneous reflux. If other pathology is suspected, a full-column technique with distension of the esophageal wall can rule out extrinsic compression of the esophagus, and a fully distended esophagogastric region is necessary to identify narrowing from a ring, stricture, or obstructing lesion (Fig. 8.2).

Therefore, the videoesophagram is the first diagnostic and preoperative test in patients with GERD or the suspicion of GERD, and gives the first understanding of the anatomical and functional deficits of the patients underlying disease.

Esophagogastroduodenoscopy (EGD) and Biopsy Protocol

Endoscopic evaluation is a necessary part of the preoperative evaluation for anti-reflux surgery. The endoscopy can help to better understand several symptoms such as dysphagia, odynophagia, aspiration, unexplained laryngeal symptoms, unexplained chronic cough, or asthma. Other diseases can also be ruled out or diagnosed like peptic ulcer disease, gastritis, esophageal, and gastric cancer. However, the role of endoscopy in preoperative planning differs from standard esophagogastroduodenoscopy in that it should focus on anatomic details important in surgical decision making—a task most often best performed by the surgeon. Ideally, the contrast study should be performed prior to the endoscopy in order to provide a roadmap of the esophagus, and to direct attention to concerning areas, such as diverticula, ulcers, or possible cancer.

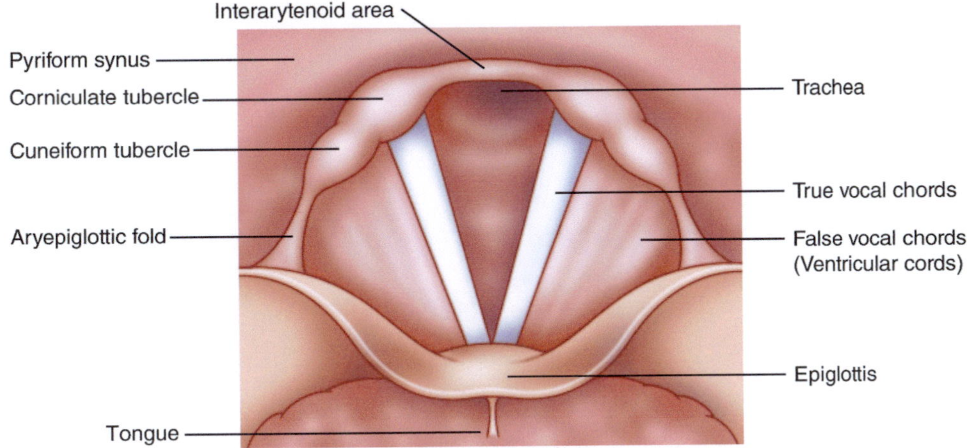

Fig. 8.3 Endoscopic view of the vocal cords

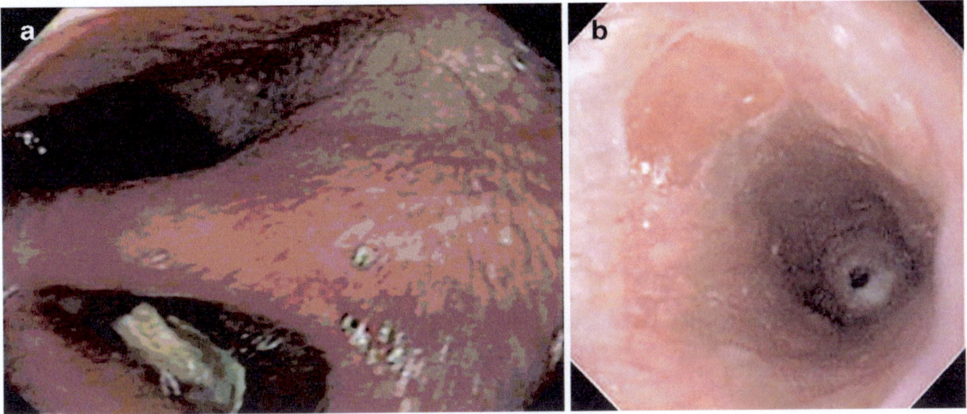

Fig. 8.4 Proximal esophageal findings that are often missed but have important relations to reflux. a Zenker's diverticulum, b gastric inlet patch

Performing a Pre-surgical EGD

After an appropriate fast, endoscopic evaluation of the esophagus starts with a careful view of the vocal cords and aryepiglottic folds (Fig. 8.3). The position of the crico-pharyngeal sphincter is best assessed on final withdrawal of the endoscope and is noted by an encroachment on the lumen as the scope is withdrawn. It is important to carefully view the entire esophagus as proximal findings are often missed (Zenker's diverticulum, gastric inlet patch, etc.) (Fig. 8.4 a, b). The presence of retained food in the esophagus or stomach is abnormal. The gastroesophageal junction is defined by where the gastric folds meet the tubular esophagus. Observations such as retained food or saliva, strictures, rings, webs, candidiasis and esophagitis are particularly relevant for patients with dysphagia and should be documented (Fig. 8.5 a–e).

On entering the stomach the gastric mucosa is carefully inspected, and the scope further advanced into the duodenal bulb and second part of the duodenum to exclude other pathology. When the endoscope is retracted back into the stomach, it is retroflexed to give a view of the gastroesophageal junction. The stomach is insufflated to assess the competency of the sphincter and to grade the gastroesophageal flap valve, or musculomucosal fold at the Angle of His, according to Hill's grading [3] (Fig. 8.6). The presence of an axial hiatal or paraesophageal hernia can be appreciated and measured which may alert the surgeon to the potential of a foreshortened esophagus. Signs of relative ischemia or mucosal damage such as Cameron's Ulcer's within the hernia should be noted (Fig. 8.7). Further, the locations of the diaphragmatic crura, the gastroesophageal junction, and squamocolumnar junction are measured and documented. The mucosa on the lesser and greater curvatures and the anterior and posterior aspect of the stomach are systematically and carefully inspected for any abnormalities. The stomach is deflated before the instrument is retracted for a final viewing of the esophagus.

Careful scrutiny of the esophageal mucosa and obligatory biopsies constitute the final segment of the endoscopic examination. A minimum of 2 biopsies in the antrum (for diagnosis of Helicobacter pylori) and 4 biopsies at the

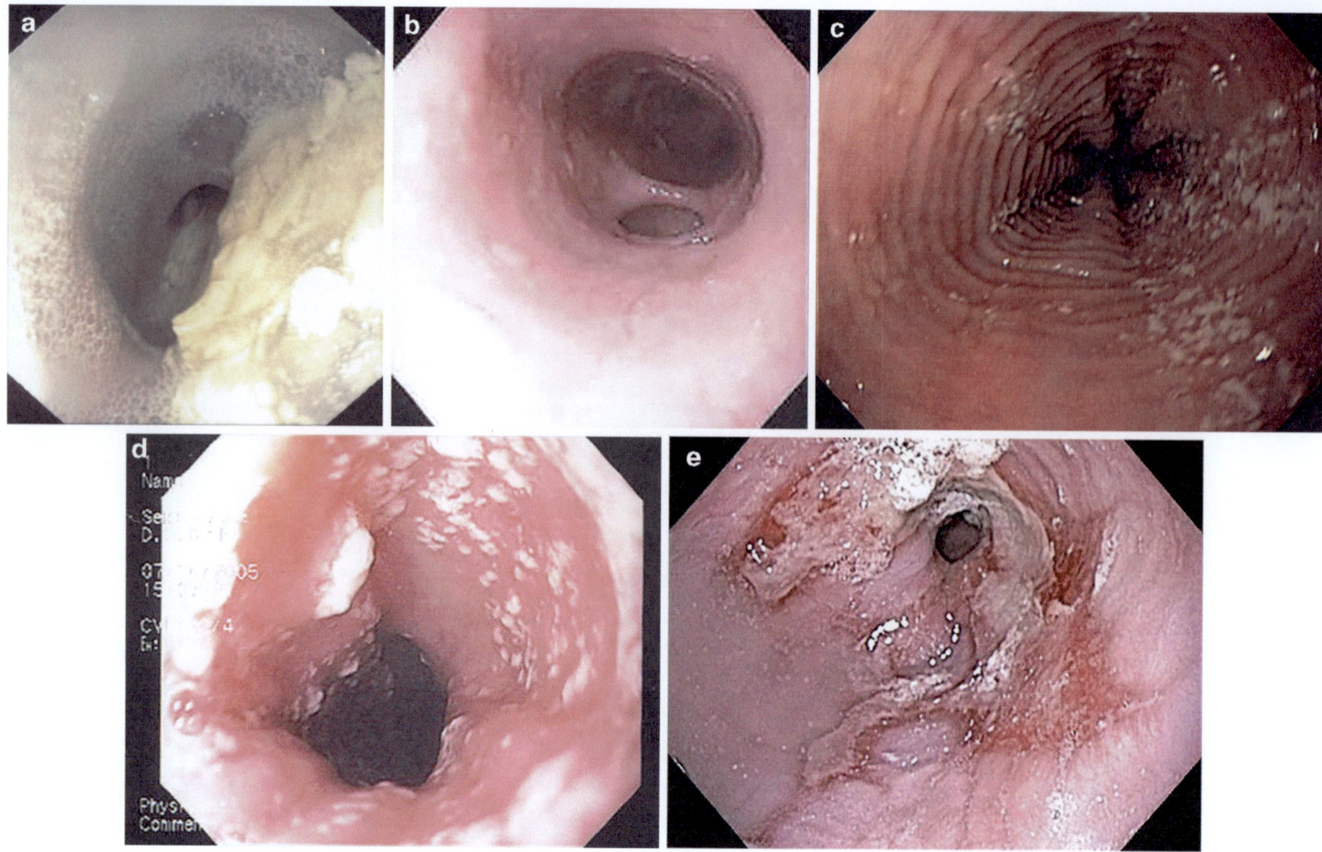

Fig. 8.5 Relevant esophageal pathologies seen on upper endoscopy: retained food (**a**) esophageal diverticulum (**b**), ringed mucosal appearance of eosinophilic esophagitis (**c**), candidiasis (**d**), severe erosive esophagitis with distal stricture (**e**)

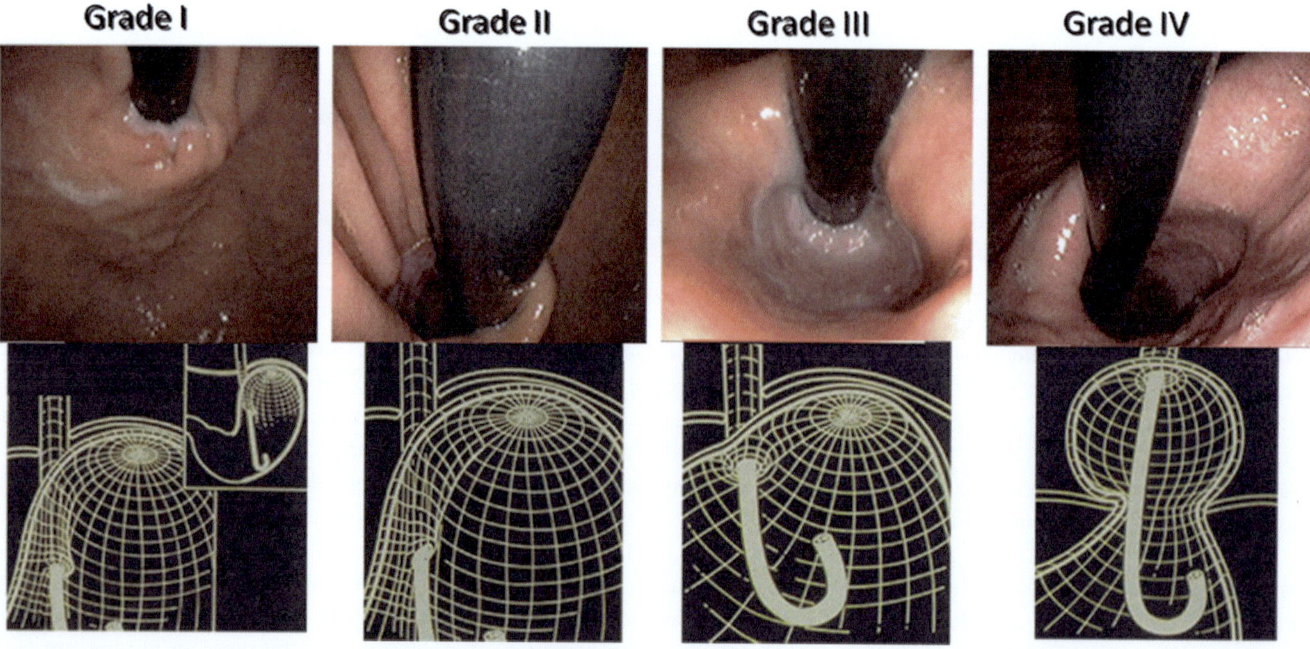

Fig. 8.6 Gastroesophageal flap valve grading according to Hill

squamocolumnar junction are mandatory. Discrepancy between the location of the squamocolumnar junction (SCJ) and the gastroesophageal junction (defined as the top of the rugal folds) indicates the presence of columnar lined metaplasia. Examination, under both white light and narrow band imaging (or equivalent), can help define subtle differences and is especially helpful in evaluating Barrett's (Fig. 8.8). Biopsies at the SCJ are required to confirm or refute the presence of intestinal metaplasia (Barrett's Esophagus) even if there is no measurable segment of columnar lined esophagus. If there is more that 1 cm difference between the SCJ and the GEJ, standard Barrett's surveillance biopsies should be taken in 4 quadrants starting in the retroflex view of the gastro-esophageal junction and the esophagus every 1–2 cm until the normal squamous mucosa is reached. It is important to obtain these biopsies prior to anti-reflux surgery because the surgery will alter the anatomy at the GEJ and may make it more difficult to evaluate in the future. Any suspicious areas should also be biopsied. In case of suspicion of candida esophagitis or eosinophilic esophagitis, biopsies of the more proximal esophagus are recommended.

Endoscopy is truly the essential part in the preoperative work-up in patients with GERD, as it can assess esophageal and gastric anatomy, function, and obtain histology in form of multiple biopsies.

Esophageal Function Testing

To determine if a surgical approach is appropriate, and, if so, which one, the surgeon depends upon the expertise of the esophageal function laboratory to provide esophageal manometry (conventional or high-resolution with impedance), esophageal pH monitoring, and multichannel intraluminal impedance testing.

The surgeon who treats benign esophageal diseases has a different mindset than the surgeon who merely excises the organ because it harbors a malignancy or is otherwise destroyed by disease. The former has to improve the function of the esophagus without removing it. Success in restoring function depends upon correct analysis of the underlying pathophysiology. The principal tool to aid the surgeon in this analysis is esophageal manometry. Manometry is critical in order to rule out achalasia or other motility disturbances (such as IEM, non-relaxing LES, or esophageal spasm) which may predispose to dysphagia after surgery.

Conventional esophageal manometry has undergone very few changes in conduct or interpretation since the 1960s. However, in the past few years, several newer methods of

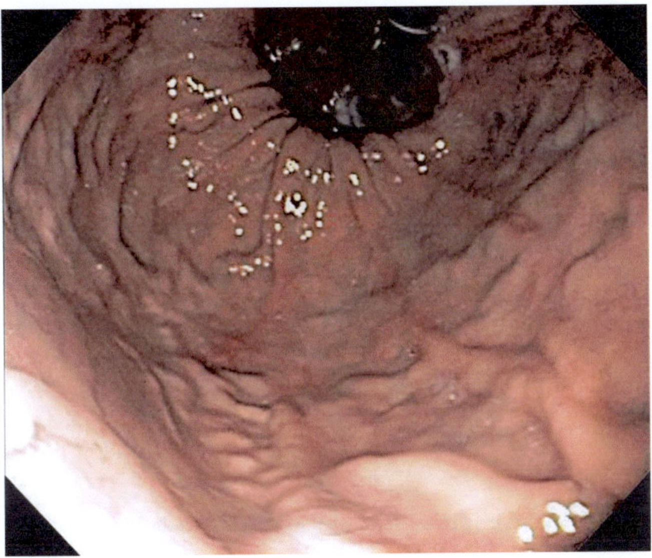

Fig. 8.7 Cameron's ulcers are often seen in large hiatal hernias. Note the linear gastritis and ulceration at the hiatal brim

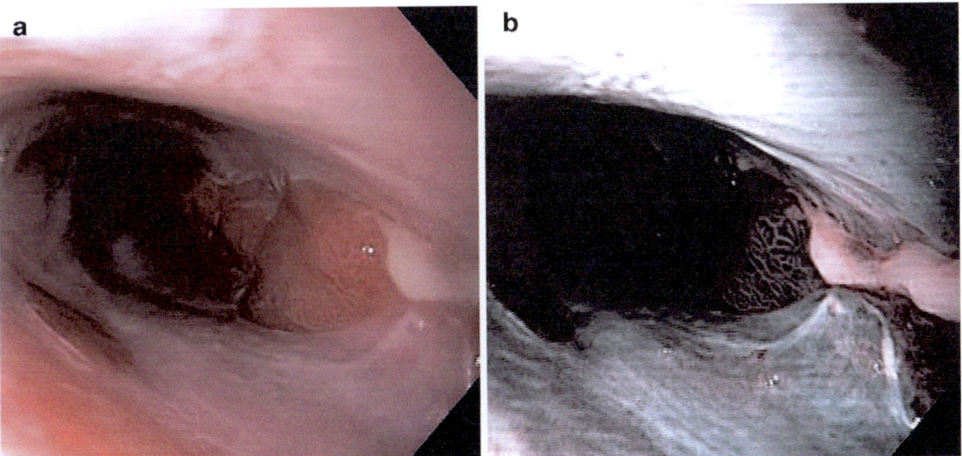

Fig. 8.8 Narrow Band imaging (NBI) is helpful in delineating esophageal pathologies like Barrett's. A non-circumferential segment of Barrett's with ulceration is shown here in white light (**a**) and NBI (**b**)

studying esophageal function have been introduced: these include High-Resolution Manometry (HRM) and Multi-channel Intraluminal Impedance (MII). Further improvement of the HRM called high-definition manometry, in which the pressure transducers grouped in banks and rings are even closer spaced is in development to assess in even greater detail the characteristics of the lower esophageal sphincter, and the esophageal motility.

Esophageal Water-Perfused Motility

Pharyngeal and esophageal motor function disorders are a common cause of symptoms, particularly dysphagia, chest pain, and those associated with gastroesophageal reflux. Motor function can be assessed by a variety of recording techniques including radiology, scintigraphy, manometry, and most recently intraluminal electrical impedance monitoring. The gold standard, however, for the assessment of motor disorders remains manometry. Manometric measurement of esophageal pressure is the most direct method for assessment of motor function. Esophageal manometry is typically performed with a catheter with five pressure transducers placed 5 cm apart (Fig. 8.9). A typical catheter is 4–5 mm in diameter and contains eight channels oriented round the circumference, each 0.6–0.8 mm in diameter, and perfused at a rate of 0.3–0.6 ml/min in order to record esophageal pressure waves with sufficient fidelity.

Only manometry can give information on the strength of contractions. Performance of technically adequate manometric recordings and interpretation of the findings requires considerable background knowledge. Perfused manometric systems rely on the transmission of the intraluminal pressures to external pressure transducers along manometric assemblies perfused with distilled water. Performance of accurate and high-fidelity manometric recordings requires a thorough understanding of how the manometric system operates as well as careful attention to technique. Poor-quality recordings inevitably lead to erroneous interpretation.

The major elements of the analysis of pharyngoesophageal manometry are the degree of upper esophageal sphincter relaxation, the integrity of pharyngeal peristalsis, and intrabolus pressure. The major elements of the analysis of esophageal motor function are the integrity of esophageal peristalsis, the assessment of the lower esophageal sphincter (LES), and the degree of lower esophageal relaxation (Fig. 8.10). A structured and systematic assessment of these elements should lead to a manometric diagnosis. In GERD the important assessment is the LES, and measurements should be obtained of the overall length, the abdominal length, and the location of the respiratory inversion point. The measurements of each of these components from each transducer are expressed as an average. A mechanically defective sphincter is identified by a presence of 1 or more of the following

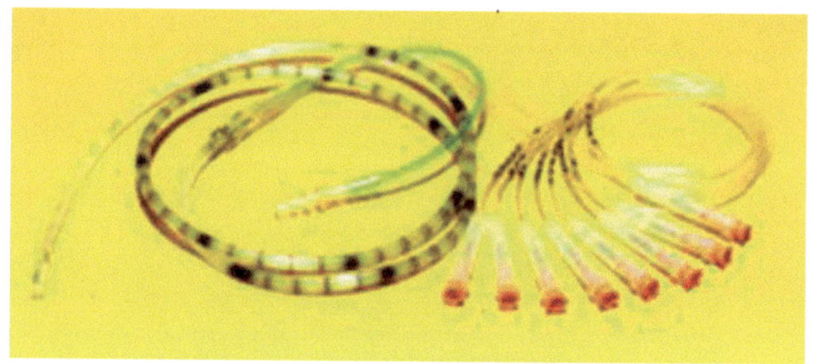

Fig. 8.9 Water-perfused Esophageal Manometry catheter

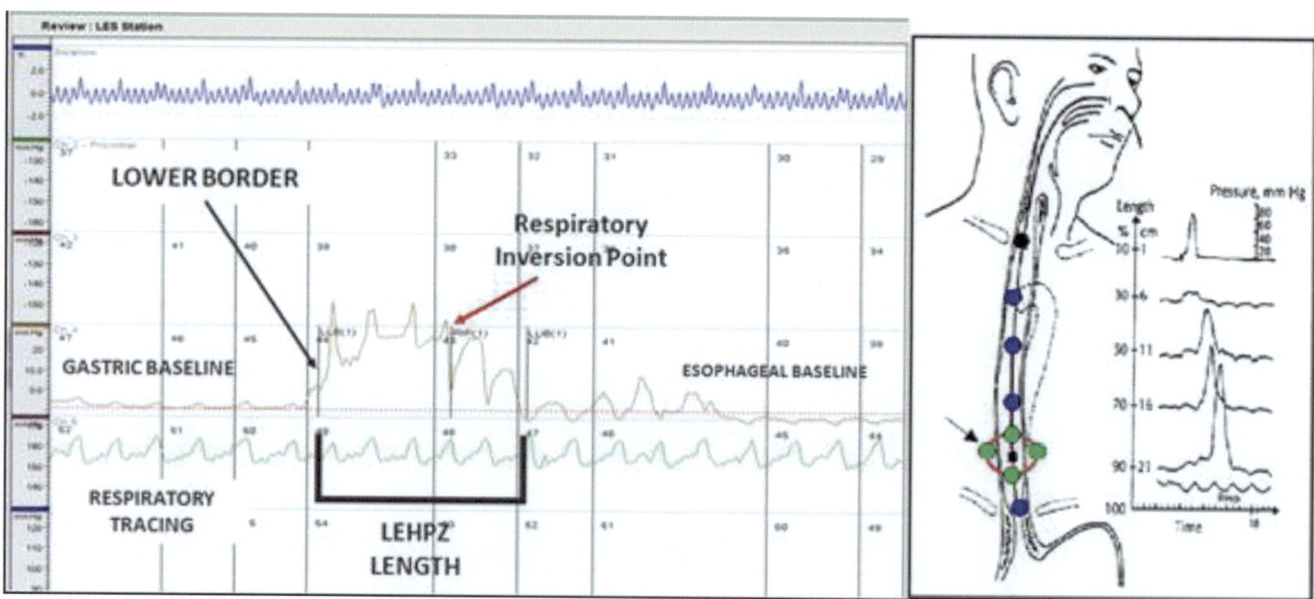

Fig. 8.10 Conventional water-perfused manometry tracing

Fig. 8.11 High-resolution
manometry tracing

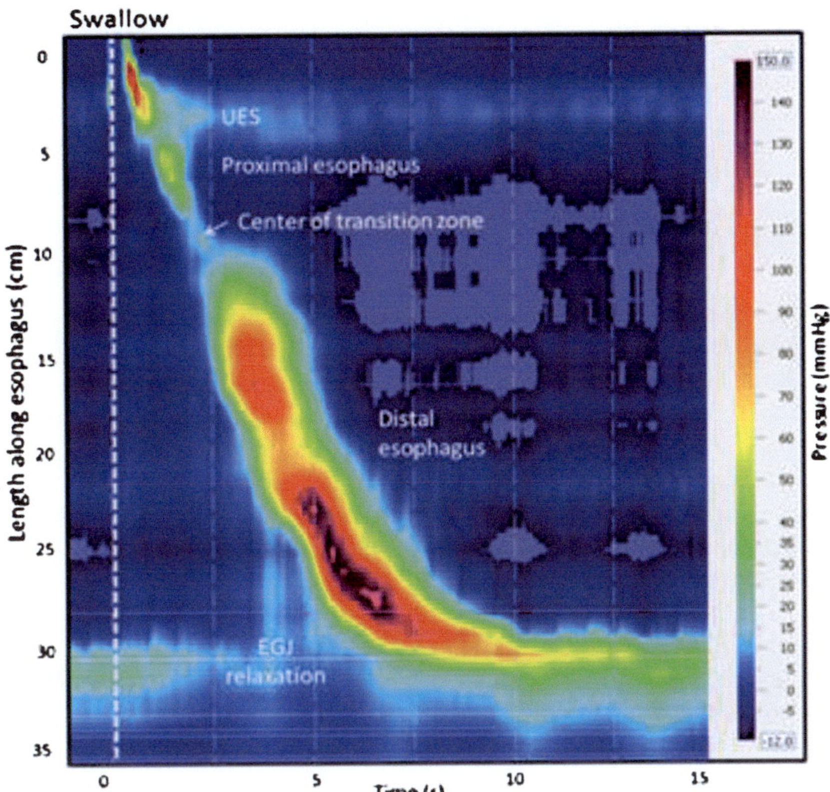

characteristics: (1) an average LES pressure of <6 mmHg, (2) an average abdominal length of <1 cm, (3) an average overall length of <2 cm. A defect in 1 or even 2 components of the LES may be compensated by good esophageal function, but with all 3 components defective excessive esophageal acid exposure is inevitable. Body motility is assessed and if 3 or more out of 10 wet swallows are abnormal, the body motility is considered impaired. The assessment of the body motility is critical for surgeons that are tailoring the fundoplication depending on the esophageal function.

High-Resolution Manometry

The development of powerful computer acquisition systems, along with high-fidelity multichannel perfusion pumps and manometric catheters, has enabled high-resolution measurement and display of esophageal motility. It differs from conventional manometry in recording pressures by 12 solid state micro transducers arranged circumferentially and spaced every centimeter of esophageal length. Sensors display the data in pseudo-three dimensional format using a topographic plot where esophageal pressures within a given range are represented by different colors (Fig. 8.11). The large amount of data and the capacity to analyze and display it intuitively has afforded many new insights into esophageal dysfunction [4]. Among these insights are the ability to distinguish three different subtypes of achalasia and predict their response to therapy, better understanding of the relationship between the lower esophageal sphincter (LES) and the crural diaphragm, the development of novel quantitative parameters to understand the nature of the dysfunction in non-specific esophageal motor disorders (NSEMD), and the elucidation of a newly described motility disorder characterized by failure of peristalsis at the transitional zone between the upper skeletal muscle and the more distal smooth muscle portion of the esophagus. Though water-perfused manometry was the gold standard for more than 3 decades, it has been widely replaced by high-resolution manometry because the testing is less cumbersome, quicker, and more comfortable for patients. Additionally, the analysis of the esophageal topography output is visually appealing and intuitively comprehensible. Regardless of the technique used, esophageal manometric testing remains an important part of the preoperative evaluation for anti-reflux surgery.

Esophageal pH Monitoring

Since its inception in the 1970s, esophageal pH monitoring remains the definitive diagnostic test to confirm abnormal gastroesophageal reflux by objectively quantifying the amount of acid present in the esophagus over a prolonged time period. It is used to diagnose GERD, to determine the severity of the disease, to assess the effectiveness of anti-acid medications or the effectiveness of surgical treatment of GERD. The development of 24 h pH monitoring was a major advance in the unraveling of the pathophysiology of

Table 8.1 Six components of pH monitoring (for the DeMeester score)

1.	% time pH < 4	Total
2.	% time pH < 4	Upright
3.	% time pH < 4	Supine
4.	Number of episodes pH < 4	
5.	Number of long episodes (>5 min) pH < 4	
6.	Time (min) longest episode	

GERD. This test is the gold standard for the diagnosis of GERD, because it has the highest sensitivity and specificity of all tests currently available. It is indicated in any patient with symptoms of GERD. It is essential in patients considered for anti-reflux surgery, but can be omitted in patients with a large hiatal hernia, Barrett's esophagus, or severe esophagitis. Another indication is atypical presentation of GERD. Ideally, medications such as H2 blockers, prokinetics, and proton pump inhibitors should be stopped 1–2 weeks before pH monitoring because of their long-lasting action. Current society guidelines recommend that all patients undergo pH monitoring off antacid medications but the test is also frequently used to determine the effectiveness of a patient's acid suppression on medication.

A typical recording collects data regarding the frequency and duration of reflux events, their relationship to meals and position (upright or supine) as well as the association of reflux events with symptoms. The patient is instructed to carry out normal activities but to avoid strenuous exertion. He or she is asked to remain in upright position while awake during the day, lying down supine only at night while sleeping, and to ingest two meals at the usual time. The patient notes in a diary the times of meals, retiring for sleep, and rising the following morning as well as the presence and duration of any symptoms.

Esophageal acid exposure is best assessed by measuring the six components of the DeMeester Score (Table 8.1). The score is a composite of values of each of the six components to give a single assessment of esophageal acid exposure. Normal acid exposure is defined as a DeMeester Score of less than 14.72 which is based on delineating the upper limits of normal as the 95th percentile derived from recordings 5 cm above the LES in 50 asymptomatic controls [5].

Catheter Based 24 h pH Monitoring

This study is performed by passing a thin plastic catheter, measuring a sixteenth of an inch in diameter, through one nostril, down the back of the throat, and into the esophagus as the patient swallows. The tip of the catheter contains a sensor that detects pH. The sensor is positioned in the esophagus so that it is exactly 5 cm above the previously determined manometric upper border of the lower esophageal sphincter. In this position the sensor records each reflux event—defined as a drop in the pH level below 4.0. The cath-

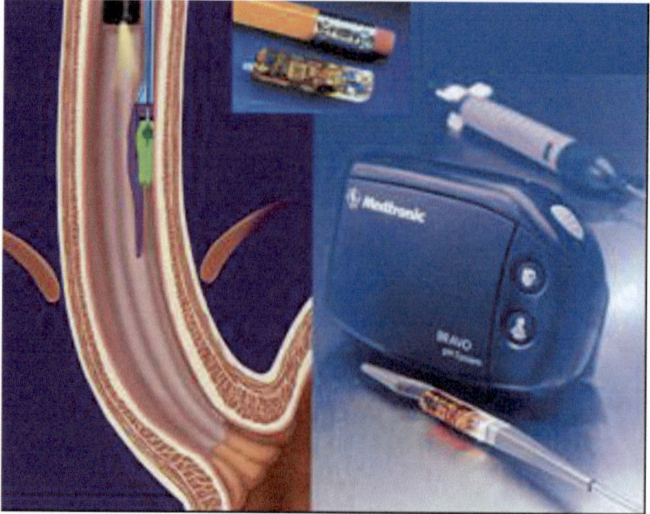

Fig. 8.12 Wireless pH monitoring capsule (Bravo) and location in esophagus

eter protrudes from the nose is connected directly to a recorder. The patient is sent home with the catheter and recorder in place and returns the next day to have them removed. During the 24 h that the catheter is in place, the patient goes about his or her usual activities, for example, eating, sleeping, and working. Meals, periods of sleep, and symptoms are recorded by the patient in a diary and/or by pushing buttons on the recorder. After the catheter is removed, the recorder is attached to a computer so that the data it has gathered can be downloaded into the computer where it is analyzed and put into graphic form.

Wireless pH Monitoring

The most recently developed device for monitoring esophageal pH uses a wireless pH capsule (BRAVO, Given Imaging, Israel). The capsule is introduced into the esophagus using a specialized deployment catheter passed through the nose or mouth. The capsule contains two wells into which the esophageal mucosa is gathered by applying suction to the catheter. A pin is then deployed across the wells and through the mucosal tissue thereby attaching the device to the lining of the esophagus. If placed through the nose after manometry the capsule is positioned 5 cm above the upper limit of the LES [6, 7]. If placed through the mouth by endoscopy, the capsule is positioned 6 cm above the squamocolumnar junction. The capsule contains an acid sensing probe, a battery, and a transmitter (Fig. 8.12). The probe monitors the acid in the esophagus and transmits the information to a recorder that is worn by the patient on a belt (Fig. 8.13). The capsule transmits for 2 days, and after 5–7 days the capsule is passed naturally.

The major advantage of the capsule device is patient comfort by avoiding a catheter in the back of the throat and convenience in the absence of a catheter in the back of patients

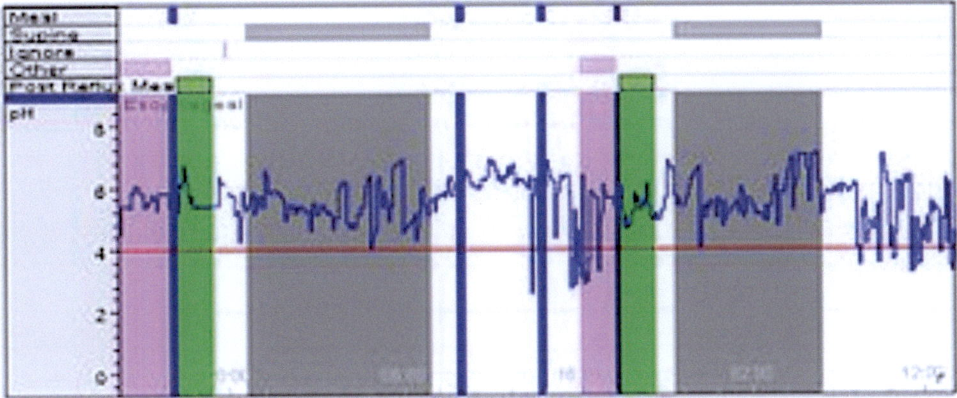

Fig. 8.13 pH monitoring and tracing

are more likely to go to work and do more normal activities without feeling self-conscious about the appearance of the catheter to others. The disadvantages of the capsule are that it cannot be used in the pharynx or in the proximal esophagus due to discomfort.

Therefore, 24 h pH monitoring or 48 h Bravo capsule pH monitoring is an essential part of the preoperative evaluation in patients with GERD, to establish objectively the diagnosis of reflux disease. Only in patients with severe reflux in combination with esophagitis or Barrett's esophagus, or in patients with large hiatal or paraesophageal hernias with symptoms, this test can be omitted.

Multichannel Intraluminal Impedance

Multichannel intraluminal impedance (MII) is a method of detecting intraesophageal bolus movement of liquid or gas regardless of pH. This method is based on measuring the resistance to alternating current (i.e., impedance) of the content of the esophageal lumen. When a pair of electrodes, separated by an isolator (i.e., catheter), is placed inside the esophagus, the electrical circuit is closed by electrical charges (i.e., ions) present in the esophageal mucosa that surround the catheter. The conductivity of the empty esophageal lumen is relatively stable, with the electrical circuit registering values around $2{,}000\text{--}4{,}000\,\Omega$. The appearance of a liquid bolus in the impedance-measuring segment is recognized as a rapid drop in impedance as the increased ionic content of the bolus improves the electrical conductivity between the two electrodes (Fig. 8.14). The impedance will remain low as long as the bolus is present between the two electrodes and will start rising once the bolus is cleared from the segment by a contraction. The presence of gas in the impedance-measuring segment is recognized by a rise in impedance typically above $5{,}000\,\Omega$, as there are no electrical charges to close the circuit when the two electrodes are suspended in air. Impedance will return to the baseline values once the air bolus has passed and the electrodes are back in contact with

the esophageal mucosa. The presence of a mixed (i.e., gas–liquid, liquid–gas) bolus is recognized by impedance changes indicating air and liquid presence.

Impedance testing is most commonly used to assess persistent symptoms in patients with adequate acid suppression. In these situations, correlation of reflux events, either non-acid or acidic, with symptoms can be helpful. Abnormal impedance is defined as more than 48 reflux events in a 24-h period regardless of composition. Impedance monitoring is performed in conjunction with 24 h pH testing and current combination catheters are available with varying sensor configurations.

Gastric Emptying Study

Delayed gastric emptying from gastric outlet obstruction or gastroparesis as a cause of secondary gastroesophageal reflux is becoming more widely recognized. Gastric emptying tests should be obtained in all reflux patients with significant symptoms of gas bloat, nausea, or vomiting (as opposed to positional reflux) prior to surgery to rule out gastroparesis. Testing should also be considered in patients with isolated non-acid reflux and regurgitation. Testing options include a 4 h nuclear gastric emptying scintigraphy [8] or via the wireless motility capsule (Smart Pill, Given Imaging, Haifa, Israel). Gastric emptying scintigraphy methods vary widely between centers which can lead to diagnostic errors. Common variations include substitution of the 4-h study with T1/2, using non-standardized test meals and inconsistent patient physical activity between time points. A consensus report outlines the recommended standard gastric emptying scintigraphy protocol that should be followed to decrease these errors [8–10]. The protocol, often referred to as the Tougas protocol, defines a standardized radiolabeled low-fat egg white meal with imaging at 0, 1, 2, and 4 h after meal ingestion. Abnormal values for quantitative emptying are >90, >60, >30, and >10 % of retained meal at each time point respectively.

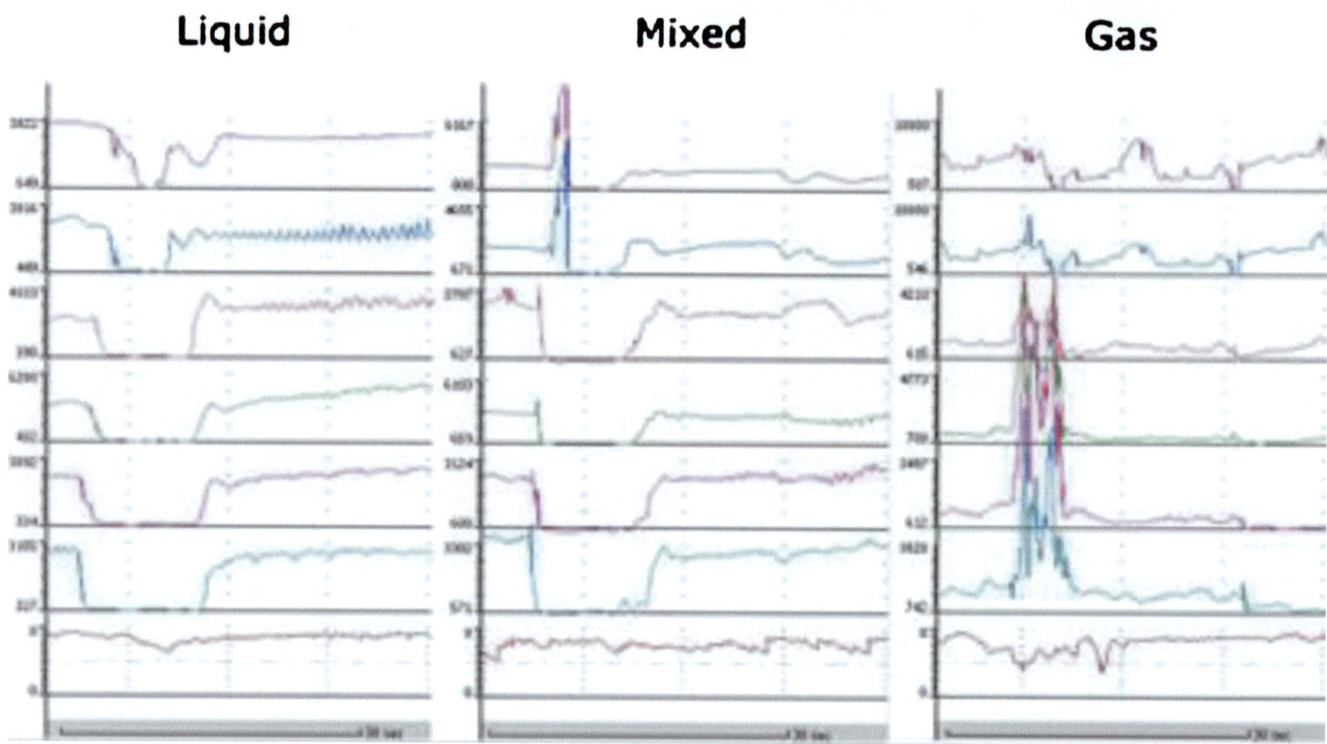

Fig. 8.14 Multichannel impedance tracing

Summary

Patients presenting with symptoms suggestive of gastro-esophageal reflux may have a myriad of associated conditions that greatly impact surgical planning. Comprehensive esophageal diagnostic testing is imperative to fully understand the pathophysiology underlying the patient's symptoms. When contemplating anti-reflux surgery, thoughtful and detailed testing will help avoid pitfalls and mis-diagnosis which may lead to poor outcomes.

References

1. Fuller L, Huprich JE, Theisen J, et al. Abnormal esophageal body function: radiographic–manometric correlation. Am Surg. 1999;65(10):911–4.
2. Dodds WJ. 1976 Walter B. Cannon Lecture: current concepts of esophageal motor function: clinical implications for radiology. AJR Am J Roentgenol. 1977;128(4):549–61.
3. Hill LD, Kozarek RA, Kraemer SJ, et al. The gastroesophageal flap valve: in vitro and in vivo observations. Gastrointest Endosc. 1996;44(5):541–7.
4. Ayazi S, Hagen JA, Zehetner J, et al. The value of high-resolution manometry in the assessment of the resting characteristics of the lower esophageal sphincter. J Gastrointest Surg. 2009;13(12): 2113–20.
5. Johnson LF, DeMeester TR. Development of the 24-hour intraesophageal pH monitoring composite scoring system. J Clin Gastroenterol. 1986;8 Suppl 1:52–8.
6. Ayazi S, Hagen JA, Zehetner J, et al. Day-to-day discrepancy in Bravo pH monitoring is related to the degree of deterioration of the lower esophageal sphincter and severity of reflux disease. Surg Endosc. 2011;25(7):2219–23.
7. Ayazi S, Lipham JC, Portale G, et al. Bravo catheter-free pH monitoring: normal values, concordance, optimal diagnostic thresholds, and accuracy. Clin Gastroenterol Hepatol. 2009;7(1):60–7.
8. Abell TL, Camilleri M, Donohoe K, Hasler WL, Lin HC, Maurer AH, et al. Consensus recommendations for gastric emptying scintigraphy: a joint report of the American Neurogastroenterology and Motility Society and the Society of Nuclear Medicine. Am J Gastroenterol. 2008;103(3):753–63.
9. Tougas G, Chen Y, Coates G, Paterson W, Dallaire C, Pare P, et al. Standardization of a simplified scintigraphic methodology for the assessment of gastric emptying in a multicenter setting. Am J Gastroenterol. 2000;95(1):78–86.
10. Tougas G, Eaker EY, Abell TL, Abrahamsson H, Boivin M, Chen J, et al. Assessment of gastric emptying using a low fat meal: establishment of international control values. Am J Gastroenterol. 2000;95(6):1456–62.

Part II

Techniques of Antireflux Surgery

Complete Fundoplications: Indications and Technique

Cecilia Engström and Lars Lundell

Introduction

There are many names used for the most common procedure in anti-reflux surgery. Rudolf Nissen serendipitously discovered the utility of a complete 360-degree fundoplication while operating on a 16-year-old patient in 1956. Following a partial esophagectomy, Dr. Nissen used the gastric fundus to protect the anastomosis and found that it also prevented reflux. Nissen described the procedure as "a simple operation to influence reflux esophagitis," and named it a "fundoplication." Today, it is generically referred to as a "complete," "total," or a "360° fundoplication" [1] (Fig. 9.1). Over the last 50 years, the original procedure has evolved and improved in parallel with increased understanding of the pathophysiology of gastroesophageal reflux disease (GERD) and its association with hiatal herniation, the function of the lower esophageal sphincter (LES), and its connection with the function of the foregut as a whole [2].

It was discovered early on that the proper function of a Nissen fundoplication depends on it being well and precisely constructed. The goal is to restore the reflux barrier at the gastroesophageal junction (GEJ) without causing esophageal outlet obstruction. The fundoplication reinforces the LES pressure by increasing the resting pressure and the relaxation (nadir) pressure [3, 4] and by inhibiting its effacement thereby maintaining sphincter length. It is also recognized that even an otherwise normal appearing valve becomes dysfunctional when it is herniated into the mediastinum. Therefore it is mandatory after the reduction of the hiatal

hernia that the esophageal hiatus be closed around the esophagus. It is also important to minimize axial tension in order to prevent herniation or disruption. While this is usually accomplished by mediastinal mobilization, on occasion a lengthening procedure (Collis gastroplasty) needs to be performed. Other contributors to the function of the Nissen valve include exposure to a positive intra-abdominal pressure and a better synchronization and overlap of the intrinsic and extrinsic sphincters including the crural pressure. Fundoplication also works by reducing the number of transient LES relaxations by decreasing the compliance of the gastric cardia [5]. Finally, a Nissen creates an obviously mechanical "flap valve" that is visible and gradable endoscopically (Fig. 9.2).

However, the Nissen results in a somewhat supracompetent valve, which tends to affect the other two functions of the gastroesophageal junction: swallowing and belching. Accordingly, the main side-effects of Nissen fundoplications are impaired swallowing (dysphagia) and gas-related symptoms caused by inability to vent air from the stomach ("bloating") [4]. In many studies up to 20 % of patients present with early post-fundoplication dysphagia, albeit this is largely temporary and diminishing with time [6, 7] (Table 9.1). It is unusual for a Nissen not to have some dysphagia postoperatively and for that reason most surgeons restrict solid intake for a period of weeks or months. Rarely dysphagia will persist for longer and at some point an endoscopy and dilation is indicated (6 weeks to 3 months after surgery are common recommendations). Failure to respond to such a dilation indicates the need for a complete physiology evaluation and consideration for revision. Likewise, inability to belch is common immediately after Nissen but should resolve after a few months. As reflux disease is often associated with aerophagia, the period of not belching can be more or less miserable for the patient and they should be warned ahead of time of this transient side effect. If gas-related problems persist beyond 6 months, consideration of dilating the wrap to promote belching or referring to a swallowing therapist may be needed [9].

C. Engström, MD, PhD
Department of Surgery, Sahlgrenska University Hospital,
Dehr Dubbsgatan, Goteburg 413 45, Sweden
e-mail: cecilia.engstrom@surgery.gu.se

L. Lundell, MD, PhD (✉)
Gastrocentrum Surgery, Karolinska University Hospital,
Stockholm S141 86, Sweden
e-mail: lars.lundell@karolinska.se

L.L. Swanstrom and C.M. Dunst (eds.), *Antireflux Surgery*,
DOI 10.1007/978-1-4939-1749-5_9, © Springer New York 2015

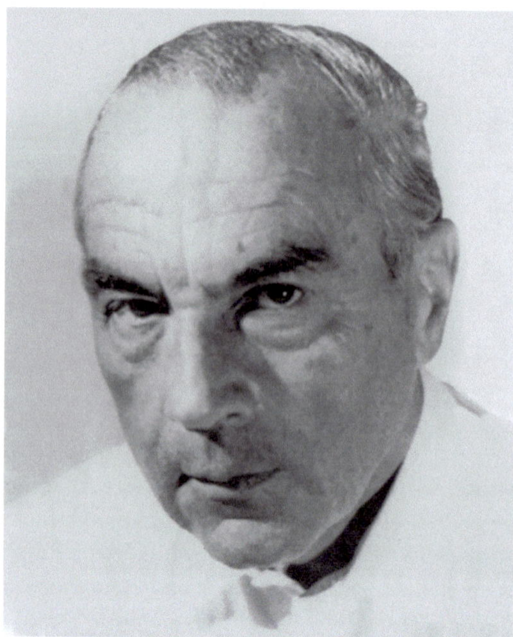

Fig. 9.1 Original case report published by Rudolf Nissen in 1956. "Rudolf Nissen (1896–1981)-Perspective" (from *Journal of Gastrointestinal Surgery*)

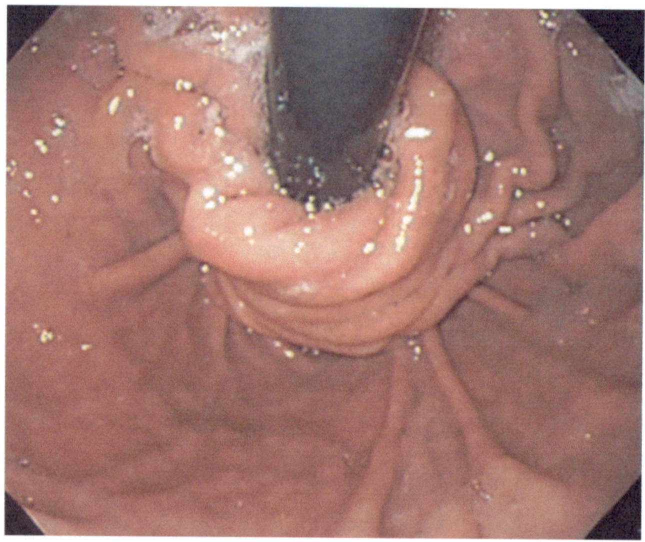

Fig. 9.2 Endoscopic retroflexed view of a normal Nissen fundoplication

Table 9.1 Post-operative symptoms at short- and long-term follow-up after laparoscopic Nissen [8]

$N = 82$	3 weeks (2–4 weeks) (%)	13 months (5–17 months) (%)
Dysphagia	9	2
Heartburn	3	1
Reflux	1	0
Gas bloat (gas issues requiring intervention)	1	0
Early satiety	96	5
Bloating	78	15
Nausea	15	5
Hyperflatulence	82	28
Diarrhea	26	8
Odynophagia	5	

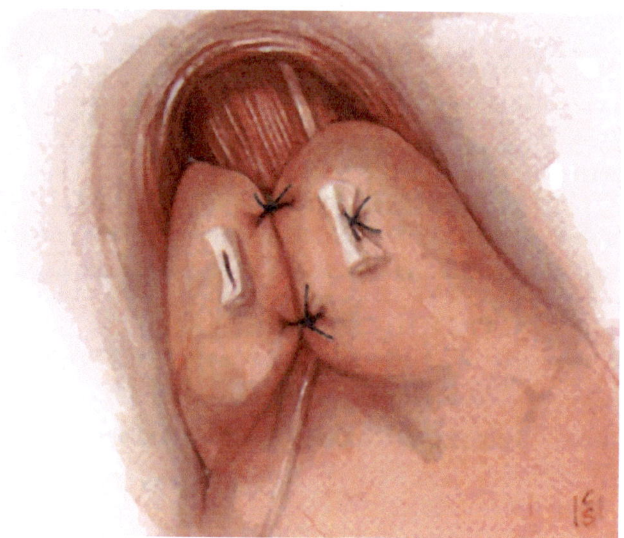

Fig. 9.3 The classic short, floppy wrap described by Donahue and DeMeester

Originally, Nissen described a long wrap utilizing the posterior and anterior wall of the stomach. Nissen fundoplication has subsequently been modified several times, especially by the work of Donahue and DeMeester who introduced the concept of reducing the length of the fundic wrap and the tightness of the encircled fundus to create a "floppy" Nissen [10, 11]. The more modern procedure includes mobilization of the distal esophagus, division of the short gastric vessels, posterior repair of the crural diaphragm, and wrapping of the fundus of the stomach around the esophagus, incorporating its entire circumference (Fig. 9.3). A short and "floppy" wrap is considered important to minimize the post-operative side-effects outlined above.

After its first description in 1991, the laparoscopic approach for Nissen fundoplication has rapidly replaced the conventional open approach. The original idea behind the introduction of the laparoscopic approach was to reduce morbidity while maintaining the established long-term effectiveness of the Nissen. During the last decade, studies have been performed with long-term follow-up to compare laparoscopic with conventional Nissen fundoplications and have confirmed that the laparoscopic approach provides substantial patient benefit without compromising outcomes [12]. The impact of the surgeons' experience and hospital volume on the results of laparoscopic Nissen fundoplication has also been well established, with consequences for the intra- and post-operative outcomes, the short-term results concerning reflux control as well as long-term clinical outcomes [13].

Most recently, the introduction of robot-assisted laparoscopy generated some enthusiasm and even opinions that this might replace the standard laparoscopic approach for procedures like the Nissen. Subsequent outcome analyses however did not justify the use of this surgical approach due to higher costs not counterbalanced by better outcomes [14].

Patient Selection for Nissen

The classical indications for Nissen fundoplication are;
- Patients with an incomplete response to pharmacological therapy with proton pump inhibition.
- Documented reflux by pH, impedance or endoscopic findings.
- Unwillingness to take lifelong medication.
- Extra-esophageal manifestations of gastro-esophageal reflux disease (caution).
- Adequate esophageal motility to overcome the outflow resistance created by the valve.

Outcomes of Nissen have been described as being better if patients are not morbidly obese [15] have typical symptoms have good response to medical therapy [16] and who have not had previous anti-reflux surgery [17, 18].

Upper endoscopies performed in chronic GERD, as part of the workup for possible surgery, have shown that at most only half of the patients will have erosive reflux disease. The majority of reflux patients today have no visibly active esophagitis [19, 20]. Ambulatory 24-h pH monitoring with symptom association analysis is therefore a gold standard test to diagnosed GERD in absence of esophageal erosions. Patients can be divided into isolated upright, isolated supine, and bi-positional reflux based on the body position in which pathological reflux occurs during pH monitoring. Traditionally those with isolated supine and bi-positional reflux are considered the best candidates for reflux surgery, as this finding indirectly indicates a mechanical defect of the LES and is associated with more severe disease. Isolated upright reflux disease is often associated with less typical manifestations of reflux disease and sometimes indicative of maladaptive behaviors. Therefore fundoplication tends to be withheld from these patients. However, well-controlled studies comparing upright refluxers with those having reflux in supine and bi-positional body positions have revealed that patients with all three reflux patterns responded equally well to Nissen fundoplication over the long-term [21, 22]. Another important predictor of outcomes is the presence of both a pathological acid exposure time and a positive symptom reflux correlation during pH monitoring. Patients with clearly pathological esophageal acid exposure benefit from a total fundoplication, irrespective whether they have a negative or a positive symptom reflux correlation [23]. There remains a question as to whether the 10–15 % of patients with GERD who have a positive symptom association in spite of normal acid exposure (so called "sensitive esophagus") are good candidates for a reflux surgery. Relatively few short-term studies have been published that would support that patients with esophageal acid hypersensitivity alone would benefit from a Nissen fundoplication to the same degree as those with abnormal clearly pathological acid reflux [24]. This patient group clearly has to be better researched.

Endoscopy negative reflux disease has traditionally been regarded as a mild form of GERD and sometimes considered to represent a relative contraindication for a total fundoplication. However, during the latest two decades studies have demonstrated that the impairment of quality of life and severity of symptoms are similar in the endoscopy negative GERD group (non-erosive reflux disease, NERD) compared with the endoscopy positive one (erosive reflux disease, ERD). Studies have carefully evaluated the effect of Nissen fundoplication on NERD and ERD patients [25]. When doing so, subjective and objective outcome measures, after total fundoplication and reoperation rates, were very comparable [26]. Therefore, at present it can be concluded that the absence of erosions on endoscopy in patients with chronic GERD symptoms and with pathological acid reflux variables on testing is not a reason to refrain from an anti-reflux operation.

Predicting Failures

It is important to define predictors of less favorable outcomes after total fundoplication. It has been assumed that patients with esophageal dysmotility, as diagnosed with esophageal manometry, are more likely to develop post-operative dysphagia. Many centers have therefore advocated a tailoring concept, meaning that a partial wrap should be done in similar situations to minimize the risk for obstructive symptoms postoperatively [27, 28]. However, randomized clinical trials have failed to demonstrate that the outcome after total fundoplication is worse in patients with poor motility compared to those with normal esophageal function [29–32]. The majority of practitioners who use Nissen may slightly modify it (e.g., use a larger dilator or make it shorter in length) but would not avoid it in mild and moderate dysmotility. The complete absence of motility on the other hand is widely considered a "red flag" and often an indication for a partial wrap.

Variations on a Theme

It is well known that the proper creation of a full 360-degree fundoplication is paramount to its success and poorly performed fundoplications can lead to disastrous outcomes.

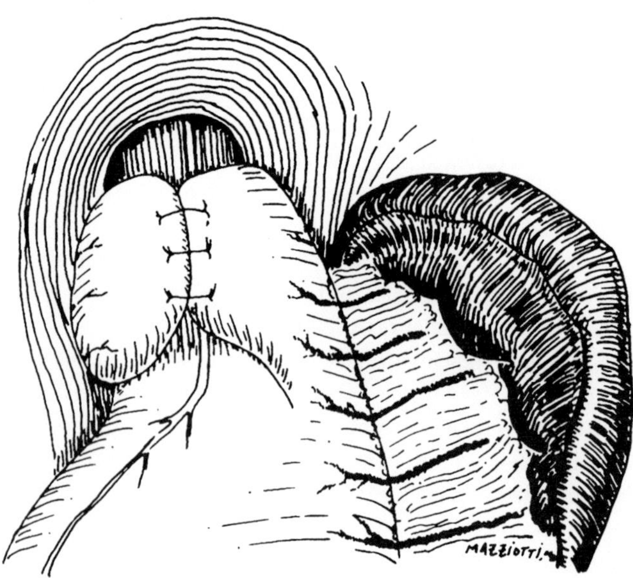

Fig. 9.4 Configuration of a Rosetti–Nissen repair with apposition of anterior gastric wall to anterior gastric wall

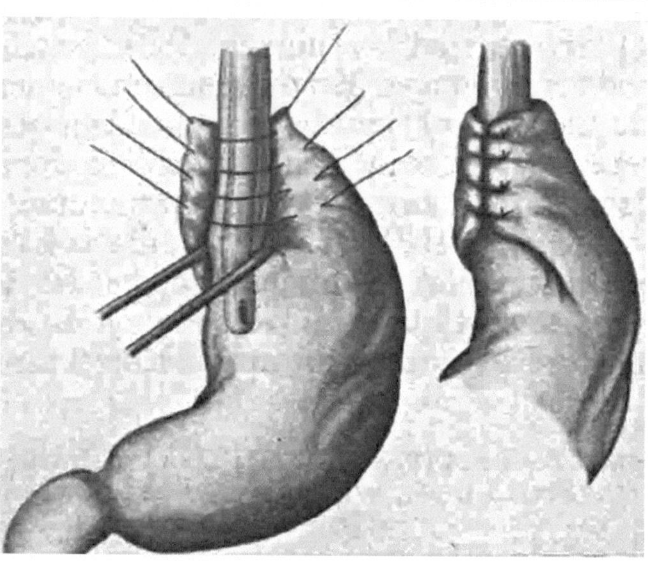

Fig. 9.5 Nissen's original description and illustration show the esophagus imbricated into the gastric fundus (anterior gastric wall to posterior gastric wall). Nissen R. [A simple operation for control of reflux esophagitis]. Schweiz Med Wochenschr. 1956;18;86(Suppl 20):590–2. [Article in German]

Despite attempts to standardize the technique, there are numerous minor variations to the "Nissen" added by practitioners based on their own experience. Some of these variations are evidence based and some are not. The *Nissen–Rossetti* variation is one of the oldest alternatives. While it still includes mobilization of the distal esophagus and posterior crural repair, it differs significantly in that the short gastric vessels are not divided and the fundoplication is created using the anterior wall of the stomach only. [33] (Fig. 9.4). Several studies seem to indicate that in the hands of experts, there are no differences in the short- or the long-term outcomes between the original Nissen and the Nissen–Rossetti modified fundoplications [34, 35].

In the early days of laparoscopic fundoplication, many surgeons avoided the division of the short gastric vessels, as it was tedious to clip or tie them individually. After early reports describing increased problems not dividing them, [36] and with the availability of new energy devices that made division quick and reliable, [37] routine division became the norm as it was for the open procedure. Still, there is little to objectively support the need to divide them. Two randomized studies have shown no significant difference in outcomes between Nissens with fundic mobilization and without [38]. Whereas in the open era of fundoplication, closure of the hiatus was considered optional, and in fact was seldom done for all but the largest hiatal hernias, it was rapidly found that reduction of any resident hiatal hernia sac and a secure hiatal closure is mandatory for laparoscopic repairs [39]. This may be because of the relative lack of adhesions resulting from laparoscopic approaches that result in a more mobile stomach that is able to easily migrate into the mediastinum. Other elements of hiatal closure remain highly controversial and include type of suture used (heavy woven permanent suture being the preferred choice), pattern of closure (simple sutures, figure of 8, pledgeted, etc.), use or avoidance of mesh, and posterior versus anterior closure. Regarding the latter, while common practice is to close the hiatus posteriorly, there is level-one evidence that supports anterior closure as equivalent [40].

Another hallmark of the open Nissen was the mandatory use of a large esophageal dilator. After incidences of bougie perforations during laparoscopic fundoplication (incidence of 0.8 % in meta-analysis) many advocated against its routine use [41, 42]. There is some evidence that wrapping over a large dilator may decrease dysphagia rates but there is no doubt that it adds time and some risk to the procedure. The only randomized study would seem to indicate a lower short- and long-term dysphagia rate with bougie use [43]. Use of a bougie therefore varies widely from center to center, with perhaps slightly more favoring not using one over its routine use [44].

The number and type of the sutures creating the Nissen probably has the most variation from center to center. Most laparoscopic practitioners prefer use of a permanent suture—most typically a woven synthetic of 0 or 2–0 gauge. The key sutures are the ones that bring the left and right wrap edges together. These range from 2 to 4 in number. There is large variation regarding the inclusion of the anterior esophageal wall with these Nissen sutures. Use of reinforcing pledgets for the fundic sutures has mostly fallen out of favor mostly due to their awkwardness in placement as well as some concern with erosion. The majority of esophageal surgeons feel that some sort of fixation is needed to prevent slipping of the wrap onto the upper stomach. The use of some sort of gastropexy sutures, either posterior to the closed hiatus, or anterior to the crura, is common but unproven [45].

In general, there are two popular methods of creating a fundoplication. The first is based on the original work of Nissen who describes his technique as an invagination of the distal esophagus into the gastric fundus: much like a Witzel's gastrostomy (Fig. 9.5). This technique maintains the orientation of the greater curvature of the fundus at 3 o'clock and pulls an equidistant point of both the anterior and posterior walls of the fundus into apposition at the 9 o'clock position on the GEJ. In this technique, the posterior wall becomes the "right wrap" and the anterior wall becomes the "left wrap" (Fig. 9.6a). The second technique involves grasping the top of the greater curvature and pulling it behind the esophagus to become the "right wrap." This point is then secured to the greater curvature remaining on the patient's left side (the "left wrap") (Fig. 9.6b). In either case, care must be taken to avoid twisting the GEJ which can generally be avoided if the first grasping point is approximately 3 cm from the GEJ along the greater curve and the second is approximately 8 cm distal (12 cm from the GEJ) along the greater curvature. A standard shoeshine maneuver between these points should be done to confirm symmetry of the wrap and a stationary GEJ (Fig. 9.7). Both techniques have been used to create a full wrap for thousands of our patients. These variations in the technique of Nissen make its performance more of an art form than a "science" and are a source of concern regarding the reproducibility of quality outcomes. Efforts have been made to "standardize" the technique based on expert consensus. This has mostly been done in the context of multicenter prospective studies.

For example, the LOTUS trial made an effort to "standardize the Nissen procedure for the trial experience. Below find a summary of the consensus document published by the LOTUS participants regarding the recommended way to perform the Nissen [46].

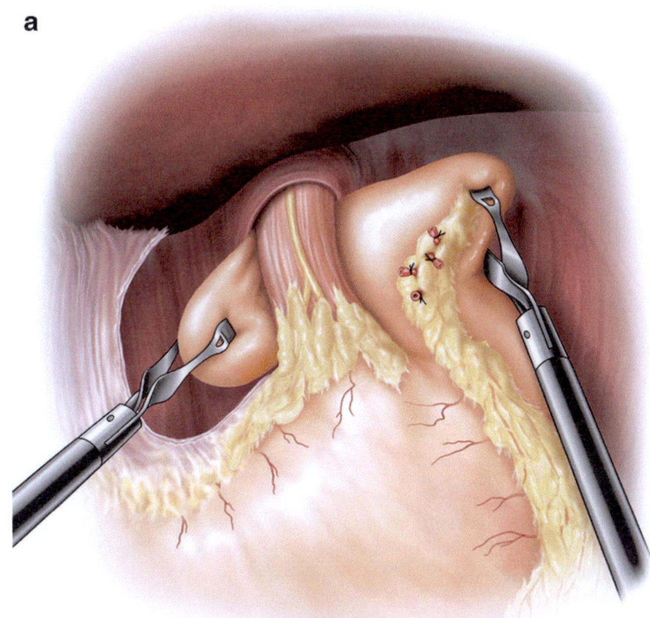

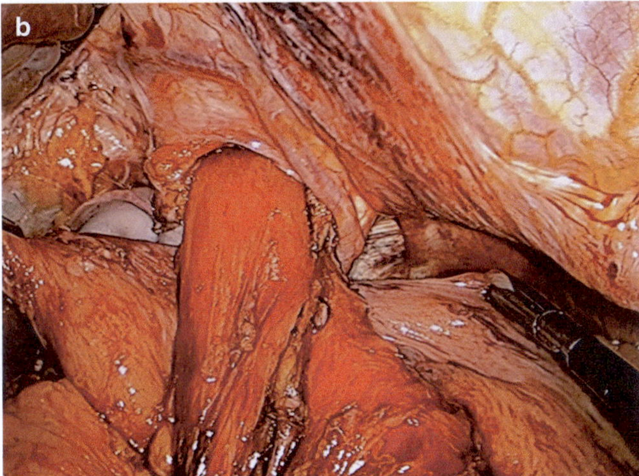

Fig. 9.7 The shoeshine maneuver ensures symmetry within the wrap without twisting. (**a**) Illustrates the maneuver in the greater curve to greater curve technique, as marked by the divided short gastric vessels. (**b**) Shows the maneuver in live tissue

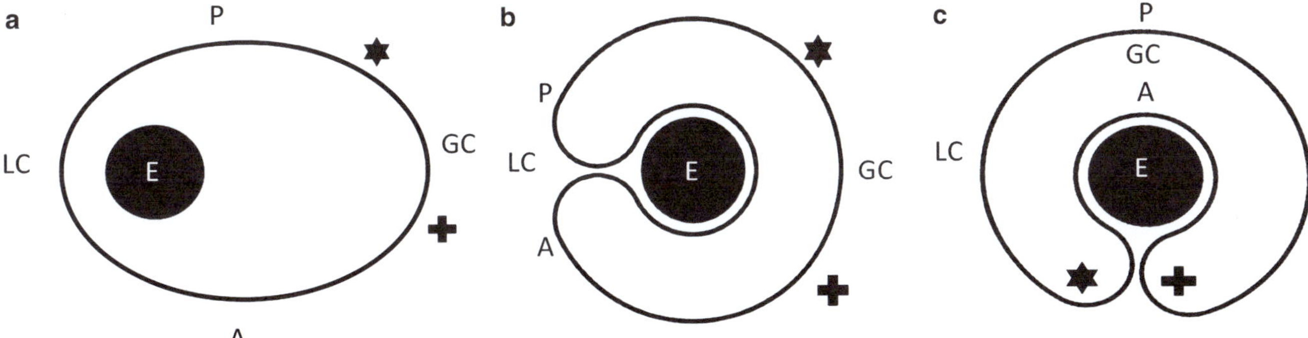

Fig. 9.6 Common variations of Nissen creation. (**a**) Normal anatomy (**b**) Anterior–posterior wrap (**c**) Greater curvature wrap LC=lesser curvature, E=esophagus, A=anterior wall of stomach, P=posterior wall of stomach, GC=greater curvature, STAR=greater curvature about 3 cm from the angle of His, CROSS=greater curvature about 6–7 cm from the angle of His

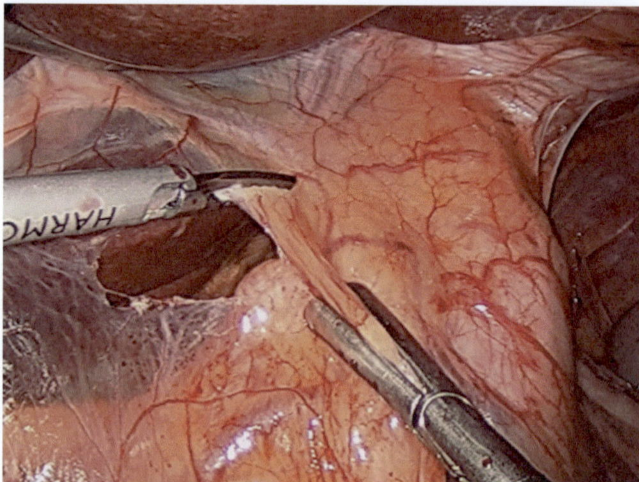

Fig. 9.8 Nissen dissection starts by opening the gastro-hepatic ligament along the caudate lobe to expose the right crus. Vagal branches and accessory hepatic vessels are preserved if possible

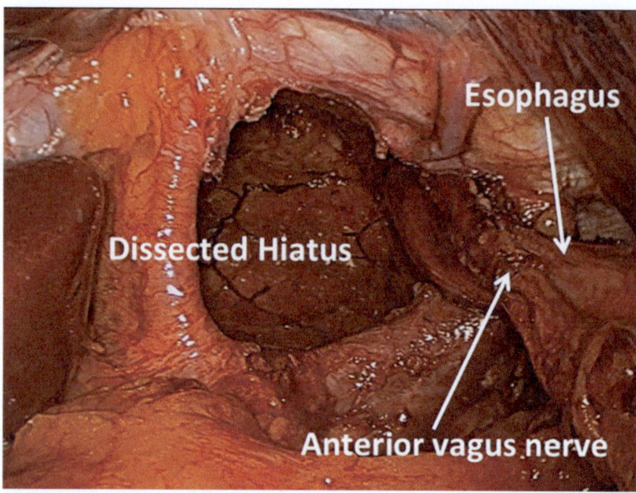

Fig. 9.9 Mediastinal esophageal mobilization is performed to achieve a tension-free, 3 cm length of intra-abdominal esophagus seen here in the setting of a large hiatal hernia

1. Open the phreno-esophageal ligament to approach the hiatus and the distal esophagus from the left to the right (Fig. 9.8).
2. Attempts should be made to preserve the hepatic branch of the anterior vague nerve.
3. Both crura should be carefully and completely dissected, all the way posteriorly to where the right and left crura connect.
4. A generous transhiatal mobilization of the esophagus should be completed to allow approximately 3 cm of the distal esophagus to be positioned within the abdominal cavity without tension (Fig. 9.9).

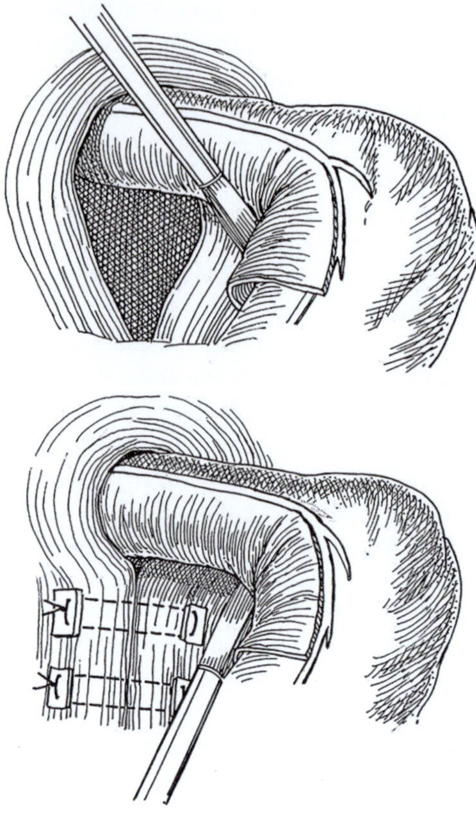

Fig. 9.10 Posterior hiatal closure with permanent sutures is critical. Sutures can be in any pattern: interrupted, figure of 8, pledgeted, etc.—but should not be strangulating

5. Short gastric vessels should be left intact if possible. They may be divided if necessary to create a tension-free wrap.
6. A posterior crural repair is always added using non-absorbable sutures. In case of a very large hiatus defect, the addition of a few anterior crural sutures can be allowed (Fig. 9.10).
7. The total wrap should be created by bringing the right and left portion of the mobile funds around the distal esophagus and sutured together in front of the anterior part of the abdominal portion of the esophagus. The length of the wrap should be 1.5–2 cm and the most distal suture (non-absorbable) should incorporate the anterior musculature wall of the esophagus. The number of sutures used should be recorded, with 2–4 sutures recommended in order to prevent a telescoping of the wrap into the thoracic aperture "slipped fundoplication" (Fig. 9.11).
8. At the time of the construction of the wrap the introduction of a large (55–60 French) bougie through the esophagus is recommended, but not defined as essential.

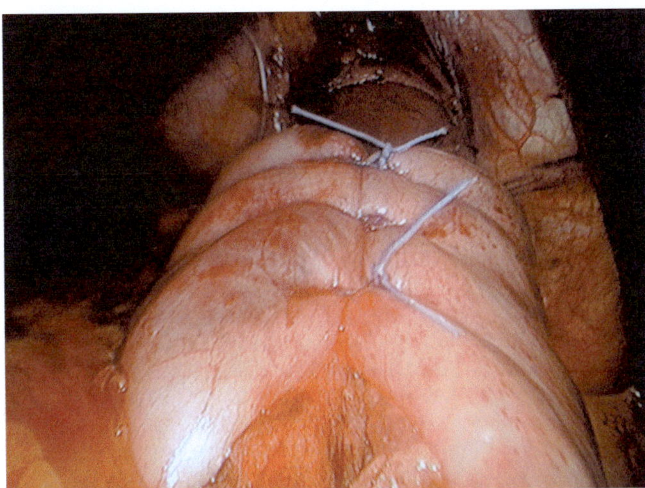

Fig. 9.11 The final result of a laparoscopic Nissen fundoplication is a 2–3 cm, well-secured loose fundoplication

Conclusions

Laparoscopic Nissen Fundoplication is the current gold standard anti-reflux procedure. It is highly effective as it addresses multiple mechanisms of physiologic defects that lead to GER. Unfortunately this "super-physiologic" valve is not patient friendly for a period of time. While there are a multitude of slight variations in how a Nissen is technically performed, we outline key items that must be accomplished to make a long lasting and tolerable reflux barrier.

References

1. Nissen R. Eine eifache Opertion zür Beeinflussung der reflux Oesophagitis. Schweiz Med Wochenschr. 1956;86:590.
2. Lord RV, DeMeester SR, Peters JH, Hagen JA, Elyssnia D, Sheth CT, DeMeester TR. Hiatal hernia, lower esophageal sphincter incompetence, and effectiveness of Nissen fundoplication in the spectrum of gastroesophageal reflux disease. J Gastrointest Surg. 2009;13(4):602–10.
3. Rydberg L, Ruth M, Lundell L. Mechanism of action of the antireflux procedure. Br J Surg. 1999;86:405–10.
4. Engström C, Blomqvist A, Dalenbäck J, Lönroth H, Ruth M, Lundell L. Mechanical consequences of short gastric vessel division at the time of laparoscopic total fundoplication. J Gastrointest Surg. 2004;8:442–7.
5. Johansson F, Holloway RH, Irelande AC, et al. Effect on transient lower esophageal relaxations and gasreflux. Br J Surg. 1997;84:686–9.
6. Watson DI, Jamieson GG. Antireflux in the laparoscopic era. Br J Surg. 1998;85(9):173–84.
7. Mardani J, Lundell L, Engström C. Total and posterior fundoplication in the treatment of GERD. Results of a randomised trial after two decades of follow up. Ann Surg. 2011;253(5):875–8.
8. Swanstrom LL, Wayne R. Spectrum of gastrointestinal symptoms after laparoscopic fundoplication. Am J Surg. 1994;167(5):538–41.
9. Lin DC, Chun CL, Triadafilopoulos GD. Evaluation and management of patients with symptoms after anti-reflux surgery. 2013
10. Donahue PE, Samelson S, Nyhus LM, et al. The floppy Nissen fundoplication. Arch Surg. 1985;120:663–8.
11. DeMeester TR, Bonnavina L, Albertucci M. Nissen fundoplication for gastroesophageal reflux disease. An evaluation of primary repair in 100 consecutive patients. Ann Surg. 1986;204:9–20.
12. Chrysos E, Tsiaoussis J, Athanasakis E, Zoras O, Vassilakis JS, Xynos E. Laparoscopic vs open approach for Nissen fundoplication. A comparative study. Surg Endosc. 2002;16(12):1679–84.
13. Luostarinen MES, Isolauri JO. Surgical experience improves the long-term results of Nissen fundoplication. Scand J Gastroenterol. 1999;34:117–20.
14. Morino M, Pellegrino L, Giaccone C, Garrone C, Rebecchi F. Randomized clinical trial of robot-assisted versus laparoscopic Nissen fundoplication. Br J Surg. 2006;93(5):553–8.
15. Tekin K, Toydemir T, Yerdel MA. Is laparoscopic antireflux surgery safe and effective in obese patients? Surg Endosc. 2012;26(1):86–95.
16. Campos GM, Peters JH, DeMeester TR, Oberg S, Crookes PF, Tan S, DeMeester SR, Hagen JA, Bremner CG. Multivariate analysis of factors predicting outcome after laparoscopic Nissen fundoplication. J Gastrointest Surg. 1999;3(3):292–300.
17. Lamb PJ, Myers JC, Jamieson GG, Thompson SK, Devitt PG, Watson DI. Long-term outcomes of revisional surgery following laparoscopic fundoplication. Br J Surg. 2009;96(4):391.
18. Salminen P, Gullichsen R, Ovaska J. Subjective results and symptomatic outcome after fundoplication revision. Scand J Gastroenterol. 2008;43(5):518–23.
19. Hungin APS, Modlin I. NERD: a new approach in managing reflux symptoms. Oxf J Med Family Pract. 2008;25(6):397–9.
20. Grande M, Sileri P, Attina' GM, Villa M, de Luca E, Ciano P, Ciangola CI, Cadeddu F. Nonerosive gastroesophageal reflux disease and mild degree of esophagitis: comparison of symptoms, endoscopic, manometric and Ph-metric atterns. World J Surg Oncol. 2012;10(1):84.
21. Broeders JA, Draaisma WA, Bredenoord AJ, Smout AJ, Broeders IA, Gooszen HG. Long-term Nissen fundoplication in non-erosive and erosive gastro-oesophageal reflux disease. Br J Surg. 2010;97(6):845–52.
22. Hong D, Swanstrom LL, Khajanchee YS, Pereira N, Hansen PD. Postoperative objective outcomes for upright, supine, and bipositional reflux disease following laparoscopic Nissen fundoplication. Arch Surg. 2004;139(8):848–52.
23. Long JD, Orlando RC. Nonerosive disease. Minerva Gastroenetrol Dietol. 2007;53(2):127–41.
24. Broeders JA, Draaisma WA, Bredenoord AJ, de Vries DR, Rijnhart-de Jong HG, Smout AJ, Gooszen HG. Oesophageal acid hypersensitivity is not a contraindication to Nissen fundoplication. Br J Surg. 2009;9:1023–30.
25. McDougall NI, Johnston BT, Kee F, Collins JS, McFarland RJ, Love AH. Natural history of reflux oesophagitis: a 10 year follow up of its effect on patient symptomatology and quality of life. Gut. 1996;38:481–6.
26. Fasas R, Fennerty B, Vakil N. Nonerosive reflux disease-current concepts and dilemmas. Am J Gastroenterol. Feb;96:303–14.
27. Wescher GJ, Glaser K, Wieschmeyer T, et al. Tailored antireflux surgery fo gastro oesophageal reflux disease: effectiveness and risk of postoperative dysphagia. Worl J Surg. 1997;21:605–10.
28. Alexiou C, Beggs D, Myers JC, et al. A tailored approach for gastro oesophageal reflux disease: the Nottingham experience. Eur J Cardiothorac Surg. 2000;17:389–95.
29. Baigre RJ, Watson DI, Myers JC, et al. Outcome of laparoscopic Nissen fundoplication in patients with disordered preoperative peristalsis. Gut. 1997;40:381–5.
30. Rydberg L, Ruth M, Abrahamson H, et al. Tailoring antireflux surgery: a randomized clinical trial. Worl J Surg. 1999;23:612–8.
31. Watson A. Update: total versus partial laparoscopic fundoplication. Dig Surg. 1998;15:172–80.

32. Strate U, Emmermann A, Fibbe C, Layer P, Zornig C. Laparoscopic fundoplication Nissen versus Toupet two years outcome of a prospective randomized clinical study of 200 patients regarding preoperative esophageal motility. Surg Endosc. 2008;22(1):21–30.

33. Rosetti M, Hell K. Fundoplication in the treatment of gastroesophageal reflux in hiatal hernia. World J Surg. 1977;1:439–44.

34. Lundell L, Abrahamsson H, Ruth M, Rydberg L, Lönroth H, Olbe L. Long-term results of a prospective randomised comparison of total fundic wrap (Nissen–Rossetti) or semifundoplication (Toupet) for gastro-esophageal reflux. Br J Surg. 1996;83:830–83.

35. Hagedorn C, Lönroth H, Rydberg L, et al. Long-term efficacy of total (Nissen–Rossetti) and posterior partial (Toupet) fundoplication: result of a randomized clinical trial. J Gastrointest Surg. 2002;6:540–5461.

36. Hunter JG, Swanstrom L, Waring JP. Dysphagia after laparoscopic antireflux surgery. The impact of operative technique. Ann Surg. 1996;224(1):51–7.

37. Swanstrom LL, Pennings JL. Laparoscopic control of short gastric vessels. J Am Coll Surg. 1995;181(4):347–51.

38. Engström C, Jamieson GG, Devitt PG, Watson DI. Meta-analysis of two randomised clinical trials to identify long-term symptoms after division of the short gastric vessels during Nissen fundoplication. Br J Surg. 2011;98:1063–7.

39. Soper NJ, Dunnegan D. Anatomic fundoplication failure after laparoscopic antireflux surgery. Ann Surg. 1999;229(5):669–76.

40. Chew CR, Jamieson GG, Devitt PG, Watson DI. Prospective randomized trial of laparoscopic Nissen fundoplication with anterior versus posterior hiatal repair: late outcomes. World J Surg. 2011;35(9):2038–44.

41. Lowham AS, Filipi CJ, Hinder RA, Swanstrom LL, Stalter K, dePaula A, Hunter JG, Buglewicz TG, Haake K. Mechanisms and avoidance of esophageal perforation by anesthesia personnel during laparoscopic foregut surgery. Surg Endosc. 1996;10(10):979–82.

42. Bochkarev V, Iqbal A, Lee YK, Vitamvas M, Oleynikov D. One hundred consecutive laparoscopic Nissen's without the use of a bougie. Am J Surg. 2007;194(6):866–70.

43. Patterson EJ, Herron DM, Hansen PD, Ramzi N, Standage BA, Swanström LL. Effect of an esophageal bougie on the incidence of dysphagia following Nissen fundoplication: a prospective, blinded, randomized clinical trial. Arch Surg. 2000;135(9):1055–61. discussion 1061–2.

44. Jarral OA, Athanasiou T, Hanna GB, Zacharakis E. Is an intraoesophageal bougie of use during Nissen fundoplication? Interact Cardiovasc Thorac Surg. 2012;14(6):828–33.

45. Tsimogiannis KE, Pappas-Gogos GK, Benetatos N, Tsironis D, Farantos C, Tsimoyiannis EC. Laparoscopic Nissen fundoplication combined with posterior gastropexy in surgical treatment of GERD. Surg Endosc. 2010;24(6):1303–9.

46. Attwood SE, Lundell L, Ell C, Galmiche JP, Hatlebakk J, Fiocca R, Lind T, Eklund S, Junghard O, LOTUS Trial Group. Standardization of surgical technique in antireflux surgery: the LOTUS Trial experience. World J Surg. 2008;32(6):995–8.

Posterior Partial Fundoplications: Indications and Technique

Michael Ujiki and Benjamin D. Shogan

Introduction

Troubled by the high incidence of dysphagia in patients undergoing the Lortat-Jacob or Nissen antireflux procedure, the French surgeon André Toupet started experimenting on cadavers [1]. In 1963, after practice on 1,000 cadavers, yet performing the procedure on only four living patients, Toupet published his original description of a partial posterior fundoplication (PPF) that now bears his name [2] (Fig. 10.1). Received with widespread criticism by the surgical community, Toupet would never again publish his technique in a scientific journal and would perform a mere 20 hiatal hernia operations in his surgical career [1].

Various types of partial fundoplications were described throughout the mid twentieth century, all having the goal of reducing postoperative dysphagia, gas bloat, and other side-effects which were common in patients having undergone a complete fundoplication. Initially, the partial wraps gained popularity more in the European countries, while the Nissen (complete 360° fundoplication) held international popularity. Although impossible to know exact numbers, it is generally thought that a Nissen procedure remains the most popular treatment for gastroesophageal reflux disease (GERD) worldwide with partial fundoplications as a primary antireflux surgery, being much less common. Most surgeons perform partial fundoplications only for specific indications such as for patients with severe esophageal motility disor-

ders or for achalasia following myotomy. However, there seems to be a trend in the literature suggesting that partial fundoplications are being performed for an expanded list of indications. In this chapter, we review the indications, technique, and outcomes for the PPF.

Indications

A comprehensive description of the indications for antireflux surgery appears elsewhere in this textbook, and a review of PPF versus other types of fundoplication in specific situations will be discussed later in this chapter. Briefly, as with other types of fundoplications, including the Nissen, PPF is indicated in patients with documented GERD or after reduction of a hiatal hernia (Table 10.1). Most surgeons give preference to a partial fundoplication over a complete wrap after a Heller myotomy performed for achalasia, or a myotomy and fundoplication after resection of an epiphrenic diverticulum. Additionally, patients whom have had a previous gastric resection or who have a tubular stomach may benefit from partial wraps due to lack of sufficient fundus to perform a full 360° wrap.

Patients with Esophageal Dysmotility

It is widely taught that partial fundoplication is superior to complete wraps in patients with severe esophageal dysmotility. To investigate, a surgical group in the UK stratified 127 reflux patients into effective and ineffective esophageal motility groups based on preoperative manometry, followed by randomization for either a Nissen or PPF [3]. At 1 year after surgery, patients who had a Nissen fundoplication had increased dysphagia scores and chest pain when eating compared to those who had a PPF. Interestingly, after the 1-year follow-up, they reported no difference in dysphagia, reflux related symptoms, or chest pain between the normal and abnormal motility patient groups, regardless of the type of fundoplication. Furthermore, they reported that there were

M. Ujiki, MD, FACS (✉)
Department of General Surgery, Minimally Invasive Surgery, NorthShore Center for Simulation and Innovation, NorthShore University HealthSystem, 2650 Ridge Avenue, NCSI Suite B665, Evanston, IL 60201, USA
e-mail: mujiki@northshore.org

B.D. Shogan, MD
Department of Surgery, General Surgery Resident, University of Chicago Medical Center, 5841 S. Maryland Avenue, Chicago, IL 60637, USA
e-mail: benjamin.shogan@uchospitals.edu

L.L. Swanstrom and C.M. Dunst (eds.), *Antireflux Surgery*, DOI 10.1007/978-1-4939-1749-5_10, © Springer New York 2015

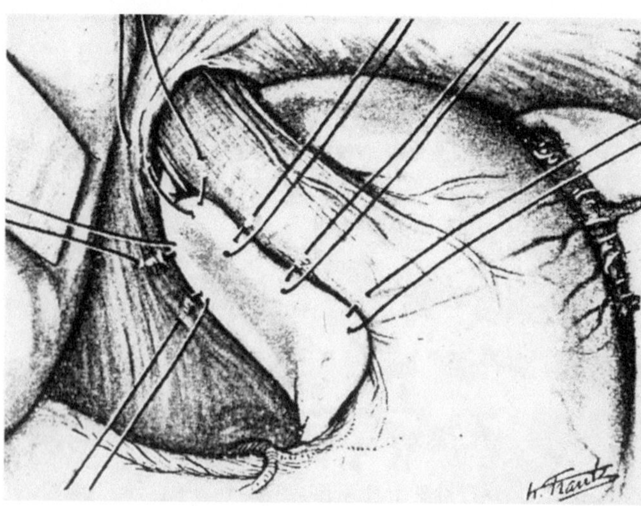

Fig. 10.1 Creation of Toupet fundoplication with key posterior gastropexy sutures and right fundoplication sutures to the esophagus. Left sided esophagopexy fundoplication sutures not shown

Table 10.1 Fundoplication indications

Indications for complete or partial fundoplication	GERD
	After reduction of hiatal hernia
Indications that favor partial fundoplication	Achalasia, after myotomy
	Epiphrenic diverticulum, after myotomy
	Previous gastric resection
	Tubular stomach

no significant differences in dysphagia rates between effective and ineffective motility groups who had a total fundoplication (28.6 vs. 16.7 %, p=0.361). Similarly, Shaw and colleagues conducted a randomized, prospective trial of 100 patients with 5-year follow-up, and reported that preoperative esophageal dysmotility had no influence over the outcome regardless of a complete or partial fundoplication [4]. Other randomized trials have demonstrated similar results [5–7]. Finally, Fein and Seyfried reviewed nine randomized trials comparing laparoscopic Nissen with various partial fundoplications. They concluded the preoperative non-specific esophageal motility disorders have no effect on the results of antireflux surgery no matter the type of fundoplication [8]. Although this goes against common surgical teaching, we conclude that the literature does not support an increased role of partial fundoplication in most cases of preoperative dysmotility ("tailored approach").

Surgical Technique

The common surgical goals of any fundoplication are to augment the lower esophageal sphincter with a gastric collar, restoration of the angle of His and the abdominal segment of

Table 10.2 Key steps in partial posterior fundoplication

Technique key points
Optimal laparoscopic position is supine with steep reverse Trendelenburg
Circumferential hiatal dissection in a clockwise fashion starting with the right crus and avoiding the vagus nerves to maximize intra-abdominal esophageal length
Fundoplication after division of short gastric vessels
Posterior and anterior gastropexy

esophagus, and repair of a hiatal hernia if present (Table 10.2). When performed correctly, the fundoplication patient will have limited dysphagia, minimal reflux symptoms, and permanent repair. Many variations have been described since Toupet's original description of an 180° posterior wrap. This original wrap, which did not close the hiatus or mobilize the fundus, had a high failure rate both from wrap herniation and incomplete reflux control. The "Toupet" was subsequently modified to make it more permanent and a better reflux barrier. Major variations included increasing the degree of fundic wrap and closing the hiatus to prevent mediastinal migration. Today the most common type of partial posterior wrap is a 270° to 340° wrap with posterior hiatal closure, which will be described below [9].

Open Verses Laparoscopic

Minimally invasive surgery has been described as the greatest surgical advance of the last century. Due to difficult hiatal exposure during a laparotomy, gastric fundoplication was an early candidate to benefit from laparoscopy. Since its introduction by Dallemagne et al. in 1991, the question of the safety and efficacy of laparoscopic fundoplication has been irrefutably answered. To date, at least 19 trials comparing open verses laparoscopic fundoplication have been performed, 12 of which were randomized-controlled trials and recently compiled into a systematic review and meta-analysis. The results clearly showed that patients whom had undergone laparoscopic fundoplication were discharged from the hospital ~2.5 days earlier, returned to normal activity 8 days earlier, and had a 65 % reduction in the relative odds of postoperative complications compared with patients having undergone an open technique [10]. On follow-up, either by questionnaire or by pH monitor, both cohorts had a similar decrease in GERD symptomatology. Importantly, despite a decreased complication rate and equal treatment failure rate, the laparoscopic cohort had a significantly higher incidence of repeat surgery, perhaps reflecting the patient's willingness to undergo a better-tolerated operation rather than a higher absolute failure rate.

A few investigators have looked specifically at laparoscopic verses open PPF fundoplication [11]. In a prospective randomized trial of nearly 200 patients, a laparoscopic approach decreased hospital length of stay and overall complication rate, despite having a similarly decreased patient-assessed symptom score on 1 and 3-year follow-up. Dissimilar to the above-mentioned meta-analysis, however, there were no differences between reoperation rates, although for the open cohort, the indication was most commonly incisional hernia, while for the laparoscopic group it was for recurrent disease.

Taken together, the literature supports laparoscopic fundoplication as a safe and effective alternative to an open technique and we recommend it in the majority of patients. Remaining indications for performing an open fundoplication include inexperience with laparoscopy, intra-operative complications that are unable to be repaired using laparoscopic measures, and patient preference. Some authorities recommend an open technique when performing a reoperation after a previous fundoplication, especially if the original operation was performed in an open fashion. Others have reported good results using laparoscopy on reoperation and thus this question is best left up to the surgeon and dependent on their laparoscopic experience.

Laparoscopic PPF

Preparation begins prior to the day of surgery. Patients with a profound esophageal motility disorder, such as achalasia, should be placed on a clear liquid diet 24 h prior to surgery. Good communication with the anesthesiologist is important to avoid a potentially lethal aspiration event as most patients with GERD or poor esophageal motility are at high-risk for aspiration and therefore rapid sequence induction and intubation is recommended.

Patient Position

The patient is positioned on the operating room table in supine position. The patient's arms can either be tucked or outstretched to ~80° and secured on padded arm boards. We prefer to abduct the legs on flat-padded split leg boards to minimize the possibility of neurovascular injury. The patient should be well secured in order to achieve steep reverse trendelenburg, which will help in displacing organs from the hiatus. The surgeon can either stand between the patient's legs, or on the patient's left depending on preference. When only one assistant is available, we find that it is best for the surgeon to stand on the patient's left with the first assistant in between the patient's legs (Fig. 10.2).

Laparoscopic Port Sites

The initial port site is placed 12 cm below the xiphoid process and 2.5 cm to the left of the midline using either an open or closed technique of entry as per surgeon preference (Fig. 10.3). It is important that this port not be placed too inferior or the mediastinum may be difficult to visualize. This initial port is typically a 10–12 mm for entry of a 10 mm

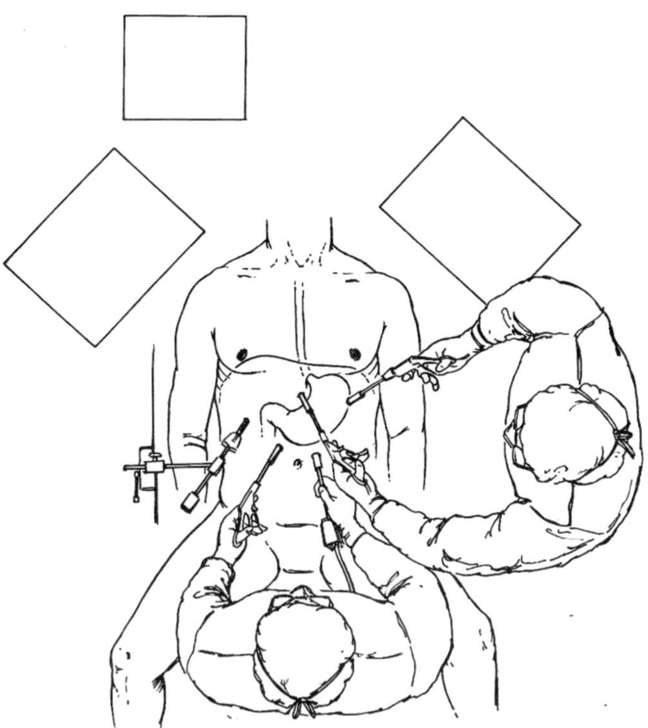

Fig. 10.2 Laparoscopic positioning

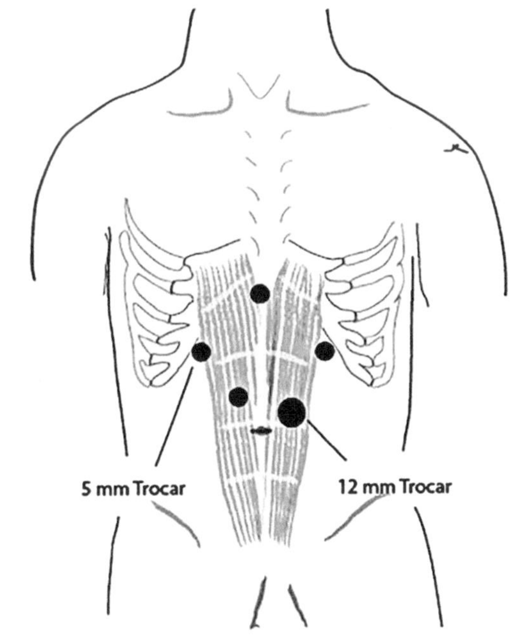

Fig. 10.3 Laparoscopic port site positioning

30–45° laparoscope. We prefer a 10 mm scope for optimal visualization. After entry, the abdomen is explored looking for iatrogenic injury and presence of intra-abdominal adhesions that would hinder subsequent port placement. A 5 mm port is then placed 15 cm from the xiphoid and 2–3 cm inferior

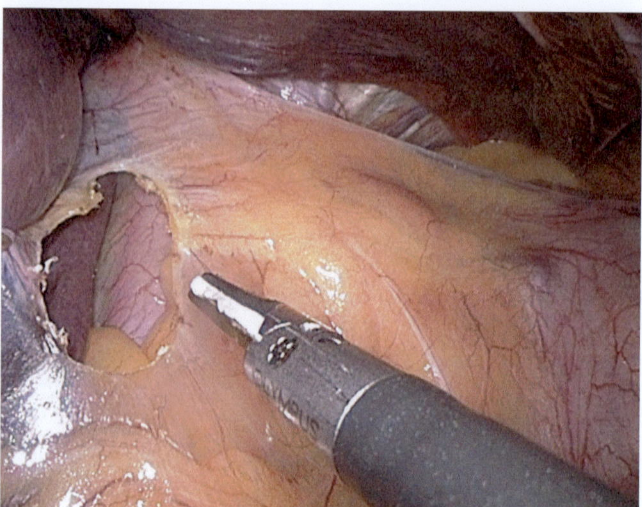

Fig. 10.4 Division of the gastrohepatic ligament

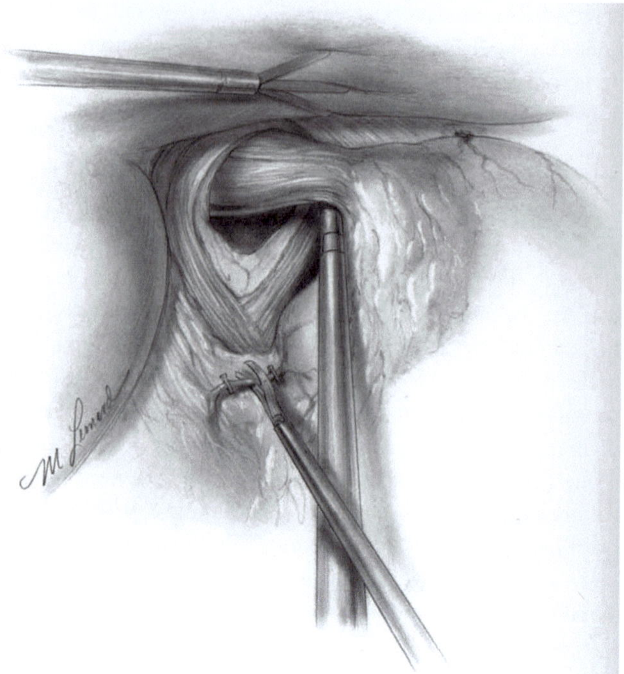

Fig. 10.5 Retrogastroesophageal junction dissection with sweep of vagus nerve anteriorly with the esophagus

to the right costal margin for the liver retractor. The left lobe of the liver is retracted anteriorly using the preferred liver retractor of the surgeon and secured to the operating room table. A 5 mm port is then placed between the first two ports and used by the assistant to retract for the surgeon. With the liver retracted, a 5 mm port is placed just inferior to the xiphoid and will serve as the surgeon's left hand. Lastly, a 5 mm port is placed 10 cm from the xiphoid and 3 cm below the left costal margin for the surgeon's right hand.

Hiatal Dissection

Using an atraumatic grasper, the assistant surgeon grasps the anterior epigastric fat pad and retracts the stomach downward and towards the left lower quadrant. The surgeon divides the hepatogastric ligament along the edge of the caudate lobe, preserving the nerve of Laterjet, and any aberrant left hepatic arteries if present, using ultrasonic or bipolar shears (Fig. 10.4). If a giant paraesophageal hernia is present, it is often better to gain access to the mediastinum anteriorly in order to avoid structures, such as the left gastric artery, that may be herniated just inside the right crus. The right anterior phrenoesophageal ligament and peritoneum overlying the anterior abdominal esophagus is fully divided staying superficial in order to avoid injury to the anterior vagus and esophagus. Careful mediastinal dissection is then performed by sweeping the esophagus away from the right crus. At this point, it is important to identify the posterior vagus and sweep it towards the esophagus, often best achieved by the surgeon retracting the right crus laterally with his or her left hand (Fig. 10.5). The left hand can then elevate the anterior crus and the mediastinal dissection is continued circumferentially in a clockwise fashion until the left and right crural limbs are freed anteriorly and posteriorly. This mediastinal dissection is performed with a combi-

nation of sharp and blunt dissection until 3–4 cm of tension-free intra-abdominal esophagus is freed. Meticulous attention is needed to avoid inadvertent vagal or esophageal injury. The hiatus is then closed posteriorly with interrupted permanent suture. Hiatal closure can be tight when repairing a large hiatal or paraesophageal hernia, or preferably somewhat lax when performing a fundoplication, particularly in a patient with a motility disorder such as achalasia.

Fundoplication

The short gastric vessels are ligated along the upper third of the gastric fundus (from the inferior pole of the spleen proximally, or approximately 10–15 cm inferior to the Angle of His) allowing free rotation of the gastric fundus without tension. A retroesophageal window is created and the posterior wall of the fundus is grasped and dragged behind the posterior vagus and posterior distal esophagus. A "shoeshine" maneuver is performed to confirm that no twisting of the esophagus is present (Fig. 10.6). If the fundus is grasped and pulled correctly, it should lie to the right of the esophagus without retracting back when let free. The assistant now grasps the gastric fundus retracting it towards midline, which in turn retracts the esophagus, exposing the posterior hiatus (Fig. 10.7). A posterior gastropexy is performed by suturing the posterior fundus to the inferior crus with one to three interrupted permanent sutures. A bougie is then placed carefully and under laparoscopic vision if desired. The size of the bougie will vary based on the diameter of the esophagus and

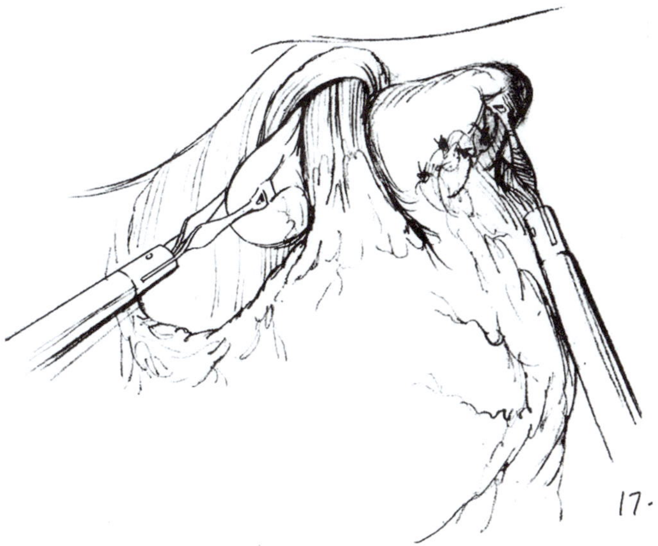

Fig. 10.6 "Shoe shine" maneuver

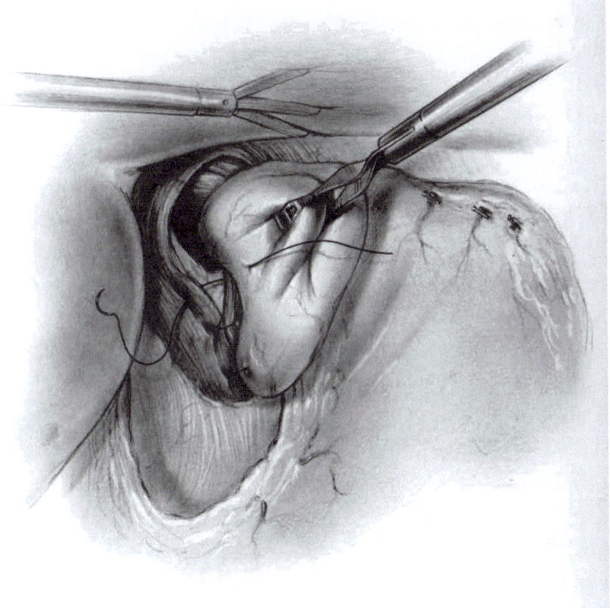

Fig. 10.7 Posterior gastropexy sutures with crural closure

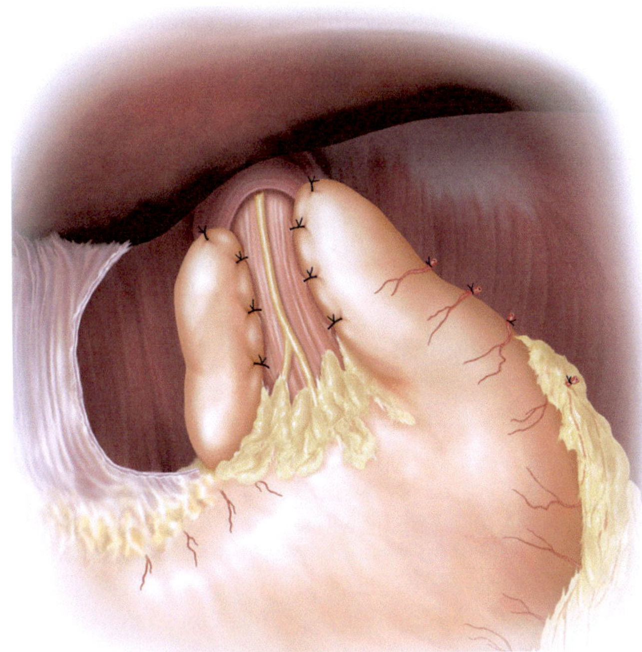

Fig. 10.8 Completed posterior partial fundoplication

Open PPF Technique

Patient Position

The patient is positioned on the operating room table in supine position, with their arms tucked. After intubation and induction of general anesthesia, a urinary catheter is placed and an upper midline incision is made from subxiphoid to supraumbilical. The surgeon may use any retraction system they prefer with the goal of optimal exposure by retraction of the xiphoid and inferior ribcage forward. As with any laparotomy, retraction is needed to separate the abdominal fascia and wound edges. Raising the head of the bed 20°–30° helps to cause the small intestine and omentum to fall inferiorly creating maximum hiatal exposure.

Technique

Hiatal dissection begins by retraction of the left lobe of the liver forward to expose the esophageal hiatus. At this point it may be necessary to divide the left triangular ligament of the liver. The phrenoesophageal ligament, comprising a superficial peritoneum and deeper fibrous layer is incised circumferentially around the esophagus to display the edges of the two hiatal pillars. Attention to detail is required during this dissection to prevent injury to the left and right vagal trunks that are found anteriorly and posteriorly respectively. Additionally, the surgeon must be meticulous during this dissection to avoid iatrogenic esophageal perforation.

When the distal esophagus is thoroughly freed from its surroundings, umbilical tape or a Penrose drain is placed behind and around the esophagus to retract it anteriorly

whether or not a myotomy has been performed; with a myotomy, we tend to use a smaller bougie (48–52Fr), whereas without a myotomy, a larger size bougie (54–60Fr) can be placed based on visual estimation of the patient's esophagus and degree of dysmotility or reflux. Two coronal stitches are placed at 10 and 2 o'clock securing the shoulders of the fundus to the diaphragmatic hiatus. Next, two to three interrupted sutures are placed from the esophagus to the left and right fundus (Fig. 10.8). If a myotomy has been performed, the edges of the fundus should be sutured to the muscle edges which will in turn splay the myotomy open.

exposing the posterior hiatus. The stomach is retracted inferiorly to expose 5–6 cm of distal esophagus. The open fundoplication is performed in a similar fashion to the laparoscopic technique (see previous).

In the original description, Toupet did not include a hiatal repair or closure, but if the hiatal orifice remains too large after the technique described above is performed, we recommend placing sutures across the hiatus to prevent slippage of the fundus.

Robotic Fundoplication

Robotic surgery is the newest commonly performed minimally invasive procedure and has been increasingly utilized in the urologic and gynecologic literature. Currently, no clear indications exist in general surgery for robotic surgery. The precise manipulations and improved dexterity afforded by the use of the robot have intrigued general surgeons and have been applied to a diverse range of operations ranging from pelvic dissections to thyroid surgery.

Due to the complexity of performing a laparoscopic fundoplication, this procedure is an easy target for a novel technique. In a pilot study of six patients undergoing robot-assisted laparoscopic PPF, Wykypiel and colleagues reported no intra-operative complications, and no reflux symptoms or dysphagia on 6-month follow-up [12]. Since this early experience, seven randomized trials have been performed comparing robotic versus laparoscopic fundoplication. A recent meta-analysis and systematic review of these randomized trials confirmed no significant difference between the robotic group and laparoscopic group for hospital stay, operative complications, postoperative dysphagia, or postoperative GERD symptom relief, although there was significant increase in operative time for those patients in the robotic cohort (weighted mean difference=4.15; 95 % CI=1.93–6.38; p<0.001) [13]. As the authors suggest, although these results are limited by small sample sizes and short follow-up, it appears that robotic surgery provides no additional benefit over laparoscopic surgery and is associated with increased operative time and cost.

Postoperative Management

After the operation is completed, the patient is brought to the recovery room, and then admitted to the surgical floor. Postoperatively, the patient takes nothing per mouth and is started on intravenous fluids and narcotics/anti-emetics as needed. For patients whom had undergone laparoscopic surgery their diet can usually be advanced later the day of surgery when post anesthesia nausea has resolved. Typically, the diet is advanced to a liquid diet for one meal, and then pureed diet for 2 weeks. We then advance from pureed to a soft diet for several days until returning to a general diet. Generally, laparoscopic patients are discharged on postoperative day 1, while patients having undergone an open technique require 2–3 more days of in-hospital recovery. We advise patients to avoid retching by taking anti-emetics at the first sign of nausea. Though most important in the first 6 months after surgery, we recommend life-long avoidance by pre-emptive antiemetic use.

Outcomes

Outcomes after PPF vary depending upon the indication. Here, we review the relevant outcome literature for the most common indications, and compare PPF to Nissen and Dor (partial anterior) fundoplication.

GERD

Patient outcomes after PPF for GERD are excellent. In both the short term and in up to 10-year follow-up, laparoscopic PPF significantly improved the quality of life and decreased GERD symptoms (heartburn and regurgitation), with only ~10 % reporting subjective recurrence of reflux exposure [14]. In an extremely long-term study, open PPF has shown to have successful control of GERD symptoms after two decades of follow-up [15]. Additionally, patients appear to be happy with their choice of undergoing surgery, with greater than 85 % reporting that they would have repeat surgery or recommend fundoplication to a friend [4, 16].

Complete or Partial

Nissen fundoplication has been extensively compared to PPF. Laparoscopic Nissen fundoplication (NF) is frequently cited as the most common operation performed for GERD. Despite generally excellent long-term outcomes with laparoscopic NF, severe or persistent dysphagia can occur in 3–43 % of patients, as well as bloating and early satiety [17–19]. These unwanted side-effects are likely due to the outflow resistance from a circumferential wrap and therefore partial wraps have been proposed to provide less long-term postoperative dysphagia due to the "hinge effect" of leaving a part of the esophagus uncovered while still maintaining similar GERD symptomatic relief. Early outcome comparisons between NF and PPF have failed to confirm this advantage and instead showed that PPF was associated with increased heartburn, increased use of protein pump inhibitors, and decreased quality of life scores [20–22]. Conversely, in a recent prospective trial, 100 patients were randomized to either laparoscopic NF or laparoscopic PPF. Despite an elevated average wrap pressure in the NF group (15.2 vs. 12.0 mmHg), there was no difference in the incidence of dysphagia, GERD symptom relief, or quality of life after an average follow-up of ~55 months [4]. Similarly, other prospective randomized trials showed equal improvement in postoperative quality of life and GERD symptomatic relief, although dysphagia and inability to belch were more common after NF [23, 24]. To provide a more definitive answer, recently two independent systematic reviews and meta-analysis have been performed [25, 26]. Both groups of authors concluded that laparoscopic PPF reduced postoperative dysphagia rates, reoperation rates, and prevalence of gas-related symptoms with similar patient satisfaction and reflux control compared to laparoscopic NF. The authors did comment that the low quality of some of the included randomized control trials might bias the reported results. Taken together we conclude, as others have, that laparoscopic PPF is a safe and viable alternative to laparoscopic NF with likely lower rates of adverse consequences and reoperation rates in select patients.

Anterior or Posterior

Comparison between partial anterior fundoplication (AF) and PPF has also been studied. In a randomized-controlled single institution trial, 95 patients were randomized to PPF and AF. After 1 year of follow-up, patients who had underwent a PPF had better control of GERD symptoms although they exhibited increased dysphagia and increased acid exposure than with an anterior wrap [27]. Similarly, in a different randomized clinical trial with longer follow-up (65 months), laparoscopic PPF continued to provide better reflux symptom control and decreased reoperation rates, and at 5 years did not come at the expense of increased dysphagia [28]. Very recently this subject was addressed by a systematic review and meta-analysis of all randomized control trials comparing AF, NF, and PPF [29]. After review of 11 trials, they found posterior fundoplication to be associated with increased GERD symptom relief and decreased reoperation rate compared to anterior wraps. In the short term, less severe dysphagia is seen in patients who undergo an anterior wrap, but dysphagia scores become equivalent in the long term. This study did not include a subgroup analysis of AF vs. PPF because of the results of the previous systematic reviews showing equivalent reflux control between complete posterior and partial posterior, and thus they ultimately conclude that of the three operations, posterior partial is the operation of choice for GERD.

Achalasia

Achalasia is characterized by failure of relaxation of the distal esophageal sphincter. Partial fundoplication has classically been used in the treatment of achalasia to rebuild the reflux barrier after esophageal myotomy. The role of fundoplication after myotomy continues to be debated with some investigations showing no patient benefit, while others show that adding a fundoplication decreases postoperative GERD

[30–32]. Recently, a systematic review and meta-analysis clearly showed the benefit of some type of a fundoplication after myotomy. This review of over 7,000 patients showed that laparoscopic myotomy in combination with fundoplication provided better symptom relief (90 %) than any other surgical technique, and significantly reduced the incidence of postoperative GERD (31.5 % without fundoplication versus 8.8 % with fundoplication, p=0.003) [33]. Given this benefit and in agreement with other groups, we recommend the routine use of fundoplication after myotomy [34, 35].

The optimal type of fundoplication to combine with myotomy is less clear and no consensus exists, but all types of surgical fundoplications have been proposed. It has been theorized that because there is aperistalsis of the distal esophagus in patients with achalasia, a complete fundoplication may impede esophageal emptying causing regurgitation and dysphagia. In a large, long-term randomized trial, Rebecchi and colleagues showed this to be true [36]. In their study, 138 patients were randomized to AF or NF fundoplication. After a mean follow-up of 152 months, they reported that the incidence of dysphagia was 15 % in the NF cohort, while it was 2.8 % in the AF, although control of reflux was equivalent (p<0.001). Other groups have confirmed an unacceptably high rate of postoperative dysphagia with a complete fundoplication [37, 38]. Despite some centers reporting adequate outcomes with NF, the general agreement is that partial fundoplications are superior to full fundoplication after myotomy [39, 40].

Few studies have compared AF to PPF after myotomy, although as outlined above, PPF appears to be the superior partial fundoplication for GERD. Very recently, in one of the only studies of its kind, this was studied during a multicenter, prospective, randomized trial [41]. Sixty patients were randomized to either AF or PPF and followed for 1 year. Dysphagia and regurgitation scores, as well as postoperative quality of life scores did not significantly differ between the two surgical procedures. Abnormal reflux was more present in the AF cohort (41.7 %) compared to the PPF cohort (21 %) but this difference failed to reach significance (p=0.152). Of note, the authors did caution interpretation of these results given the small sample size and significant amount of patients lost to follow-up. It should be noted that some groups recommend AF over PPF given less disruption of hiatal anatomy and coverage and reinforcement of the esophageal mucosa with the fundus, although there is limited evidence to confirm or refute this [41]. Together, given the current literature and lack of long-term outcome data, anterior or posterior partial fundoplication after myotomy is the surgeon's preference.

Epiphrenic Diverticulum

Epiphrenic diverticulum is a rare esophageal disorder characterized by out-pouchings of the distal 10 cm of esophagus.

Patients often present with dysphagia, odynophagia, chest pain, or regurgitation, although an increasing number of patients are diagnosed incidentally having undergone radiographic or endoscopic evaluation for a different indication. While there is agreement that operative intervention is indicated in the case of severe symptoms, some authors advise surgery in asymptomatic patients to avoid aspiration risk [42]. When surgery is performed, the technique remains up for debate and open, laparoscopic, transabdominal, and transthoracic approaches have been described. Most authors advocate the use of diverticulectomy and myotomy rather than diverticulectomy alone given the link between diverticula and primary spastic esophageal motility disorders [43, 44]. Unfortunately, there is no data comparing dysphagia and GERD in patients having undergone myotomy with and without fundoplication for epiphrenic diverticulum. In a retrospective review, similar to the achalasia literature, the addition of fundoplication was shown to be associated with decreased postoperative heartburn [45]. Different than for achalasia, the treatment of diverticulum requires diverticulotomy and thus creation of a distal esophageal suture line. Albeit only 13 patients were included in their study, Del Genio et al. [44] showed that the addition of a NF increased dysphagia and resulted in a 23.1 % leak rate, possibly due to the increased esophageal pressure that a NF creates. On the other hand, Klaus et al. [45] reported excellent symptom control and no leaks in patients having undergone a PPF. Similar results have been seen with an AF or Belsey Mark IV fundoplication [43]. Given the rarity of these diseases further studies will be needed to provide a definitive answer on the optimal type of fundoplication, but given the current literature it appears that either type of partial fundoplication is warranted.

Perioperative Complications

As with all surgical procedures, fundoplication is prone to postoperative complications. Fortunately the risk of catastrophic adverse consequences is low. As described by Greenstein and Hunter [46], postoperative events can be divided into early and late complications. Early complications are rare and include ileus (<5 %), pneumothorax (1–3 %), wrap herniation (<1 %), gastric or esophageal perforation (<1 %), hemorrhage (<1 %), wound infection (<0.5 %), and mortality (<0.2 %). Importantly, Tan and colleagues noted a significantly increased rate of postoperative complications in patients undergoing PPF when performing their systematic review and meta-analysis of all randomized-controlled trials comparing NF and PPF [26]. In most of the PPF arms of the 7 included randomized trials, there were commonly 1–3 patients who had a postoperative complication including hemorrhage, pneumothorax, or plural effusion, while the NF cohort commonly reported a lack of postoperative adverse events. In each of the individual studies the complication rate between the two groups did not reach significance, but when pooled for their meta-analysis the difference was significant. The authors hypothesized that because the distal esophagus has no serosal layer, suturing the fundus directly to esophagus and diaphragm during a PPF could increase the risk of perforation.

Late complications, including dysphagia, gas-related symptoms, and GERD symptoms are more frequent and may be related to the type of fundoplication as described earlier in the text. Presentation and management of the more serious complications are worth discussing in detail:

Perforation

Likely the most feared complication after esophageal or gastric surgery is perforation or anastomotic leak, as it is well known to be associated with increased morbidity and mortality. Perforation may occur at anytime during the dissection, during use of the bougie or endoscope, during suture plication of the fundus, or may appear late as a consequence of ischemia or electrocautery injury unrecognized intraoperatively. If perforation is found during the operation, it should be repaired primarily with coverage of the suture line with the gastric fundus when possible. We feel that the routine use of closed suction drains for this type of repair is unwarranted. A perforation or leakage from a suture line found postoperatively is more troubling and is usually diagnosed by fever, leukocytosis, and possible abdominal peritoneal signs, leading to imaging and demonstration of extravasation of contrast. In this situation, treatment can include reoperation in the case of an early leak, or endoscopic stenting, antibiotic therapy, and drainage in the case of leaks later than 24–48 h.

Herniation

Herniation can occur in the immediate postoperative period when the gastric fundus herniates through the hiatus. Fortunately, acute herniation is rare, thought to occur in <1 % of patients, and is characterized by epigastric pain and tachycardia, and confirmed by a contrast study. Early herniation requires immediate reoperation, reduction, and repeat crural closure. Late herniation, which occurs years or decades after the original operation, is addressed in other parts of this text.

Dysphagia

Dysphagia is one of the more frustrating complications after antireflux surgery. Symptoms of dysphagia such as regurgitation, inability to swallow, or the feeling of food getting stuck in the patient's throat, are common in the early postoperative period, but symptoms will only persist after the first few weeks in less than 10 % of patients [47]. In this early period, symptoms are thought to arise from esophageal or gastric edema and therefore patients are advised to eat small, soft, and frequent meals, which over time will resolve their symptoms. Fortunately, only 3 % of patients will report continued dysphagia after 6 months, and this incidence appears to be lower with PPF versus a complete NF [26]. As a guideline, patients who have persistent dysphagia for more then 6–12 weeks should undergo barium swallow to assess esophageal motility and wrap placement. In patients with continued dysphagia and abnormal passage of barium through the gastro-esophageal junction, we recommend endoscopic dilation with successive dilations as needed. With a PPF, to get to the point of dilation is rarely required, and when it is performed it is likely curative [48]. Patients with chronic dysphagia, severe symptoms, or symptoms arising from herniation may require reoperation.

Summary

Despite initial criticism when it was first presented in André Toupet in the early 1960s, the PPF has now gained widespread popularity. PPF is indicated in patients with documented GERD or after reduction of a hiatal hernia, and is favorable over complete fundoplication in patients who have undergone a myotomy for treatment of achalasia or epiphrenic diverticulum. Surprisingly, the literature does not support an increased role of partial fundoplication in cases of preoperative dysmotility. For all indications, outcomes after PPF are excellent with the majority of patients reporting increased quality of life, decreased reflux related symptoms, and minimal, if any, dysphagia. Finally, the advent of laparoscopic PPF has afforded patients a safe procedure with a shorter hospital stay.

References

1. Katkhouda N, Khalil MR, Manhas S, Grant S, Velmahos GC, Umbach TW, et al. André Toupet: surgeon technician par excellence. Ann Surg. 2002;235:591–9.
2. Toupet A. La technique d'oesophagoplastie avec phrenogastropexie appliquée dans la cure radicale des hernies hiatales et comme complément de l'opération de Heller dans les cardiospasmes. Mem Acad Chir. 1963;89:394–9.
3. Booth MI, Stratford J, Jones L, Dehn TC. Randomized clinical trial of laparoscopic total (Nissen) versus posterior partial (Toupet) fundoplication for gastro-oesophageal reflux disease based on preoperative oesophageal manometry. Br J Surg. 2008;95:57–63.
4. Shaw JM, Bornman PC, Callanan MD, Beckingham IJ, Metz DC. Long-term outcome of laparoscopic Nissen and laparoscopic Toupet fundoplication for gastroesophageal reflux disease: a prospective, randomized trial. Surg Endosc. 2010;24:924–32.
5. Broeders JA, Roks DJ, Ahmed Ali U, Draaisma WA, Smout AJ, Hazebroek EJ. Laparoscopic anterior versus posterior fundoplication for gastroesophageal reflux disease: systematic review and meta-analysis of randomized clinical trials. Ann Surg. 2011;254:39–47.
6. Chrysos E, Tsiaoussis J, Zoras OJ, Athanasakis E, Mantides A, Katsamouris A, et al. Laparoscopic surgery for gastroesophageal reflux disease patients with impaired esophageal peristalsis: total or partial fundoplication? J Am Coll Surg. 2003;197:8–15.
7. Rydberg L, Ruth M, Abrahamsson H, Lundell L. Tailoring antireflux surgery: a randomized clinical trial. World J Surg. 1999;23:612–8.
8. Fein M, Seyfried F. Is there a role for anything other than a Nissen's operation? J Gastrointest Surg. 2010;14:S67–74.
9. Swanström LL. Laparoscopic Toupet fundoplication. In: Patterson GA, Pearson FG, Cooper JD, Deslauriers J, Rice TW, Luketich JD, et al., editors. Pearsons thoracic and esophageal surgery. Philadelphia: Elsevier Health Sciences; 2008.
10. Peters MJ, Mukhtar A, Yunus RM, Khan S, Pappalardo J, Memon B, et al. Meta-analysis of randomized clinical trials comparing open and laparoscopic anti-reflux surgery. Am J Gastroenterol. 2009;104:1548–61.
11. Hakanson BS, Thor KB, Thorell A, Ljunggvist O. Open vs laparoscopic partial posterior fundoplication a prospective randomized trial. Surg Endosc. 2007;21:289–98.
12. Wykypiel H, Wetscher GJ, Klaus A, Schmid T, Gadenstaetter M, Bodner J, et al. Robot-assisted laparoscopic partial posterior fundoplication with the DaVinci system: initial experiences and technical aspects. Langenbecks Arch Surg. 2003;387:411–6.
13. Markar SR, Karthikesalingham AP, Hagen ME, Talamini M, Horgan S, Wagner OJ. Robotic vs laparoscopic Nissen fundoplication for gastro-oesophageal reflux disease: systematic review and meta-analysis. Int J Med Robot. 2010;6:125–31.
14. Kamolz T, Granderath FA, Bammer T, Wykypiel Jr H, Pointer R. "Floppy" Nissen vs. Toupet laparoscopic fundoplication: quality of life assessment in a 5-year follow-up (part 2). Endoscopy. 2002;34:917–22.
15. Mardani J, Lundell L, Engstrom C. Total or posterior partial fundoplication in the treatment of GERD: results of a randomized trial after 2 decades of follow-up. Ann Surg. 2011;253:875–8.
16. Sgromo B, Irvine LA, Cushieri A, Shimi SM. Long-term comparative outcome between laparoscopic total Nissen and Toupet fundoplication: symptomatic relief, patient satisfaction, and quality of life. Surg Endosc. 2008;22:1048–53.
17. Anvari M, Allen CJ. Prospective evaluation of dysphagia before and after laparoscopic Nissen fundoplication without routine division of short gastrics. Surg Laparosc Endosc. 1996;6:424–9.
18. Perdikis G, Hinder RA, Lund RJ, Raiser F, Katada N. Laparoscopic Nissen fundoplication: where do we stand? Surg Laparosc Endosc. 1997;7:17–21.
19. Sato K, Awad ZT, Filipi CJ, Selima MA, Cummings JE, Fenton SJ, et al. Causes of long-term dysphagia after laparoscopic Nissen fundoplication. JSLS. 2002;6:35–40.
20. Farrell TM, Archer SB, Galloway KD, Branum GD, Smith CD, Hunter JG. Heartburn is more likely to recur after Toupet fundoplication than Nissen fundoplication. Am Surg. 2000;66:229–36.
21. Fein M, Bueter M, Thalheimer A, Pachmayr V, Heimbucher J, Freys SM, et al. Ten-year outcome of laparoscopic antireflux surgery. J Gastrointest Surg. 2008;12:1893–9.
22. Fernando HC, Luketich JD, Christie NA, Ikramuddin S, Schauer PR. Outcomes of laparoscopic Toupet compared to laparoscopic Nissen fundoplication. Surg Endosc. 2002;16:905–8.
23. Broeders JA, Bredenoord AJ, Hazebroek EJ, Broeders IA, Gooszen HG, Smout AJ. Reflux and belching after 270 degrees versus 360 degree laparoscopic posterior fundoplication. Ann Surg. 2012;255:59–65.

24. Koch OO, Kaindlstorfer A, Antoniou SA, Asche KU, Granderath FA, Pointer R. Laparoscopic Nissen verses Toupet fundoplication: objective and subjective results of a prospective randomized trail. Surg Endosc. 2012;26:413–22.

25. Broeders JA, Broeders JL, Mauritz FA, Ahmed Ali U, Draaisma WA, Ruurda JP, et al. Systematic review and meta-analysis of laparoscopic Nissen (posterior total) verses Toupet (posterior partial) fundoplication for gastro-oesophageal reflux disease. Br J Surg. 2010;97:1318–30.

26. Tan G, Yang Z, Wang Z. Meta-analysis of laparoscopic total (Nissen) versus posterior (Toupet) fundoplication for gastroesophageal reflux disease based on randomized clinical trials. ANZ J Surg. 2011;81:246–52.

27. Hagedorn C, Jönson C, Lönroth H, Ruth M, Thune A, Lundell L. Efficacy of an anterior as compared to a posterior laparoscopic partial fundoplication. Results of a randomized controlled clinical trial. Ann Surg. 2003;238:189–96.

28. Engstrom C, Lönroth H, Mardani J, Lundell L. An anterior or posterior approach to partial fundoplication? Long term results of a randomized trial. World J Surg. 2007;31:1221–5.

29. Broeders JA, Sportel IG, Jamieson GG, Nijjar RS, Granchi N, Myers JC, et al. Impact of ineffective oesophageal motility and wrap type on dysphagia after laparoscopic fundoplication. Br J Surg. 2011;98:1414–21.

30. Burpee SE, Mamazza J, Schlachta CM, Bendavid Y, Klein L, Moloo H, et al. Objective analysis of gastroesophageal reflux after laparoscopic Heller myotomy: an antireflux procedure is required. Surg Endosc. 2005;19:9–14.

31. Lyass S, Thoman D, Steiner JP, Phillips E. Current status of an antireflux procedure in laparoscopic Heller myotomy. Surg Endosc. 2003;17:554–8.

32. Wang PC, Sharp KW, Holzman MD, Clements RH, Holcomb GW, Richards WO. The outcome of laparoscopic Heller myotomy without antireflux procedure in patients with achalasia. Am Surg. 1998;64:515–20.

33. Campos GM, Vittinghoff E, Rabl C, Takata M, Gadenstatter M, Lin F, et al. Endoscopic and surgical treatments for achalasia: a systematic review and meta-analysis. Ann Surg. 2009;249:45–57.

34. Eckardt AJ, Eckardt VF. Current clinical approaches to achalasia. WJG. 2009;15:3969–75.

35. Stefanidis D, Richardson W, Farrell TM, Kohn GP, Augenstein V, Fanelli RD. SAGES guidelines for the surgical treatment of esophageal achalasia. Surg Endosc. 2012;26:296–311.

36. Rebecchi F, Giaconne C, Farinella E, Campaci R, Morino M. Randomized controlled trial of laparoscopic Heller Myotomy plus Dor Fundoplication versus Nissen Fundoplication for achalasia: long-term results. Ann Surg. 2008;248:1023–30.

37. Topart P, Deschamps C, Taillefer P, Duranceau A. Longterm effect of total fundoplication on the myotomized esophagus. Ann Thorac Surg. 1992;54:1046–51.

38. Chen LQ, Chugtai T, Sideris L, Nastos D, Taillefer R, Ferraro P, et al. Long-term effects of myotomy and partial fundoplication for esophageal achalasia. Dis Esophagus. 2002;15:171–9.

39. Falkenback D, Johansson J, Oberg S, Kjelin A, Wenner J, Zllling T, et al. Heller's esophagomyotomy with or without a 360 degrees floppy Nissen fundoplication for achalasia: long-term results from a prospective, randomized trial. Dis Esophagus. 2003;16:284–90.

40. Rossetti G, Brusciano L, Amato G, Maffettone V, Napolitano V, Russo G, et al. A total fundoplication is not an obstacle to esophageal emptying after Heller myotomy for achalasia: results of a long term follow-up. Ann Surg. 2005;241:614–21.

41. Rawling A, Soper NJ, Oelschlager B, Swanstrom L, Matthews BD, Pellegrini C, et al. Laparoscopic Dor versus Toupet fundoplication following Heller myotomy for achalasis: results of a multicenter, prospective, randomized-controlled trial. Surg Endosc. 2012;26:18–26.

42. Altorki N, Sunagawa M, Skinner D. Thoracic esophageal diverticula. Why is the operation necessary? J Thorac Cardiovasc Surg. 1993;105:260–4.

43. Nehra D, Lord RV, Demeester TR, Theisen J, Peters JH, Crookes P, et al. Physiologic basis for the treatment of epiphrenic diverticulum. Ann Surg. 2002;235:346–54.

44. Del Genio A, Rossetti G, Maffettone V, Renzi A, Brusciano L, Limongelli P, et al. Laparoscopic approach in the treatment of epiphrenic diverticula: long-term results. Surg Endosc. 2004;18:741–5.

45. Klaus A, Hinder RA, Swain J, Achem SR. Management of epiphrenic diverticula. J Gastrointest Surg. 2003;7:906–11.

46. Greenstein AJ, Hunter JG. Antireflux surgery in GERD. In: Tichansky DS, Morton J, Jones DB, editors. The SAGES manual of quality, outcomes, and patient safety. New York: Springer; 2012.

47. Wills VL, Hunt DR. Dysphagia after antireflux surgery. Br J Surg. 2001;88:486–99.

48. Almond LM, Wadley MS. A 5-year prospective review of posterior partial fundoplication in the management of gastroesophageal reflux disease. Int J Surg. 2010;8:239–42.

Anterior Partial Fundoplications: Indications and Technique

David I. Watson

Indications

Worldwide, the most common operation performed for the treatment of gastro-esophageal reflux disease remains the Nissen fundoplication. However, in some patients this procedure is followed by troublesome side effects, such as dysphagia, abdominal bloating, inability to belch, flatulence etc, and these can lead to the perception of a less than satisfactory outcome. Modifying a Nissen to a partial fundoplication is a strategy that can reduce the risk of these side effects. There are two competing approaches for construction of a partial fundoplication—anterior vs. posterior. When compared to Nissen fundoplication longer term follow-up within randomized controlled trials has demonstrated advantages for both of these approaches [1], although probably the lowest risk of side effects follows anterior partial fundoplication variants [2]. The placement of the gastric fundus behind the distal esophagus when constructing either a posterior partial or a Nissen fundoplication lifts the distal esophagus forward and angulates the gastro-esophageal junction which might contribute to post-fundoplication dysphagia, as well as other gas-related side effects. With anterior partial fundoplication the gastric fundus is placed in front of the esophagus, and the esophagus is not lifted forward or angulated, resulting in a more anatomically correct position.

Worldwide, the Dor fundoplication, a variant of the anterior partial fundoplication, is often added following cardiomyotomy for achalasia, in an attempt to minimize the risk of reflux following this procedure. With cardiomyotomy the lower esophageal sphincter is fully divided, and the body of the esophagus in patients with achalasia also lacks peristalsis. This is a highly refluxogenic situation. It is widely agreed that the use of an anterior partial fundoplication is appropri-

ate in these patients, and the reported clinical outcomes are generally good, with good antireflux efficacy. If an anterior fundoplication is effective in this difficult situation, it seems like it would make sense to consider wider application in the context of surgery for reflux, as an alternative to a Nissen fundoplication for example, which can minimize side effects but still achieve reflux control, would be desirable. Examples of high-risk situations where a partial fundoplication is already more widely used include patients with reflux and an aperistaltic esophagus, as well as difficult clinical situations such as reflux with atypical throat symptoms, and scenarios where the surgeon wants to control reflux but avoid adding any new post-fundoplication problems (emotionally "challenging" patients). Using an anterior partial fundoplication as a form gastropexy in patients undergoing repair of a large hiatus hernia, in whom the presenting symptoms are due to mechanical problems from the hernia, rather than gastro-esophageal reflux, also makes sense.

In the past, the absence of good long-term outcome studies led many surgeons to apply a selective approach to the use of partial fundoplications for the surgical treatment of gastro-esophageal reflux, with the Nissen fundoplication widely accepted as the "gold standard" and the expectation that partial wraps would have a compromised success rate. However, long-term outcome data at 10 or more years follow-up is now available, and this suggests overall success rates for partial wraps which are equivalent to Nissen fundoplication [3, 4]. This late follow-up data shows similar patient satisfaction with the overall outcome, but with a trade-off between the risk of recurrent reflux versus the risk of side effects. For anterior partial fundoplication, the supporting data is more robust for anterior 180° partial fundoplication [3, 5], than for anterior 90° partial fundoplication with some studies suggesting a higher rate of recurrent reflux following the latter approach [6, 7].

Hence, in clinical practice, there is now sufficient data to support the application of an anterior 180° partial fundoplication in most patients presenting for antireflux surgery. In patients with reflux and normal or relatively normal esopha-

D.I. Watson, MBBS, MD, FRACS (✉)
Flinders University, Department of Surgery, Flinders Medical Centre, Flinders Drive, Bedford Park, SA, Australia
e-mail: david.watson@flinders.edu.au

L.L. Swanstrom and C.M. Dunst (eds.), *Antireflux Surgery*,
DOI 10.1007/978-1-4939-1749-5_11, © Springer New York 2015

geal motility a discussion about the risks of side effects versus the risk of recurrent reflux following anterior 180° partial versus Nissen fundoplication is appropriate, and in my practice patients are encouraged to choose the type of fundoplication which best fits their expectations. Approximately 60 % choose an anterior 180° partial fundoplication. In addition, an anterior 180° partial fundoplication is always used for patients in whom the side effect profile needs to be minimized (scenarios described above). In patients with a large hiatus hernia, but no reflux symptoms, repair of the hernia rather than controlling reflux becomes the aim of surgery, I construct an anterior 90° partial fundoplication primarily to improve anchorage of the stomach within the abdomen, as minimization of the risk of side effects is particularly important in these patients.

Surgical Technique

When constructing an anterior partial fundoplication, the key steps are to reduce and repair any hiatal hernia, stabilize and maintain an adequate length of intra-abdominal esophagus, and create a stable flap valve by folding and anchoring the anterior fundus loosely across the front of the esophagus. Stabilization of the partial fundoplication requires anchorage to the more rigid diaphragmatic hiatus, and this new anatomical relationship needs to be stable for the long-term. To ensure this, adequately large bites of tissue must be taken with each suture—stomach, esophagus and hiatal rim. As the laparoscope magnifies the view, the tendency to be cautious and take superficial bites of all structures must be resisted. Full thickness sutures of the esophageal and gastric walls are rarely a problem, and adequate sutures ensure adequate anchorage of the fundoplication.

Hiatal Dissection and Repair

Laparoscopic port placement is as for any other laparoscopic antireflux procedure. Four ports and a Nathanson liver retractor are used for surgical access. Two 11 mm ports are placed, one supra-umbilically for the laparoscope, and the other just below the left costal margin in the mid-clavicular line as the main working port. Two 5 mm ports are also placed, one just below the right costal margin in the mid-clavicular line, and the other in the left flank. A separate 5 mm subxiphoid incision is used for the Nathanson liver retractor.

The hiatus is dissected to expose the hiatal rim and the intra-abdominal esophagus, and any associated hiatal hernia is fully reduced. My preference is to use a blunt dissection technique, supplemented by diathermy hook dissection as required. If dissection is maintained in the correct plane and the fascial coverings over the hiatal rim are preserved so that muscle fibers are not exposed, then dissection is virtually

bloodless. Troublesome bleeding indicates dissection in the wrong plane. If a very large hiatus hernia is present, the hiatal rim must be dissected first and the hernia sac removed fully from the chest before progressing to esophageal dissection.

The next step is dissection of the esophagus and the posterior hiatus. Care must be taken when dissecting behind the esophagus, as blind dissection or enthusiastic use of energy sources in this area can lead to perforation of the esophagus. The esophagus is encircled with a tape and retracted anteriorly and to the left, and dissection continues until both hiatal pillars are well displayed with the left pillar visible from behind the esophagus. The hiatus is then repaired posterior to the esophagus with interrupted non-absorbable sutures. Usually 1-3 sutures are sufficient. Care should be taken to avoid excessively narrowing the hiatus as this can cause post-operative dysphagia.

Construction of an Anterior 180° Partial Fundoplication

When constructing an anterior 180° partial fundoplication, the aim is to create a stable flap valve, and anchor the distal esophagus within the abdomen. This is done by suturing the gastric fundus to the distal esophagus and the right side of the hiatal rim. The short gastric blood vessels do not need to be divided. Before suturing, the correct piece of stomach for the construction of the partial wrap must be carefully selected (Figs. 11.1 and 11.2). When doing this, the assistant uses a grasper to retract the pericardial fat pad downwards into abdomen. This ensures that the gastro-esophageal junction and at least 4–5 cm of distal esophagus are fully reduced into

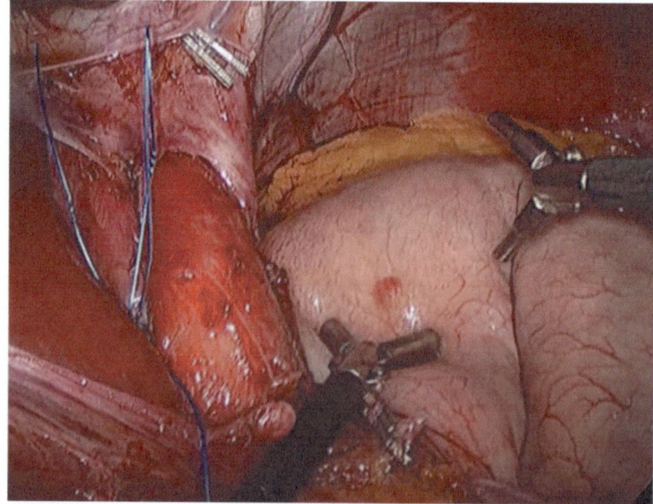

Fig. 11.1 Selection of the correct piece of anterior fundus for anterior 180° partial fundoplication. The assistant pulls the gastro-esophageal junction downwards. The correct piece of fundus is usually closer to the gastro-esophageal junction than the greater curve aspect of the fundus

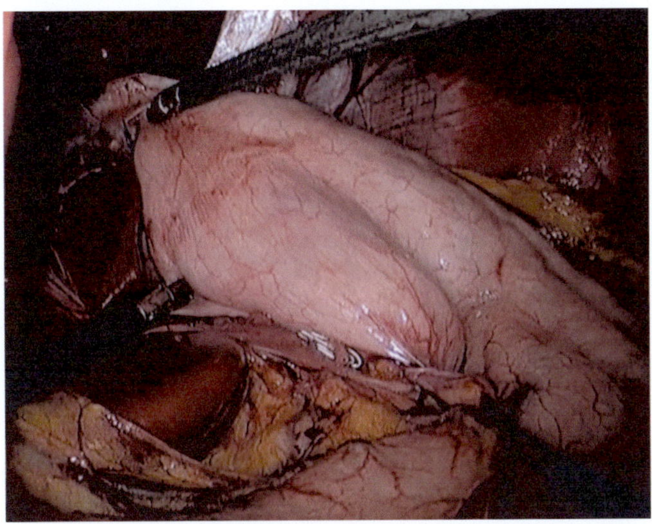

Fig. 11.2 The correct piece of anterior fundus is selected when it sits loosely across the anterior esophagus and hiatus

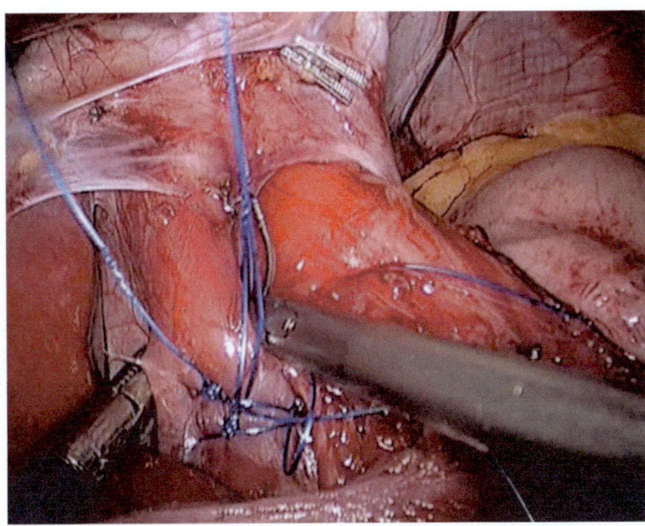

Fig. 11.4 The first suture also includes a generous bite of the right hiatal pillar at the level of the most anterior hiatal repair suture

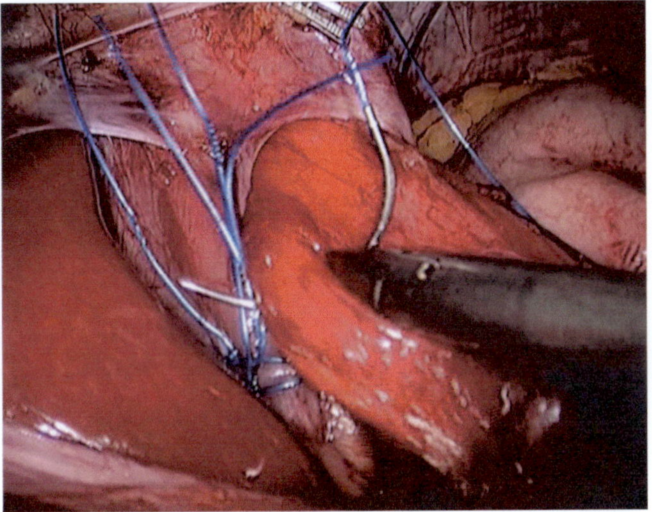

Fig. 11.3 The first suture includes the postero-lateral wall of the distal esophagus at least 2 cm proximal to the gastro-esophageal junction. To stabilize the anatomy a generous depth of tissue is included in this suture

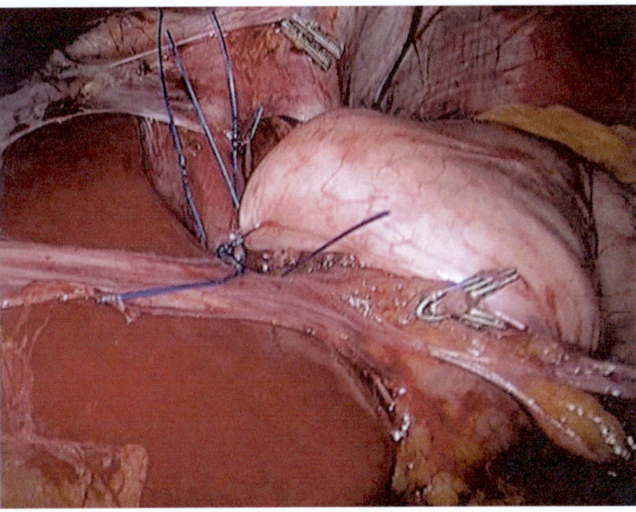

Fig. 11.5 The completed first suture anchors the anterior fundus to the right postero-lateral esophagus and the right hiatal pillar. When correctly placed this suture sets and guides the placement of the remaining sutures

the abdomen. Next, the upper part of the anterior gastric fundus is folded across the esophagus and manipulated until it sits loosely across the front of the esophagus and hiatus. This entails using the fundus approximately 1/4 to 1/3 of the way from the gastro-esophageal junction to the greater curve of the fundus, rather than the more lateral fundus, which is adjacent to insertion of the short gastric vessels.

The first fundoplication suture is critical as correct placement sets up the rest of the operation and ensures the anterior partial fundoplication is correctly constructed. This suture is placed through the gastric fundus, then the postero-lateral wall (7–8 o'clock position) of the distal esophagus at least

2 cm proximal to the gastro-esophageal junction (Fig. 11.3), and finally through the right hiatal pillar at approximately the same level as the most anterior hiatal repair suture (Figs. 11.4 and 11.5). Generous bites of the gastric and esophageal walls and the hiatal rim are included to ensure a stable fundoplication, and near full thickness bites (and perhaps occasionally actual full thickness bites) stabilize the anatomy long-term.

The second and third sutures are also placed through the gastric fundus, the distal esophagus, and the right hiatal pillar, with the second suture placed 5 mm above the first, and the third suture placed a further 5 mm proximally (Fig. 11.6). Two "crown" sutures are then placed to anchor the fundus to

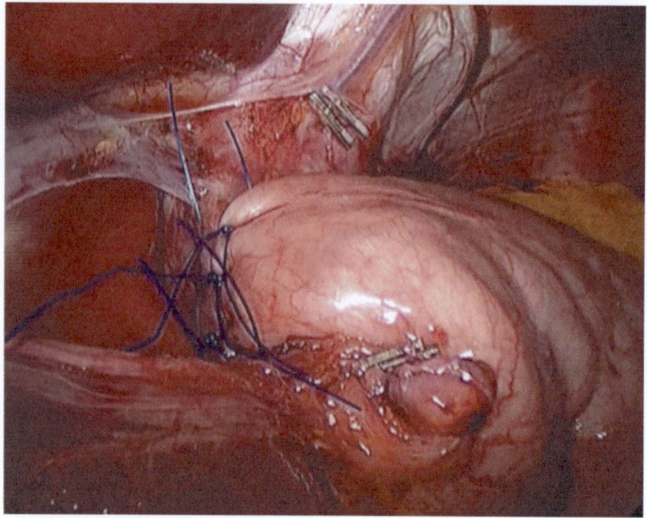

Fig. 11.6 The first three sutures all incorporate the fundus, the esophagus and the right hiatal pillar. They are placed approximately 5 mm apart and anchor the fundus loosely across the esophagus

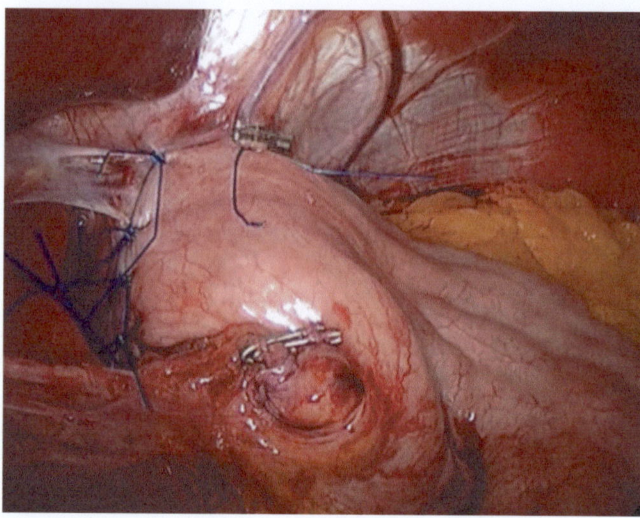

Fig. 11.8 The completed anterior 180° partial fundoplication

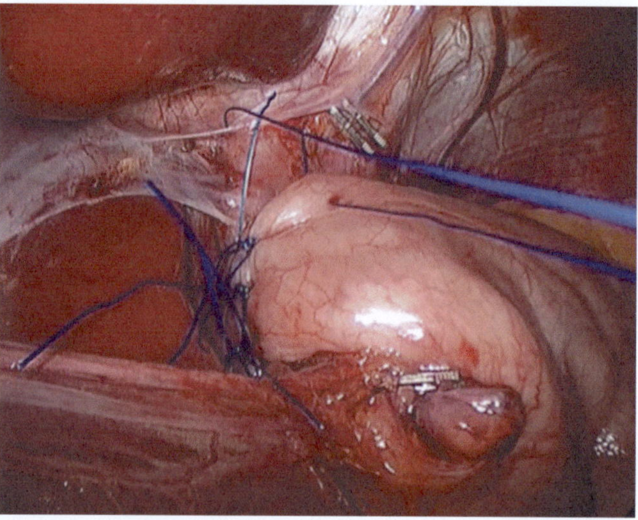

Fig. 11.7 The first "crown" suture attaches the fundus to the hiatal rim at the 11 o'clock position

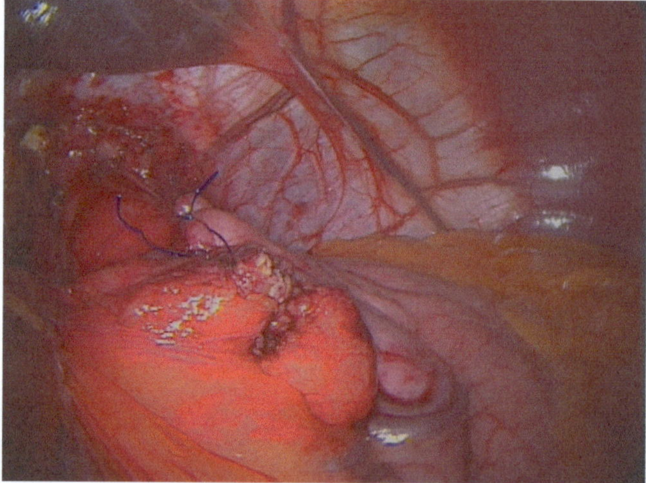

Fig. 11.9 When constructing an anterior 90° partial fundoplication, two sutures are placed to close the angle of His. The highest of these sutures incorporates the left side of the esophagus, the fundus and the left hiatal pillar

the diaphragm, closing the space across the anterior hiatus. The first of these sutures attaches the fundus to the hiatal rim at the 11 o'clock position (Fig. 11.7), and the second at the 1–2 o'clock position (Fig. 11.8). No sutures are needed on the left lateral side of the esophagus.

Construction of an Anterior 90° Partial Fundoplication

A somewhat different approach is used when constructing an anterior 90° partial fundoplication, although the aim is still to create a stable flap valve by anchoring the distal esophagus within the abdomen, and then the gastric fundus to the distal esophagus. However, the fundus is not sutured to the right hiatal rim during this procedure. The assistant still retracts the pericardial fat pad downwards into abdomen to reduce the gastro-esophageal junction and a length of distal esophagus into the abdomen.

The first suture attaches the right postero-lateral esophagus (7–8 o'clock position), at least 2 cm proximal to the gastro-esophageal junction, to the right hiatal pillar at the level of the most anterior hiatal repair suture. This attaches the esophagus to the hiatal rim—i.e., and esophagopexy. The next two sutures close the angle of His (Fig. 11.9). The gastric fundus immediately adjacent to left side of the distal esophagus is sutured to the distal esophagus. The first of these sutures attaches the left side of the esophagus (3 o'clock position,

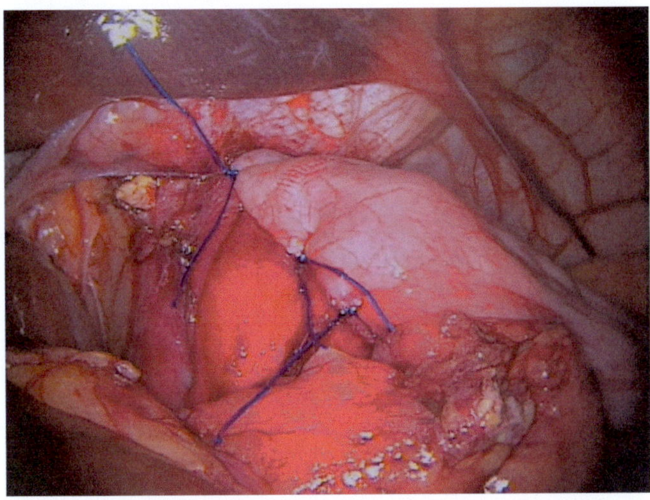

Fig. 11.10 After closing the angle of His, the gastric fundus is sutured to the anterior esophagus and to the anterior rim of the esophageal hiatus (11 o'clock position)

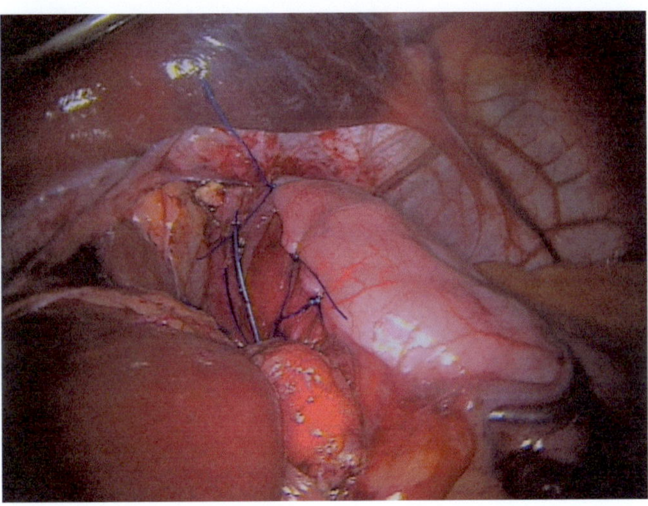

Fig. 11.11 The completed anterior 90° partial fundoplication

1–2 cm above the gastro-esophageal junction) to the gastric fundus. The second suture attaches the left side of the esophagus to the gastric fundus 1 cm proximal to the first suture, and also includes the left hiatal pillar at the 3 o'clock position. This creates a second point of anchorage to the hiatal rim.

Next the gastric fundus is rolled over the left anterior esophagus so that it sits loosely in place covering the left anterolateral aspect of the esophagus. The apex of this piece of fundus is sutured to the anterior esophagus (11–12 o'clock position) and to the anterior rim of the esophageal hiatus, at the 11 o'clock position (just to the right of the midline) (Fig. 11.10). This creates a third point of anchorage between the esophagus and the hiatal rim. The final suture is between the gastric fundus and the anterior esophagus 1 cm below the previous suture (Fig. 11.11). Again, generous bites of the gastric and esophageal walls, as well as the hiatal rim are needed to stabilize the fundoplication.

Results

The results from clinical trials as well as long-term follow-up of large prospective case series support the use of anterior partial fundoplication for the surgical treatment of gastro-esophageal reflux. Six randomized controlled trials have compared Nissen vs. anterior partial fundoplication. The first trial (from my unit) enrolled 107 patients to Nissen vs. anterior 180° partial fundoplication [5, 8, 9]. Early outcomes were reported in 1999, and at 6 months follow-up patients who underwent anterior 180° partial fundoplication had less dysphagia, were less troubled by flatus, were more likely to be able to belch normally and reported a better overall outcome [8]. A subsequent report of 5-year follow-up outcomes confirmed the early results [9], with significantly less dysphagia, less abdominal bloating, better preservation of belching, and a greater proportion of patients reporting a good overall outcome 5 years after the anterior 180° fundoplication, although this was offset by slightly better reflux control following Nissen fundoplication. At 10 years follow-up, however, the clinical outcomes for both procedures converged, and no clinically or statistically significant differences were demonstrable for Nissen vs. anterior 180° fundoplication at late follow-up [5].

Baigrie et al. [10] reported 2-year outcomes from a similar trial which enrolled 161 patients to Nissen vs. anterior 180° partial fundoplication, and showed equivalent control of reflux symptoms, and less dysphagia following anterior 180° partial fundoplication, although in this study re-operation for recurrent reflux was more common after anterior partial fundoplication. Cao et al. [11] reported 5-year outcomes from another trial that included 100 patients. Reflux control was similar for anterior 180° partial vs. Nissen fundoplication, and flatulence was less common after anterior fundoplication. Raue et al. [12] reported equivalent outcomes at 18 months follow-up in a smaller trial of 64 patients.

Two randomized trials, both coordinated from my unit, have compared laparoscopic anterior 90° partial vs. Nissen fundoplication. In the first, 112 patients were enrolled in a multicenter Australia and New Zealand trial [13]. Side effects were less common following anterior 90° fundoplication, but offset by a slightly higher incidence of recurrent reflux at early (6 months) follow-up. At 5 years outcomes were similar for side effects and overall satisfaction with the outcome, although reflux was more common after anterior 90° partial fundoplication [6]. Similar short-term outcomes, with less side effects, offset by more reflux, were reported from a parallel single-center randomized trial that enrolled 79 patients [14].

Two other randomized trials have compared anterior vs. posterior partial fundoplication. Hagedorn et al. [15] enrolled 95 patients to posterior (Toupet) vs. anterior 120° partial fundoplication, and showed better reflux control, but more side effects following posterior fundoplication. However, the clinical and objective outcomes following anterior 120°

fundoplication in this trial were significantly worse than the outcomes from other randomized studies, with the average 24 h pH monitoring acid (pH < 4) exposure time being 5.6 % following anterior 120° fundoplication. In other studies this figure has been approximately 2.5 % [8, 13], suggesting a problem with the surgical technique used for anterior 120° fundoplication in Hagedorn et al.'s study. Khan et al. [16] recently reported 6-month follow-up from a trial which enrolled 103 patients to anterior 180° vs. posterior partial fundoplication. Reflux control was also better after posterior fundoplication, but offset by more side effects.

Overall, the results from these randomized trials suggest that anterior partial fundoplication achieves satisfactory control of reflux, a reduced incidence of post-fundoplication dysphagia and other side effects, and a good overall clinical outcome. However, the reduced incidence of side effects is offset to some extent by a higher risk of recurrent reflux. More recently, we reported a much larger series of 548 patients who underwent anterior 180° partial fundoplication and were followed prospectively for up to 16 years [3]. Approximately 90 % of these patients were highly satisfied with their clinical outcome at very late follow-up, and these results compare favorably with late outcomes following Nissen fundoplication. Data from all these studies confirms that anterior partial fundoplication offers a valid alternative to other types of fundoplication and minimizes the risks of side effects. There is now sufficient data to support its acceptability as a surgical treatment of gastro-esophageal reflux.

References

1. Varin O, Velstra B, De Sutter S, Ceelen W. Total vs partial fundoplication in the treatment of gastroesophageal reflux disease: a meta-analysis. Arch Surg. 2009;144:273–8.
2. Broeders JA, Roks DJ, Ahmed Ali U, et al. Laparoscopic anterior versus posterior fundoplication for gastroesophageal reflux disease: systematic review and meta-analysis of randomized clinical trials. Ann Surg. 2011;254:39–47.
3. Chen Z, Thompson SK, Jamieson GG, et al. Anterior 180 degree partial fundoplication – a 16 year experience with 548 patients. J Am Coll Surg. 2011;212:827–34.
4. Mardani J, Lundell L, Engström C. Total or posterior partial fundoplication in the treatment of GERD: results of a randomized trial after 2 decades of follow-up. Ann Surg. 2011;253:875–8.
5. Cai W, Watson DI, Lally CJ, et al. Ten-year clinical outcome of a prospective randomized clinical trial of laparoscopic Nissen versus anterior 180° partial fundoplication. Br J Surg. 2008;95:1501–5.
6. Nijjar RS, Watson DI, Jamieson GG, et al. Five year follow-up of a multicentre double blind randomized clinical trial of laparoscopic Nissen vs. anterior 90° partial fundoplication. Arch Surg. 2010;145:552–7.
7. Shukri MJ, Watson DI, Lally CJ, et al. Laparoscopic anterior 90° fundoplication for reflux or large hiatus hernia. ANZ J Surg. 2008;78:123–7.
8. Watson DI, Jamieson GG, Pike GK, et al. Prospective randomized double blind trial between laparoscopic Nissen fundoplication and anterior partial fundoplication. Br J Surg. 1999;86:123–30.
9. Ludemann R, Watson DI, Game PA, et al. Laparoscopic total versus anterior 180° fundoplication – five year follow-up of a prospective randomized trial. Br J Surg. 2005;92:240–3.
10. Baigrie RJ, Cullis SN, Ndhluni AJ, et al. Randomized double-blind trial of laparoscopic Nissen fundoplication versus anterior partial fundoplication. Br J Surg. 2005;92:819–23.
11. Cao Z, Cai W, Qin M, et al. Randomized clinical trial of laparoscopic anterior 180° partial versus 360° Nissen fundoplication: 5-year results. Dis Esophagus. 2012;25:114–20.
12. Raue W, Ordemann J, Jacobi CA, et al. Nissen versus Dor fundoplication for treatment of gastroesophageal reflux disease: a blinded randomized clinical trial. Dig Surg. 2011;28:80–6.
13. Watson DI, Jamieson GG, Lally C, et al. Multicentre prospective double blind randomized trial of laparoscopic Nissen versus anterior 90 degree partial fundoplication. Arch Surg. 2004;139:1160–7.
14. Spence GM, Watson DI, Jamieson GG, et al. Single centre prospective randomized trial of laparoscopic Nissen versus anterior 90 degree partial fundoplication. J Gastrointest Surg. 2006;10:698–705.
15. Hagedorn C, Jonson C, Lonroth H, et al. Efficacy of an anterior as compared with a posterior laparoscopic partial fundoplication: results of a randomized, controlled clinical trial. Ann Surg. 2003;238:189–96.
16. Khan M, Smythe A, Globe J, et al. Randomized controlled trial of laparoscopic anterior versus posterior fundoplication for gastrooesophageal reflux disease. ANZ J Surg. 2010;80:500–15.

Nathan Conway and Lee L. Swanstrom

Incidence and Classification

In the world of antireflux surgery, there is gastroesophageal reflux disease (GERD)—often associated with an axial hiatal hernia—and there are paraesophageal hernias (PEH), representing a different entity altogether. PEH represent a condition where the esophageal hiatus of the diaphragm is sufficiently enlarged to allow for the migration of abdominal contents into the posterior mediastinum, most commonly the stomach. PEH are relatively rare, accounting for only approximately 5 % of the overall number of hiatal hernias, compared to the more typical axial hiatal hernia with an estimated incidence of 5 per 1,000 [1]. Despite the relative rarity of the disorder, surgical referrals for PEH are becoming increasingly common as the population ages as there are no "medical" solutions to this "mechanical" problem (Fig. 12.1).

Hiatal hernias are classified as five types based on the relative position of the gastroesophageal junction (GEJ) to the hiatus and the nature of the hernia contents. The most common is Type I, or sliding hiatal hernia, characterized by cephalad displacement of the GEJ into the mediastinum. These rarely have symptoms related to the mechanical aspects of the hernia. The remaining types are considered true PEH. The rarest is Type II hernias, characterized by cephalad displacement of the fundus through the hiatus while the GEJ remains in its normal position. Type III hiatal hernias have cephalad displacement of both the GEJ and fundus. A type IV hernia is a hiatal hernia containing another organ, such as colon, pancreas, spleen, etc. And finally, we have categorized patients with post fundoplication mediastinal herniation as "Type V" hernias (Fig. 12.2).

Etiology and Pathogenesis

A paraesophageal hernia occurs when there is anatomic disruption of the crural diaphragm with progressive migration of abdominal contents (primarily the gastric fundus) due to the pressure differential between the abdominal cavity and the chest. PEH is therefore primarily a disease of the diaphragm and the phrenoesophageal ligament as opposed to a disease of the GEJ or a result of reflux. The exact nature of the biologic defect and whether it is truly a problem with the diaphragm or the phrenoesophageal ligament (or both) is not well understood. There is published confirmation of structural differences in both the diaphragmatic muscle and the phrenoesophageal tissues with data demonstrating cellular and metabolic defects in elastin and collagen as well as distortion of metalloproteinase activity [2–4]. That PEH is a disease of the diaphragm and supportive structures are further corroborated by documented, and commonly clinically encountered, familial inheritance patterns [5].

As is common with any hernia, PEH comprises three components: the myofascial defect, the hernia sac, and the hernia contents. It is very rare for the hiatal defect to be small in primary PEH. Typically, there is a large defect with atrophy of the crural pillars. In extreme cases the defect can extend nearly to the vena cava and/or create a common opening with the aortic hiatus due to extreme effacement of the posterior crural decussation. The combination of a large horizontal defect, thin atrophic tissues, and probably an intrinsic connective tissue deficiency explain the difficulty of achieving a durable repair in PEH. Common to groin hernias, as the muscle defect enlarges, the circumferential suspensory "ligament" of the GEJ undergoes fatty degeneration and enlargement as it forms the hernia sac. The hernia sac in PEH is a complex structure and includes both an anterior and posterior component. The anterior sac is composed of the mediastinal portion of the phrenoesophageal ligament, a fibro-fatty connective tissue

N. Conway, MD
Department of Surgery, Group Health, 209 Martin Luther King Jr Way, Tacoma, WA 98405, USA
e-mail: conwaynate@gmail.com

L.L. Swanstrom, MD (✉)
Division of GI and MIS Surgery, The Oregon Clinic, Providence Portland Medical Center, 4805 SE Glisan St #6N60, Portland, OR 97213, USA
e-mail: lswanstrom@gmail.com

L.L. Swanstrom and C.M. Dunst (eds.), *Antireflux Surgery*,
DOI 10.1007/978-1-4939-1749-5_12, © Springer New York 2015

Fig. 12.1 Annual volumes of paraesophageal hernia operations in a single academic practice

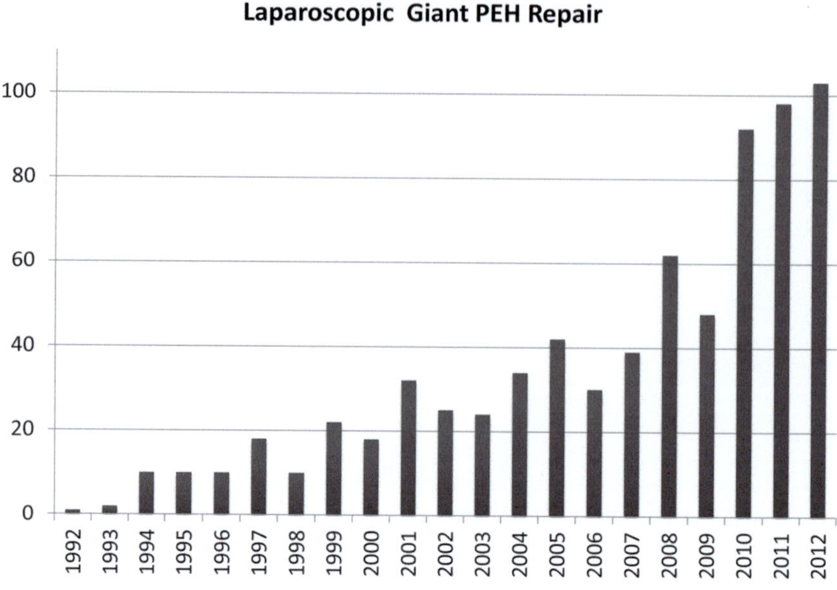

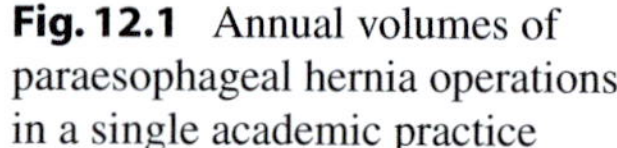

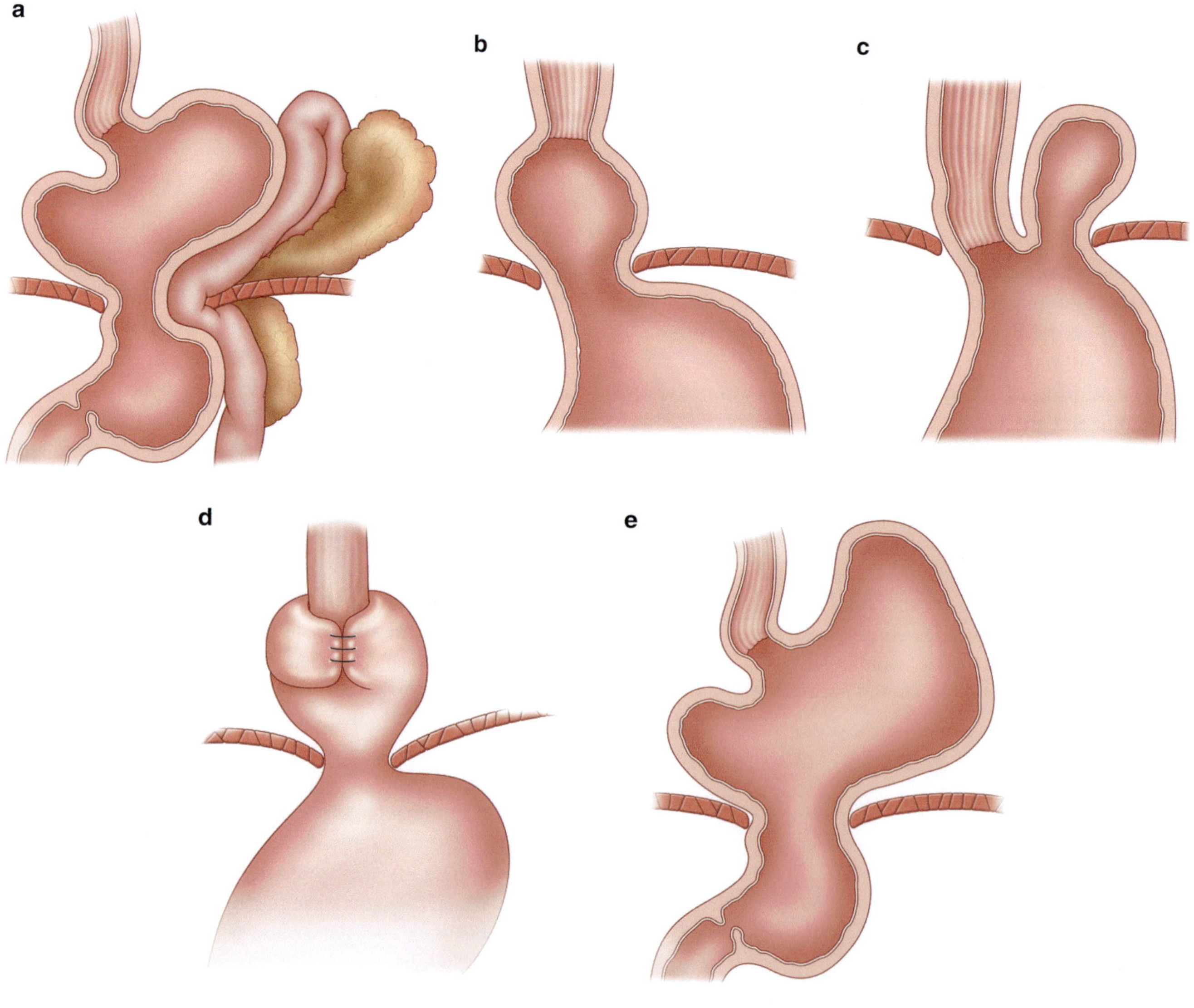

Fig. 12.2 Types of hiatal hernia: (**a**) Type 1 or sliding hernia, (**b**) Type 2 or true paraesophageal hernia, (**c**) Type 3 or complex or "giant" hiatal hernia, (**d**) Type 4 paraesophageal with other organs herniated, (**e**) Type 5, post surgical herniation

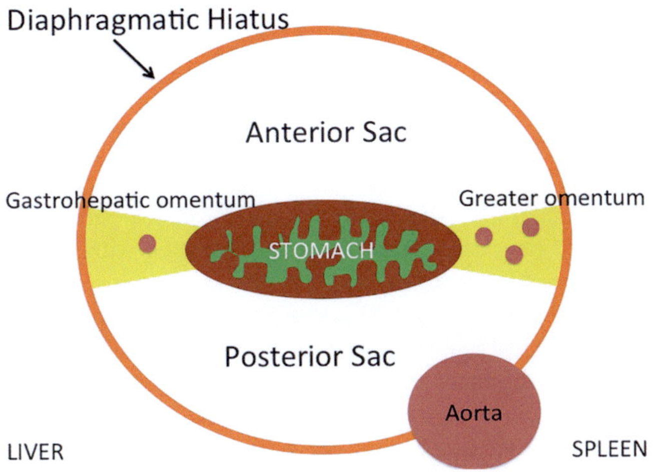

Fig. 12.3 The anatomy of the PEH is important to understand, especially the structure of the anterior and posterior hernia sack. The lateral fusion of these two hernia sacs incorporate the neurovascular supply of the lesser and greater gastric curve

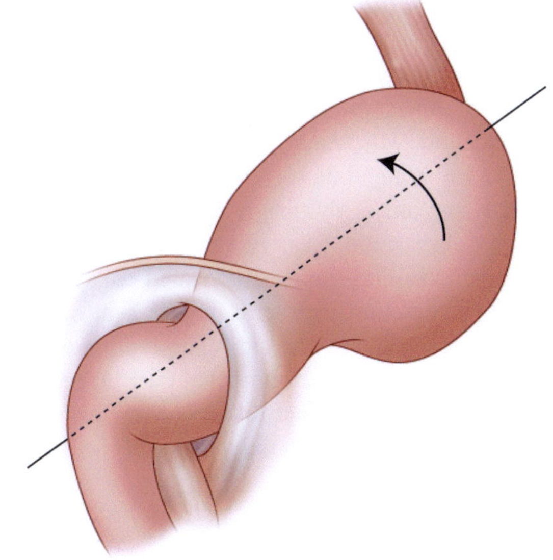

Fig. 12.4 Organoaxial volvulus

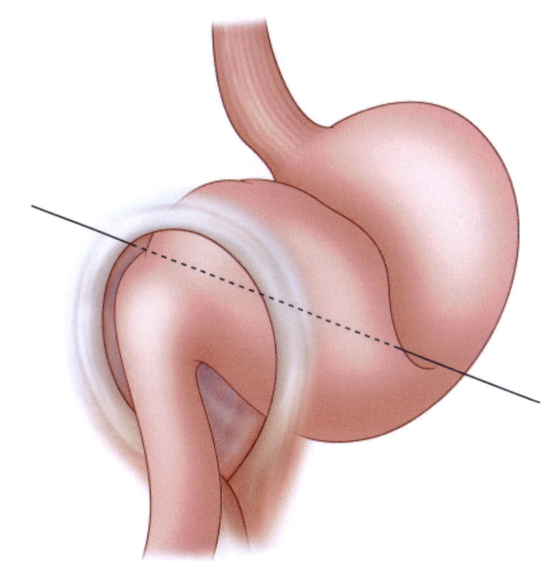

Fig. 12.5 Mesenteroaxial volvulus

layer, and the peritoneum of the abdominal cavity. The posterior sac is made of the same components but the peritoneal lining is the retroperitoneum of the lesser gastric sac. The lateral fusion of these two hernia sacs incorporates the neurovascular supply of the lesser and greater gastric curve (Fig. 12.3). The intrinsic laxity of the phrenoesophageal ligament and the other ligaments that hold the stomach in position (such as the gastrosplenic and gastrohepatic ligaments) result in mobility of the stomach, which, with the pressure differential between abdomen and chest, preferentially migrates into the mediastinum and thoracic spaces along with the degenerated ligament, forming an intrathoracic hernia sac. As the stomach herniates, the fundus may rotate around the long axis of the stomach toward the right creating the potential for an organoaxial volvulus (Fig. 12.4). Rotation around the short axis is called mesenteroaxial volvulous (Fig. 12.5) When very large, either of these rotations can result in the condition called "upside-down stomach". The herniated stomach can form adhesions in an intrathoracic position leading to incarceration and can also compress the herniated blood supply against the crura or even torse, both resulting in strangulation—a true surgical emergency [6].

Indications for Repair

PEH are frequently asymptomatic with an annual incidence of acute symptoms ranging from 0.7 to 7 % of patients [7]. Due to the potential for catastrophic, life-threatening complications, and the perceived increased risk of emergency surgery, traditional teaching has advocated repair of all identified PEH [8, 9]. However, more recent studies suggest that not all PEH mandate repair and that asymptomatic PEH can be managed expectantly and, in the surgically unfit, even delayed indefinitely [10, 11]. Sivho et al. found that need for emergency surgery was only 1.16 % per year, with a lifetime risk of 18 % at the age of 65 years. The mortality rate resulting from emergency repair of PEH is also only 2 % (compared to the historic rate of nearly 50 %) [8, 10, 12]. When emergency repair is attempted, the morbidity and mortality rates of early repair (17 and 3.4 %, respectively) are better than late repair (30 and 4.6 %, respectively), late being defined as occurring 1 or more days after presentation [13].

The presenting symptoms of PEH that indicate surgery can vary widely. Chest pain and shortness of breath, attributed both to mass effect with pulmonary or atrial compression, is a common but nonspecific symptom and underlying cardiac disease must be ruled out. Persistent or frequent non-cardiac chest pain is worrisome for incarceration and/or compromised blood flow which may lead to ulceration, bleeding, perforation, or strangulation. Another relatively common presenting symptom is dysphagia and/or vomiting due to gastric outlet obstruction. Giant PEH is frequently associated with chronic anemia—probably related to mechanical (Cameron's) ulcers. Lastly, patients may present with typical reflux symptoms of heartburn and regurgitation due to pre-existing GERD or to the development of GERD secondary to anatomic disruption of the antireflux barrier from the progressive migration of the GEJ into the chest [6].

Preoperative Evaluation

Upper Gastrointestinal Contrast Study

An upper gastrointestinal contrast study is a useful first test to evaluate patients presenting with symptoms of dysphagia or heartburn and the most important test in establishing the diagnosis when paraesophageal hernia is suggested on other studies, such as plain chest radiograph or computed tomography [14]. UGI studies are extremely valuable in delineating the anatomy of the hernia (size and type), ruling out gastric volvulus and obstruction, and for assessing for esophageal length and potential hernia reducibility (Fig. 12.6). UGI also can suggest the presence of an underlying motility disorder indicating further evaluation. Given a proper videoesophagram, functional outcomes following paraesophageal hernia repair can be predicted for those patients with esophageal dysmotility documented by manometry but who are able to clear a food bolus at contrast

esophagography [15]. Lastly, the UGI study is commonly used to evaluate recurrence of symptoms following repair.

Upper Endoscopy

Upper endoscopy should always be considered part of the extended physical exam of patients presenting with foregut problems. Its benefit in patients with known or suspected PEH is well recognized [16]. Examination will help identify the esophageal length, amount of herniated stomach, degree of gastric volvulus, and extent of venous engorgement [17] (Fig. 12.7). Furthermore, mucosal abnormalities can be identified, such as esophagitis, gastritis, erosions (Cameron's Ulcer's), Barrett's changes, or neoplasms [18].

pH Testing

Abnormal esophageal acid exposure may be present in up to 70 % of those with type III PEH [19]. For those selectively performing fundoplication with paraesophageal hernia repairs, pH testing is therefore necessary. Otherwise, we do not routinely obtain preoperative pH testing for known PEH, as it generally does not change the subsequent management (i.e., a fundoplication will routinely be added to the repair in all cases) [17, 20].

Esophageal Manometry

Though it is not universally required by all esophageal surgeons during the workup of PEH, esophageal manometry can still provide useful information and should be strongly considered. High-resolution manometry can

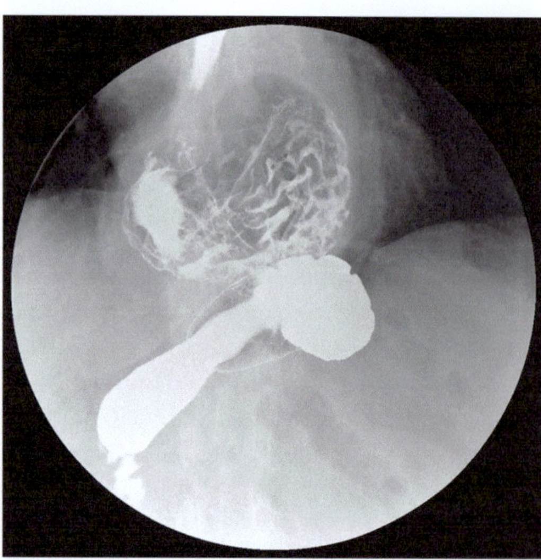

Fig. 12.6 Upper gastrointestinal contrast study demonstrating a giant paraesophageal hernia

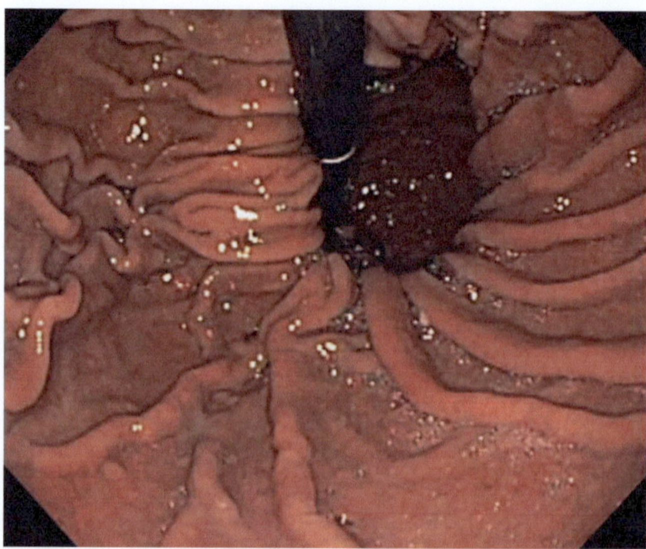

Fig. 12.7 Retroflex view of the hiatus on upper endoscopy showing a typical paraesophageal hernia

Fig. 12.8 (**a**) High-resolution manometry showing the classic "double hump" pattern created by separation of the LES and diaphragmatic hiatus in hiatal hernias. (**b**) Evidence of gastroesophageal junction outflow obstruction in PEH. This topography could be misinterpreted as simultaneous esophageal contractions with impaired LES relaxation especially in the absence of a "double hump" or other knowledge of the presence of a PEH

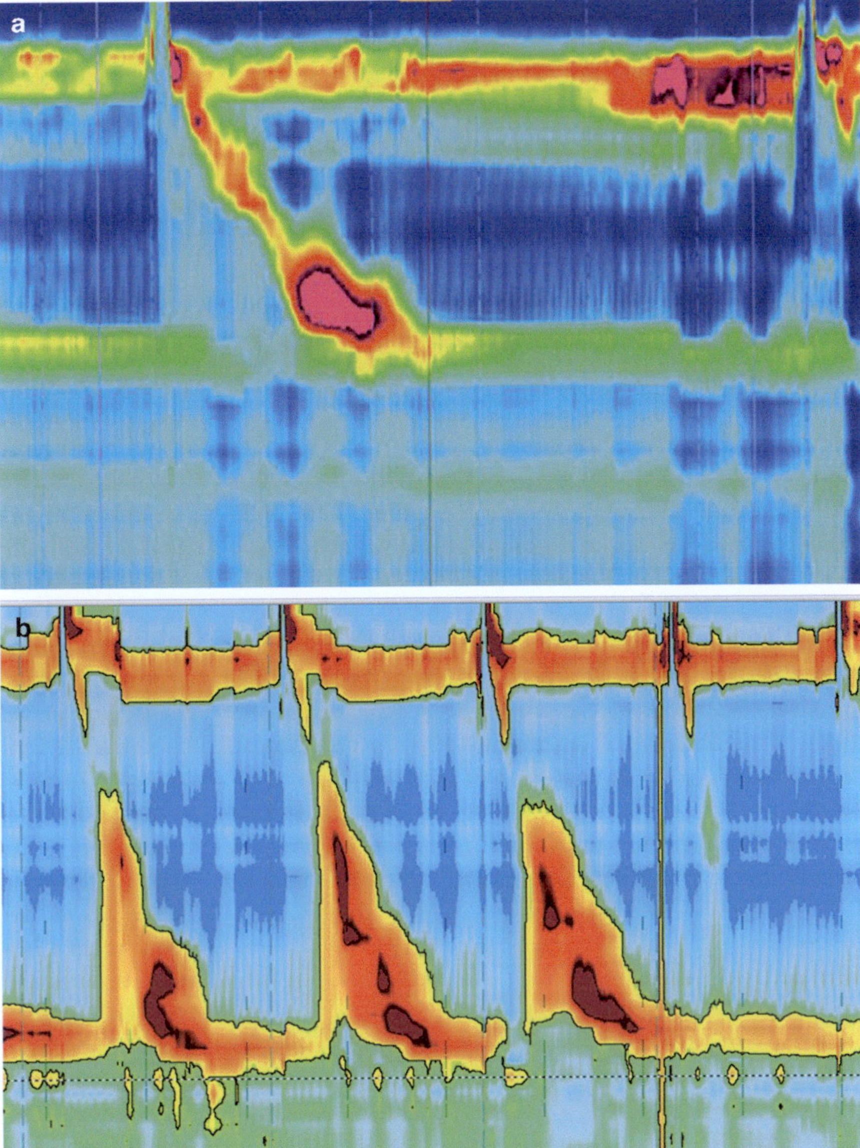

provide a very unique measurement or "map" of the hiatal hernia itself which can complement the sometimes vague information from endoscopy and X-ray studies. Presence of a large hiatal hernia does not exclude primary motility disorders like DES or even achalasia, and symptoms of dysphagia are as likely to be from dysmotility as they are from anatomic distortion. Identification of an underlying esophageal motility problem preoperatively can help guide patient expectations regarding potential persistent dysphagia despite hernia repair. Roman et al found that patients with large hiatal hernias overall had lower mean GEJ pressures, a lower distal contractile integral, slower contractile front velocity, and a shorter distal latency time [21].

Esophageal manometry in the paraesophageal hernia patient often poses unique challenges both with technically obtaining the study and with interpretation. The clas-

sic manometric finding suggestive of a hiatal hernia is the "double hump" pattern created by separation of the LES and diaphragmatic hiatus (Fig. 12.8a). However, not all manometries for PEH show a "double hump" either due to inability to pass the catheter out of the hernia and across the diaphragm or to a wide hiatus that it does not exert a measurable pressure reading on the catheter. It can be difficult to pass the catheter past the crural diaphragm in approximately half of the patients and therefore the presence of a large hiatal hernia may result in a technically imperfect study in as many as 57 % of cases [21, 22]. Evidence of GEJ outflow obstruction can also be seen in PEH due to the mass effect of the herniated stomach at the hiatus. This can lead to elevated integrated relaxation pressure (IRP) and intrabolus pressure (IBP) which may be misinterpreted as a poorly relaxing LES with simultaneous esophageal contractions (Fig. 12.8b).

Laparoscopic Operative Technique

Positioning

The patient is positioned in the supine position on a split-leg operating table with the arms outstretched and legs abducted. All pressure points are padded. The patient is secured to the table with leg and arm straps as steep reverse Trendelenburg position is used to facilitate hernia reduction and visualization of the upper abdominal cavity.

Access and Trocar Placement

After general endotracheal anesthesia is obtained, the abdomen is prepped and draped. Local anesthetic (0.25 % bupivacaine with epinephrine) is used prior to making incisions. Insufflation is obtained by the Veress needle technique in the left mid-abdomen, followed by a 10 mm dilating trocar. A 10 mm 45-degree laparoscope is inserted. The underlying intra-abdominal contents are inspected for injury and a brief survey of the surgical field is performed. The remaining trocars are placed under direct visualization with the laparoscope. In total, five ports are placed—a 10 mm one for the camera and the rest typically being 5 mm (Fig. 12.9). A liver retractor elevates the left lobe and is subsequently held by a table-mounted retractor holder allowing a more stable and less traumatic consistent exposure of the esophageal hiatus (Fig. 12.10).

Dissection

No attempt should be made to reduce the stomach (or other viscera) by direct traction as this is seldom successful and can easily cause traumatic injury as one is pulling directly against the pressure generated by the laparoscopic insufflator. The herniated stomach of a PEH is often fragile due to edema, relative devascularization, and chronic inflammation. A no touch technique will prevent grasper injuries. If the hiatal opening is packed tightly with omentum, an attempt can be made to gently reduce just the omentum but not the viscera. Dissection begins at the apex of the hiatus. The hernia sac is grasped anteriorly from within the mediastinum and everted. The hernia sac is grasped between two graspers and a small incision with an ultrasonic dissecting shear is made at the edge. This allows entry into the mediastinal space. Extra care and time should be taken during this part of the operation as identifying the correct plane is paramount to the rest of the dissection. This step should be bloodless—if not, the most likely problem is that the muscular diaphragm is being dissected and the surgeon should redirect the dissection appropriately (Fig. 12.11). Once the correct plane is identified, blunt dissection is used to sweep mediastinal tissues off the hernia sac and cautery or ultrasonic energy is used as needed to maintain a hemostatic field. It should be noted that there are several tissue planes in the mediastinum: peritoneum, retroperitoneum, mediastinal fascia, mediastinal pleura, and true pleura. If one is in the correct tissue plane—between the peritoneum/retroperitoneum and mediastinal fascial planes—it is relatively avascular and bleeding should be minimal. If one is having constant bleeding during the mediastinal dissection, it is an indication that one is too deep into the mediastinum.

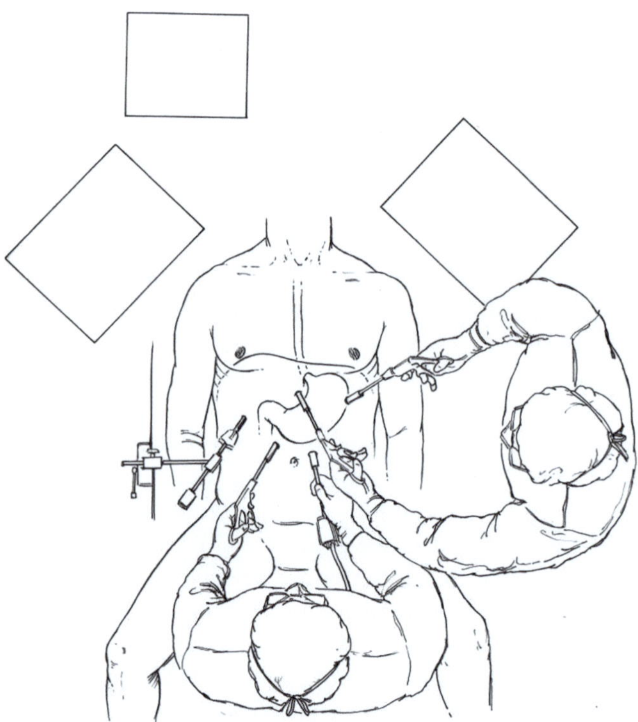

Fig. 12.9 Position of the patient and the laparoscopic ports for PEH repair

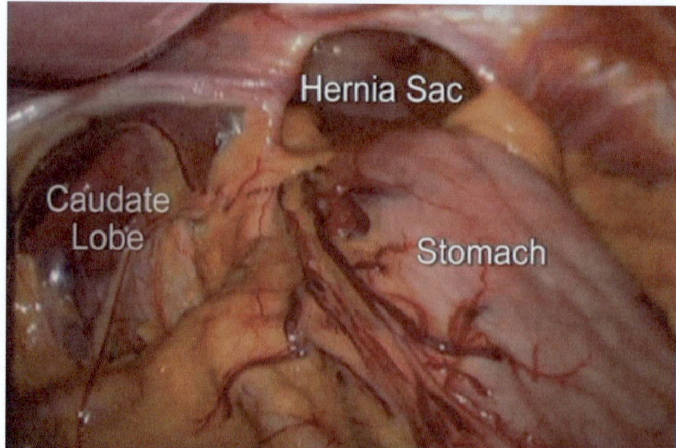

Fig. 12.10 Anatomy of the hiatus prior to dissection and reduction of the paraesophageal hernia

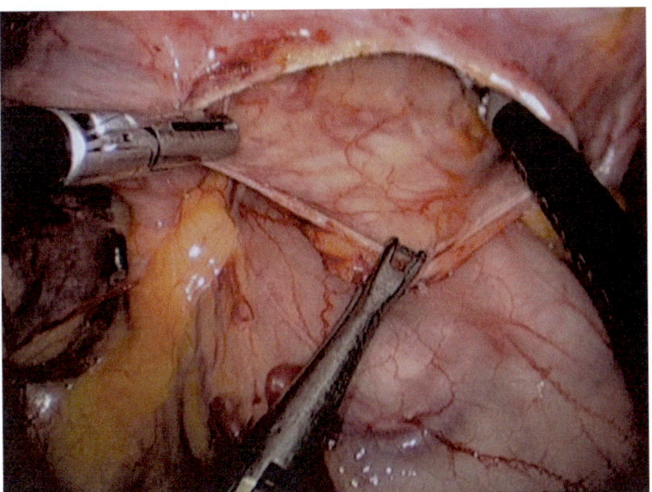

Fig. 12.11 Mobilization is focused on hernia sack dissection and starts with careful dissection at the hiatal apex to enter into the correct avascular plane

Using gentle caudal traction on the edge of the hernia sac and blunt/ultrasonic mobilization of the mediastinal portion, as well as circumferential division of the phrenoesophageal ligament from the hiatus, the hernia sac is reduced out of the mediastinum. This dissection should proceed first toward the left crus as the tissue planes along the right crus are more complex—usually including the herniated pars flacida and possibly the left gastric artery pedicle. It needs to be remembered that a type III hernia typically includes herniation of both the anterior sack (peritoneal cavity) and a posterior sack (the retroperitoneum or lesser sack), with the fusion plane between the two corresponding to the lesser and greater gastric curves and containing the short gastric vessels and lesser curve vasculature and vagus nerves (Fig. 12.3). After mobilizing the left side of the hernia and clearing the left crus (hopefully far enough posterior that the base of the right crus is seen), attention can be transferred to the right side. We recommend dividing the phrenoesophageal ligament about 1 cm from the edge of the crura to avoid denuding the crura of its peritoneal fascia since it is under tension and will retract after division. Once the left side is mobilized, the laparoscopic insufflation starts working for you as the positive pressure is now directed into the mediastinum and not inside the hernia sack, making it easier to invert and reduce the right side of the hernia sack, with all of its herniated vascular and vagal contents, and restoring a more normal anatomical picture. With the right hernia sack inverted into the abdomen by the assistant, mobilization of the right crus can then proceed by dividing the pars flacida along the caudate lobe which exposes the phrenoesophageal ligament, which can be dissected by continuing its division from the hiatal apex to its fusion posterior with the left crus.

Reduction of the hernia sack into the abdominal cavity effectively brings the stomach and GEJ into the abdomen without ever applying direct traction on the organ. An extended, or type II, mediastinal dissection is still typically required to enable adequate intra-abdominal esophageal length. This dissection can be carried high into the mediastinum, even to the level of the carina, to completely mobilize the distal esophagus and maximize intra-abdominal esophageal length. In 2–5 % of PEH cases, this extended dissection will not achieve adequate tension-free esophageal length; in which case a Collis lengthening procedure should be performed (see Chap. 19). The anterior and posterior vagus nerves should be identified early and preserved during the mobilization portion of the procedure. At this point or later, the upper gastric fundus is mobilized by dividing the short gastric arteries using bipolar or ultrasonic energy, starting at the watershed area just cephalad to the last arcade of the gastroepiploic artery usually near the lower pole of the spleen.

In most cases, a portion of the mediastinal hernia sack should be resected after the GEJ is fully reduced. This is both to better expose the anatomy of the GEJ and also because the fatty degenerated phrenoesophageal ligament that comprises the sack would be trapped between the esophagus and subsequent wrap. To resect it, the assistant can put traction on the right side of the sack, in the direction of the right lower quadrant which puts the anterior vagus on stretch making it easier to see. The left side of the sack is placed on stretch toward the left lower quadrant and the sack is divided from the gastric lesser curve caudally along (to the left of) the anterior vagus. It can then be dissected off the anterior stomach just past the greater curve and removed. One should avoid trying to completely excise the hernia sack as doing so would risk injury to the vagus nerves and even left gastric artery and the right side of the sack is not a problem for the subsequent repair. Once the left side of the GEJ is cleared, the intra-abdominal esophageal length can be reassessed and further mediastinal dissection is performed as needed to achieve at least 2–3 cm of intra-abdominal esophagus (Fig. 12.12). Intraoperative endoscopy is a useful adjunct at this point, to identify the esophagogastric junction and ensure adequate intra-abdominal esophageal length.

Diaphragm Repair

In differentiation from standard reflux disease, which is primarily a disorder of the lower esophageal sphincter mechanism, PEH is in fact a disease of the diaphragmatic hiatus. This makes the hiatal closure the most critical element of PEH treatment as well as the most tenuous. Due to its inherent need for a repair under tension, the typically thin and atrophic tissues and probably some genetic based connective tissue compromise, a simple primary closure will have a high failure rate. Likewise, a true tension-free repair using a bridging

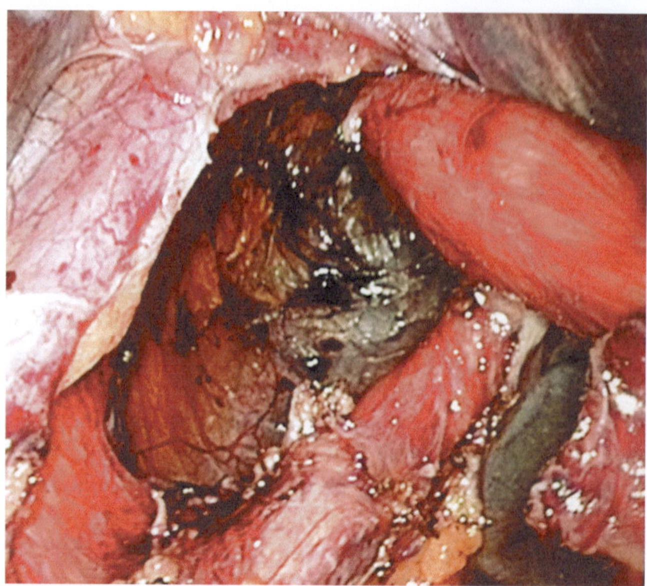

Fig. 12.12 Adequate length of the intraoperative esophagus should be determined

permanent mesh is discouraged as it results in too much unprotected mesh in contact with the constantly moving esophagus, increasing the risk of esophageal erosion. The most frequently used strategy is therefore, some sort of reinforced posterior repair. Reinforcement can be in the form of different suture patterns, the use of mesh, or both. Common reinforced suture patterns include simple figure-of-8, use of pledgets, or horizontal mattress sutures. Implantation of mesh to reinforce the diaphragmatic closure remains controversial. On one hand, permanent mesh has the lowest hernia recurrence rate in randomized studies [23]. Contrarily, erosions of permanent mesh into the esophagus can be a devastating complication [24, 25]. Biologic mesh has been shown to have a good safety profile and to improve short-term recurrence rates [26, 27]. Unfortunately it is very expensive and does not appear to improve long-term recurrence rates [28]. Because of the expense of biologics, and no definite long-term advantage, many surgeons reinforce their primary repair with a simple absorbable mesh [29]. Despite the controversies, mesh implantation is a frequently used technique for various indications. When used, mesh is usually placed as an overlay after the primary crural closure. Indications and techniques of mesh implantation at the esophageal hiatus are covered more in depth in the next chapter.

Antireflux Surgery

The majority of surgeons add a fundoplication following reduction of the hernia and hiatal repair. The rationale for this is multifactorial. First, a subset of PEH patients will have a defective antireflux barrier in addition to the hernia and will therefore benefit from an additional fundoplication. Second, the extensive hiatal dissection and requisite disruption of the phrenoesophageal ligament during PEH repair is thought to induce reflux if not accompanied by a fundoplication. Lastly, a fundoplication acts as a physical "bumper" to prevent recurrent herniation of the GEJ into the mediastinum although this has not been uniformly supported [30]. The adjunct of a fundoplication to PEH repair can be either a partial or complete wrap—a decision usually made based on clinical symptoms of concurrent reflux or dysphagia, esophageal function on manometry, or simply the surgeon's personal preference. The detailed techniques of various fundoplications are discussed in detail in other chapters. Upper endoscopy is then performed to assess the wrap. Lastly, a closed suction drain is left through the hiatus into the mediastinal dissection space at the conclusion of the operation in order to evacuate fluid and gas and collapse the dead space.

Postoperative Care

Anti-nausea medications are used liberally to avoid vomiting. Patients remain *nil per os* until an upper GI water soluble contrast study is performed on postoperative day one to rule out acute herniation. In our practice, drain amylase is checked daily. If both are normal, patients are progressed to liquids followed by a pureed diet as tolerated. The drain is removed just prior to discharge. Patients are typically discharged in 1–3 days. All medications are crushed or converted to liquid form until their diet progresses to regular consistency. Proton pump inhibitors are discontinued.

Follow-Up

Patients are discharged on a pureed diet for two weeks. Patients are seen in 3–4 weeks postoperatively and allowed to advance to a solid diet as tolerated. Routine pH and manometry and a barium esophagram are scheduled at 12 months postoperatively. Because of their high risk of recurrence, we have recommended follow-up every 3 years with a barium esophagram or endoscopy.

Results

Paraesophageal hernia repair has evolved from an open transthoracic operation to a predominantly laparoscopic procedure with the inherent benefits of minimally invasive surgery but PEH repair should not be considered simply a "big Nissen" operation. The underlying pathophysiology is fundamentally different with more complex anatomy, more

Table 12.1 Paraesophageal hernia outcomes

	Patients	Technique	Morbidity (%)	Mortality (%)
Allison [34]	95	Open	31	0.3
Pearson et al. [35]	53	Open TT	19	2
Swanstrom et al. [36]	52	Laparoscopic	12	0
Orringer et al. [37]	240	Open	~15	1.7
Low and Unger [38]	72	Open	23.6	0
Luketich et al. [39]	662	Laparoscopic	NR	1.7
Mittal et al. [40]	73	Mixed	35.6	1.4
Zehetner [41]	146	Mixed	25	0
Bhayani et al. [13]	224	Mixed	31	5

difficult dissections, and typically older patients. As a result the operations take longer (1–2 h for a typical lap Nissen vs 2–4 h for a PEH). Furthermore, "emergency" fundoplication surgery is virtually unheard of in comparison to PEH surgery, which carries an average mortality rate of 8–16 % compared to <1 % for elective repairs [31, 32]. The morbidity and mortality rates are minimal with a straightforward fundoplication compared to PEH repair (<1 vs 18 % and 18 %) (Table 12.1). Despite the risks, PEH repair significantly improves patients' quality of life [33].

When defined as a hiatal hernia > than 2 cm, recurrence rates are almost always reported to be higher following PEH repair. A meta-analysis done in 2007 showed a 25.5 % recurrence when measured by objective testing at a mean of 1 year [42]. When looking specifically at laparoscopic PEH repair, recurrence rates are about the same (Table **12.2**). Fortunately recurrences are mostly radiographic or endoscopy diagnoses and were seldom symptomatic. Reoperation for symptomatic recurrence is uniformly rare (<3 %). These facts are leading some to question whether the definition of >2 cm is clinically relevant or should be revised, though there are few studies that detail the natural history and outcomes of these small hernias over time.

Conclusions

PEH represent a condition where the esophageal hiatus of the diaphragm is sufficiently enlarged to allow for the migration of abdominal contents into the posterior mediastinum, most commonly the stomach. PEH is associated with varying degrees of compressive symptoms and/or torsion. Laparoscopic paraesophageal hernia repair is a technically difficult procedure that is best addressed by experienced specialists. By the nature of the disease, it will always have a tendency to recurrence—a problem that no one has totally resolved through technique or technical adjuncts. Still, PEH repair provides significant benefit to symptomatic patients by preventing complications and improving their quality of life.

Table 12.2 Recurrence rates after laparoscopic PEH repair

Series	Recurrence rate (%)
Swanstrom et al. [36]	8
Wu et al. [43]	23
Weichmann et al. [44]	7
Khaitan et al. [45]	40
Jobe et al. [46]	32
Mattar et al. [47]	33
Diaz et al. [48]	20
Targarona et al. [49]	20
Aly et al. [50]	30
Gangopadhyay et al. [51]	24
Lubezky et al. [52]	55
Zaninotto et al. [53]	20
Rathore et al. [54]	12
Luketich et al. [39]	16
Dallemagne et al. [55]	66
Oelschlager et al. [28]	54
	Mean = 30 %

References

1. Pierre AF, Luketich JD, Fernando HC, Christie NA, Buenaventura PO, Litle VR, Schauer PR. Results of laparoscopic repair of giant paraesophageal hernias: 200 consecutive patients. Ann Thorac Surg. 2002;74(6):1909–15.
2. Fei L, del Genio G, Rossetti G, Sampaolo S, Moccia F, Trapani V, Cimmino M, del Genio A. Hiatal hernia recurrence: surgical complication or disease? Electron microscope findings of the diaphragmatic pillars. J Gastrointest Surg. 2009;13(3):459–64.
3. Curci JA, Melman LM, Thompson RW, Soper NJ, Matthews BD. Elastic fiber depletion in the supporting ligaments of the gastroesophageal junction: a structural basis for the development of hiatal hernia. J Am Coll Surg. 2008;207(2):191–6.
4. Melman L, Chisholm PR, Curci JA, Arif B, Pierce R, Jenkins ED, Brunt LM, Eagon C, Frisella M, Miller K, Matthews BD. Differential regulation of MMP-2 in the gastrohepatic ligament of the gastroesophageal junction. Surg Endosc. 2010;24(7):1562–5.
5. Carré IJ, Johnston BT, Thomas PS, Morrison PJ. Familial hiatal hernia in a large five generation family confirming true autosomal dominant inheritance. Gut. 1999;45(5):649–52.

6. Oelschlager BK, Eubanks TR, Pellegrini CA. Hiatal hernia and gastroesophageal reflux disease. In: Townsend, et al (editors). Sabiston textbook of surgery. 18th ed. 2007.

7. Peters JH. Esophagus and diaphragmatic hernia. In: Brunicardi FC, et al. editors. Schwartz's principles of surgery, 9th ed. 2010.

8. Skinner DB, Belsey RH. Surgical management of esophageal reflux and hiatus hernia. Long-term results with 1,030 patients. J Thorac Cardiovasc Surg. 1967;53(1):33–54.

9. Haas O, Rat P, Christophe M, Friedman S, Favre JP. Surgical results of intrathoracic gastric volvulus complicating hiatal hernia. Br J Surg. 1990;77(12):1379–81.

10. Stylopoulos N, Gazelle GS, Rattner DW. Paraesophageal hernias: operation or observation? Ann Surg. 2002;236:492–501.

11. Floch NR. Paraesophageal hernias: current concepts. J Clin Gastroenterol. 1999;29:6–7.

12. Sihvo EI, Salo JA, Räsänen JV, Rantanen TK. Fatal complications of adult paraesophageal hernia: a population-based study. J Thorac Cardiovasc Surg. 2009;137(2):419–24.

13. Bhayani NH, Kurian AA, Sharata AM, Reavis KM, Dunst CM, Swanstrom LL. Wait only to resuscitate: early surgery for acutely presenting paraesophageal hernias yields better outcomes. Surg Endosc. 2013;27(1):267–71.

14. Schieman C, Grondin SC. Paraesophageal hernia: clinical presentation, evaluation, and management controversies. Thorac Surg Clin. 2009;19(4):473–84.

15. D'Alessio MJ, Rakita S, Bloomston M, Chambers CM, Zervos EE, Goldin SB, Poklepovic J, Boyce HW, Rosemurgy AS. Esophagography predicts favorable outcomes after laparoscopic Nissen fundoplication for patients with esophageal dysmotility. J Am Coll Surg. 2005;201(3):335–42.

16. Spivak H, Lelcuk S, Hunter JG. Laparoscopic surgery of the gastroesophageal junction. World J Surg. 1999;23(4):356–67.

17. Banki F, DeMeester T. Paraesophageal Hiatal Hernia. In: Cameron JL, Cameron AM, editors. Current surgical therapy. 10th ed. Philadelphia: Elsevier Saunders; 2011. p. 33–8.

18. Critchlow J. Paraesophageal herniation. In: Fischer JE (editor). Mastery of Surgery, 5th ed. Lippincott Williams & Wilkins. 2007. pp. 641–9 (Fuller CB, Hagen JA, DeMeester TR, et al. The role of fundoplication in the treatment of type II paraesophageal hernia. J Thorac Cardiovasc Surg 1996;111:655–61).

19. Fuller CB, Hagen JA, DeMeester TR, et al. The role of fundoplication in the treatment of type II paraesophageal hernia. J Thorac Cardiovasc Surg. 1996;111:655–61.

20. Wolf PS, Oelschlager BK. Laparoscopic paraesophageal hernia repair. Adv Surg. 2007;41:199–210.

21. Roman S, Kahrilas PJ, Boris L, Bidari K, Luger D, Pandolfino JE. High-resolution manometry studies are frequently imperfect but usually still interpretable. Clin Gastroenterol Hepatol. 2011;9(12):1050–5.

22. Hashemi M, Peters JH, DeMeester TR, Huprich JE, Quek M, Hagen JA, Crookes PF, Theisen J, DeMeester SR, Sillin LF, Bremner CG. Laparoscopic repair of large type III hiatal hernia: objective followup reveals high recurrence rate. J Am Coll Surg. 2000;190:553–60.

23. Granderath FA, Carlson MA, Champion JK, Szold A, Basso N, Pointner R, Frantzides CT. Prosthetic closure of the esophageal hiatus in large hiatal hernia repair and laparoscopic antireflux surgery. Surg Endosc. 2006;20(3):367–79.

24. Stadlhuber RJ, Sherif AE, Mittal SK, Fitzgibbons Jr RJ, Michael Brunt L, Hunter JG, Demeester TR, Swanstrom LL, Daniel Smith C, Filipi CJ. Mesh complications after prosthetic reinforcement of hiatal closure: a 28-case series. Surg Endosc. 2009;23(6):1219–26.

25. Parker M, Bowers SP, Bray JM, Harris AS, Belli EV, Pfluke JM, Preissler S, Asbun HJ, Smith CD. Hiatal mesh is associated with major resection at revisional operation. Surg Endosc. 2010;24(12):3095–101.

26. Goers TA, Cassera MA, Dunst CM, Swanström LL. Paraesophageal hernia repair with biomesh does not increase postoperative dysphagia. J Gastrointest Surg. 2011;15(10):1743–9.

27. Oelschlager BK, Pellegrini CA, Hunter J, Soper N, Brunt M, Sheppard B, Jobe B, Polissar N, Mitsumori L, Nelson J, Swanstrom L. Biologic prosthesis reduces recurrence after laparoscopic paraesophageal hernia repair: a multicenter, prospective, randomized trial. Ann Surg. 2006;244(4):481–90.

28. Oelschlager BK, Pellegrini CA, Hunter JG, Brunt ML, Soper NJ, Sheppard BC, Polissar NL, Neradilek MB, Mitsumori LM, Rohrmann CA, Swanstrom LL. Biologic prosthesis to prevent recurrence after laparoscopic paraesophageal hernia repair: long-term follow-up from a multicenter, prospective, randomized trial. J Am Coll Surg. 2011;213(4):461–8.

29. Parsak CK, Erel S, Seydaoglu G, Akcam T, Sakman G. Laparoscopic antireflux surgery with polyglactin (vicryl) mesh. Surg Laparosc Endosc Percutan Tech. 2011;21(6):443–9.

30. van der Westhuizen L, Dunphy KM, Knott B, Carbonell AM, Smith DE, Cobb 4th WS. The need for fundoplication at the time of laparoscopic paraesophageal hernia repair. Am Surg. 2013;79(6):572–7.

31. Ballian N, Luketich JD, Levy RM, Awais O, Winger D, Weksler B, Landreneau RJ, Nason KS. A clinical prediction rule for perioperative mortality and major morbidity after laparoscopic giant paraesophagealhernia repair. J Thorac Cardiovasc Surg. 2013;145(3):721–9.

32. Polomsky M, Jones CE, Sepesi B, O'Connor M, Matousek A, Hu R, Raymond DP, Litle VR, Watson TJ, Peters JH. Should elective repair of intrathoracic stomach be encouraged? J Gastrointest Surg. 2010;14(2):203–10.

33. Louie BE, Blitz M, Farivar AS, Orlina J, Aye RW. Repair of symptomatic giant paraesophageal hernias in elderly (>70 years) patients results in improved quality of life. J Gastrointest Surg. 2011;15(3):389–96.

34. Allison PR. Hiatus hernia: (a 20-year retrospective survey). Ann Surg. 1973;178(3):273–6.

35. Maziak DE, Todd TR, Pearson FG. Massive hiatus hernia: evaluation and surgical management. J Thorac Cardiovasc Surg. 1998;115(1):53–60.

36. Swanstrom LL, Jobe BA, Kinzie LR, Horvath KD. Esophageal motility and outcomes following laparoscopic paraesophageal hernia repair and fundoplication. Am J Surg. 1999;177(5):359–63.

37. Patel HJ, Tan BB, Yee J, Orringer MB, Iannettoni MD. A 25-year experience with open primary transthoracic repair of paraesophageal hiatal hernia. J Thorac Cardiovasc Surg. 2004;127(3):843–9.

38. Low DE, Unger T. Open repair of paraesophageal hernia: reassessment of subjective and objective outcomes. Ann Thorac Surg. 2005;80(1):287–94.

39. Luketich JD, Nason KS, Christie NA, Pennathur A, Jobe BA, Landreneau RJ, Schuchert MJ.Outcomes after a decade of laparoscopic giant paraesophageal hernia repair. J Thorac Cardiovasc Surg. 2010;139(2):395–404, 404.e1. doi: 10.1016/j.jtcvs.2009.10.005. Epub 2009.

40. Mittal SK, Bikhchandani J, Gurney O, Yano F, Lee T. Outcomes after repair of the intrathoracic stomach: objective follow-up of up to 5 years. Surg Endosc. 2011;25(2):556–66. doi: 10.1007/s00464-010-1219-3. Epub 2010 Jul 10, Dec 11.

41. Zehetner J, Demeester SR, Ayazi S, Kilday P, Augustin F, Hagen JA, Lipham JC, Sohn HJ, Demeester TR. Laparoscopic versus open repair of paraesophageal hernia: the second decade. J Am Coll Surg. 2011;212(5):813–20. doi:10.1016/j.jamcollsurg.2011.01.060. Epub 2011 Mar 23.

42. Rathore MA, Andrabi SI, Bhatti MI, Najfi SM, McMurray A. Metaanalysis of recurrence after laparoscopic repair of paraesophageal hernia. JSLS 2007;11(4):456–60.

43. Wu JS, Dunnegan DL, Soper NJ. Clinical and radiologic assessment of laparoscopic paraesophageal hernia repair. Surg Endosc. 1999;13(5):497–502.

44. Wiechmann RJ, Ferguson MK, Naunheim KS, McKesey P, Hazelrigg SJ, Santucci TS, Macherey RS, Landreneau RJ. Laparoscopic management of giant paraesophageal herniation. Ann Thorac Surg. 2001;71(4):1080–6. discussion 1086–7.

45. Khaitan L, Houston H, Sharp K, Holzman M, Richards W. Laparoscopic paraesophageal hernia repair has an acceptable recurrence rate. Am Surg. 2002;68(6):546–51. discussion 551–2.

46. Jobe BA, Aye RW, Deveney CW, Domreis JS, Hill LD. Laparoscopic management of giant type III hiatal hernia and short esophagus. Objective follow-up at three years. J Gastrointest Surg. 2002;6(2):181–8. discussion 188.

47. Mattar SG, Bowers SP, Galloway KD, Hunter JG, Smith CD. Long-term outcome of laparoscopic repair of paraesophageal hernia. Surg Endosc. 2002;16(5):745–9. Epub 2002 Feb 8.

48. Diaz S, Brunt LM, Klingensmith ME, Frisella PM, Soper NJ. Laparoscopic paraesophageal hernia repair, a challenging operation: medium-term outcome of 116 patients. J Gastrointest Surg. 2003;7(1):59–66. discussion 66–7.

49. Targarona EM, Novell J, Vela S, Cerdán G, Bendahan G, Torrubia S, Kobus C, Rebasa P, Balague C, Garriga J, Trias M. Mid term analysis of safety and quality of life after the laparoscopic repair of paraesophageal hiatal hernia. Surg Endosc. 2004;18(7):1045–50. Epub 2004 Jun 10.

50. Aly A, Munt J, Jamieson GG, Ludemann R, Devitt PG, Watson DI. Laparoscopic repair of large hiatal hernias. Br J Surg. 2005;92(5):648–53.

51. Gangopadhyay N, Perrone JM, Soper NJ, Matthews BD, Eagon JC, Klingensmith ME, Frisella MM, Brunt LM. Outcomes of laparoscopic paraesophageal hernia repair in elderly and high-risk patients. Surgery. 2006;140(4):491–8. discussion 498–9. Epub 2006 Sep 6.

52. Lubezky N, Sagie B, Keidar A, Szold A. Prosthetic mesh repair of large and recurrent diaphragmatic hernias. Surg Endosc. 2007;21(5):737–41. Epub 2007 Feb 16.

53. Zaninotto G, Portale G, Costantini M, Fiamingo P, Rampado S, Guirroli E, Nicoletti L, Ancona E. Objective follow-up after laparoscopic repair of large type III hiatal hernia. Assessment of safety and durability. World J Surg. 2007;31(11):2177–83. Epub 2007 Aug 29.

54. Rathore MA, Andrabi I, Nambi E, McMurray AH. Intermediate-term results of laparoscopic repair of giant paraesophageal hernia: lack of follow-up esophagogram leads to detection bias. JSLS. 2007;11(3):344–9.

55. Dallemagne B, Kohnen L, Perretta S, Weerts J, Markiewicz S, Jehaes C. Laparoscopic repair of paraesophageal hernia. Long-term follow-up reveals good clinical outcome despite high radiological recurrence rate. Ann Surg. 2011;253(2):291–6.

The Hill Antireflux Operations Repair and Its Variants

Ralph W. Aye and Aditya Gupta

Introduction

When Lucius D. Hill introduced the antireflux operation that bears his name to the American Surgical Association in 1967 it set a new standard in antireflux surgery [1]. Basing his operation on detailed anatomic dissections and incorporating the regular use of pre-op and intra-operative esophageal manometry and pH testing, Hill added an element of science and objectivity to a field that was in early development, setting standards that continue to the present day. The principles upon which the operation is based are sound, and the operation has proven to be highly effective and durable [2, 3]. The surgeon who learns the procedure and incorporates it into his or her repertoire is rewarded with expanded surgical options in both straightforward and complex cases, and a far better understanding of the function and anatomy of antireflux procedures.

Advantages of the Hill Repair

1. The most anatomically accurate and complete reconstruction of the antireflux barrier.
2. A very low incidence of gas bloat and long-term dysphagia.
3. Inferior fixation of the gastroesophageal junction (GEJ) without reliance on a fundoplication, greatly reducing herniation and wrap slippage.
4. Intra-operative manometric control over final lower esophageal sphincter (LES) pressure.
5. Suitability for patients with ineffective esophageal motility [4].
6. No need for an esophageal lengthening procedure, even in cases of short esophagus [5].
7. Suitability for complex re-operative cases, or following partial gastrectomy or gastric bypass, as it does not rely on a fundoplication.
8. Proven durability [6, 2].
9. No need to take the short gastric vessels.

Principles of Repair

There are three anatomic concepts behind the Hill repair: (1) intra-abdominal posterior fixation of the GEJ; (2) the central role of the collar sling musculature of the LES in the proper reconstruction of the GEJ; and (3) the importance of the gastroesophageal valve (GEV) for the competence of the antireflux barrier. In addition, the Hill repair accomplishes the other established goals of antireflux surgery, including closure of the crura, establishment of an intra-abdominal segment of distal esophagus, and re-establishment of the length and pressure of the LES.

All three primary components of the repair are accomplished through the Hill repair sutures, which anchor the anterior and posterior aspects of the collar sling musculature of the LES to the preaortic fascia just superior to the celiac trunk. It is helpful to understand the anatomy of the LES in order to appreciate the proper placement and function of the Hill sutures. This anatomy has been delineated by Liebermann-Meffert [7] and consists of the clasp fibers of the lesser curvature of the LES which inter-digitate with the collar sling musculature of the oblique gastric muscle layer, formed as a horseshoe surrounding the anterior, posterior, and greater curvature (angle of His) aspects of the GEJ (Fig. 13.1). As four Hill sutures are used, this allows progressive tightening of the sling fibers and emphasis of the angle

R.W. Aye, MD, FACS (✉)
Thoracic and Esophageal Surgery, Thoracic Oncology,
Swedish Medical Center and Cancer Institute,
1101 Madison Street, Suite 900, Seattle, WA 98104, USA
e-mail: Ralph.Aye@swedish.org

A. Gupta, MD
Foregut and Thoracic Surgery, Swedish Thoracic Surgery,
Swedish Medical Center and Cancer Institute,
1101 Madison Avenue, Suite 850, Seattle, WA 98104, USA
e-mail: adi_dec17@yahoo.com

L.L. Swanstrom and C.M. Dunst (eds.), *Antireflux Surgery*,
DOI 10.1007/978-1-4939-1749-5_13, © Springer New York 2015

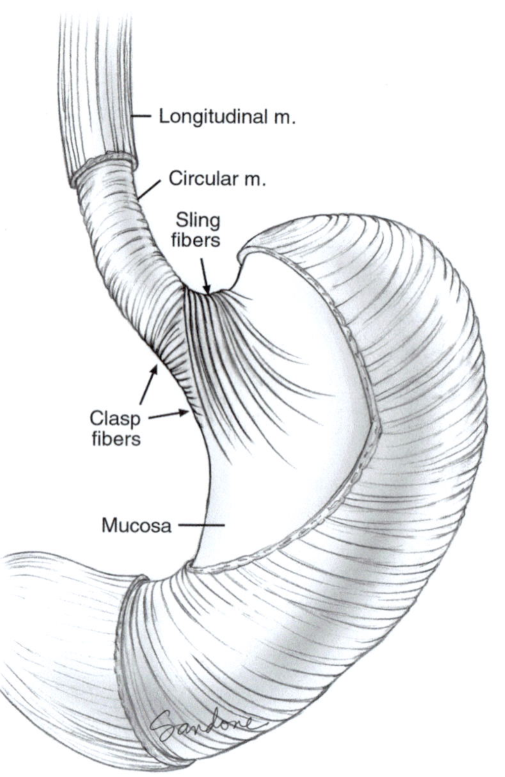

Fig. 13.1 Diagrammatic illustration of the Collarsling Musculature. ©2001 Corinne Sandone. Reproduced with permission of illustrator

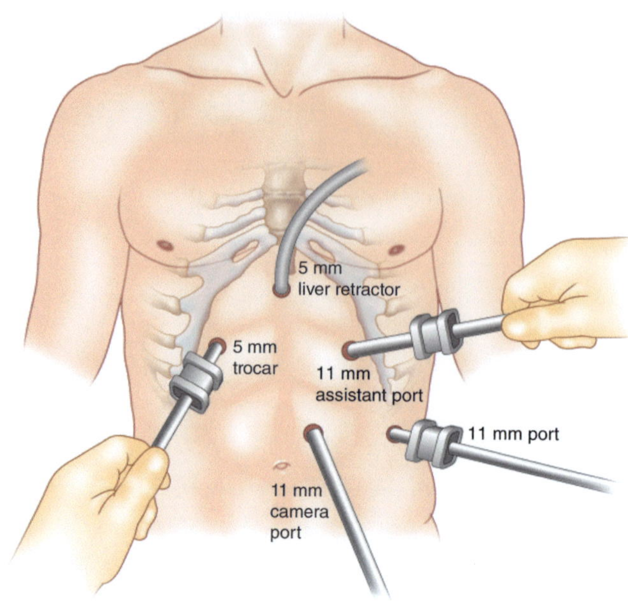

Fig. 13.2 Trocar placement for laparoscopic Hill repair

of His. It is not always needed to tie all four or to tie them particularly tightly which explains the need for intra-operative manometry to allow more accurate tailoring of the valve to the individual.

Hill Repair Technique

Our standard positioning is low dorsal lithotomy with both arms out, the surgeon between the legs, the assistant on the patient's left and the camera operator on the right, or using a robotic arm for camera fixation (Stryker Endoscopy; Wingman Scope Holder; 240-240-000). Prior to beginning the operation, the manometric equipment is prepared. The catheter is a water perfused, single use 8 channel esophageal manometry catheter, with four pressure ports at 0 cm from the tip, and subsequent ports at 5 cm intervals (Sierra Scientific Instruments, Catalog # 9012P1222). The manometric catheter is placed through a clear 48 Fr dilator (Cook Medical, Winston-Salem, NC), with the pressure port 10 cm beyond the tapered tip of the dilator, and taped together at the upper end. This arrangement is passed through the esophagus to 30 cm at the beginning of the case by the surgeon or an experienced anesthesiologist, taking care that the manometric catheter leads the way and does not fold under. The distal channel is connected to a transducer and anesthesia

monitor at pulmonary artery catheter settings, or to a dedicated esophageal manometry system.

Five trocars are used for the operation. It is noteworthy that a 10–11 mm assistant port is placed just below the left costal margin in the mid-clavicular line, or more medially when the costal margin is narrow. This requires placement of the surgeons' right-hand work port more inferiorly than would be typical for a Nissen repair, but the assistant port location facilitates management of the upper two untied repair sutures (Fig. 13.2). A sixth optional port for downward traction of lesser curvature fat may be added in the left lower quadrant to gain better exposure to the preaortic fascia. The left lobe of the liver is elevated with a 5 mm retractor [Nathanson: Cook medical, G26912, C-NLRS-1001 and G26913, C-NLRS-1002] and fixed to a self-retaining table-mounted system [Thompson Surgical, Cat # 90011B].

Dissection is performed with ultrasonic shears. Care is taken to dissect along the anterior aspect of the phrenoesophageal fat pad (Hill's phrenoesophageal bundle) and bring it down with the dissection, keeping it attached to the GEJ. Following dissection the anterior and posterior fat pad/bundles are trimmed as necessary to eliminate hernia sac and redundancy, while avoiding the lesser curvature and the Vagus nerves. Short gastric vessels are not routinely taken, but it is essential to free the entire posterior fundus by opening the lesser sac from left gastric artery to GEJ. This is accomplished from the lesser curvature aspect under view from the angled laparoscope and through critical exposure provided by the assistant, who lifts the posterior phrenoesophageal tissue immediately posterior to the

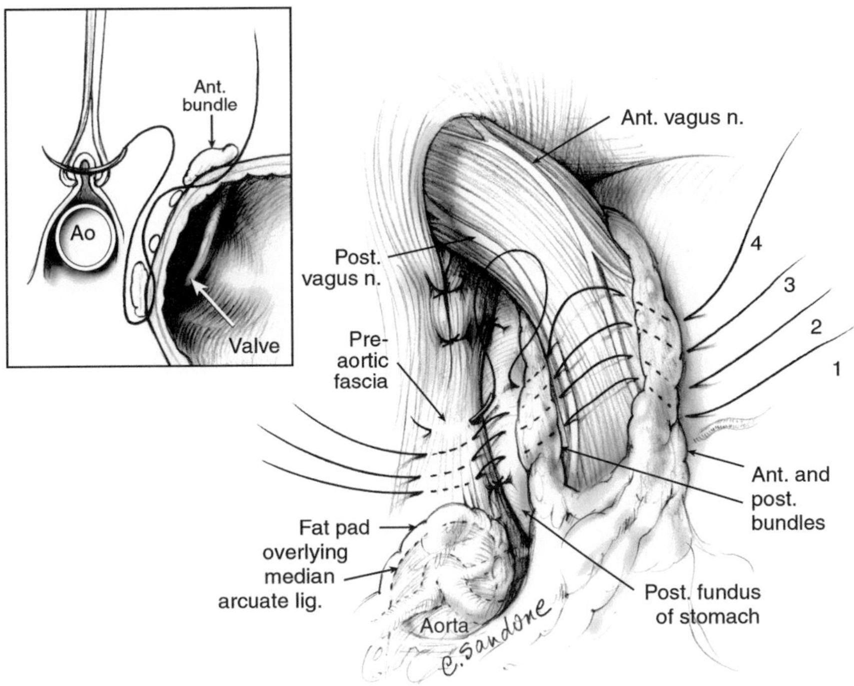

Fig. 13.3 Illustration of the Hill sutures. ©2001 Corinne Sandone. Reproduced with permission of illustrator

posterior Vagus nerve. The location of the celiac trunk should be roughly identified (though not dissected) and the preaortic fascia and overlying diaphragmatic muscle should be exposed down to this level. The preaortic fascia is a dense connective tissue layer that lies deep to the posterior fusion of the right and left crura and extends inferiorly to the celiac axis, where its inferior edge forms the median arcuate ligament.

Dissection is continued into the mediastinum to obtain adequate length of intra-abdominal esophagus. A Penrose drain is not used and would be in the way of subsequent suture placement. Following dissection the hiatus is closed posteriorly with 0-braided non-absorbable suture using an extracorporeal knot pusher or the Ti-Knot device [LSI Solutions; Ti-Knot, Catalog # TK-5]. For larger hernias, some of the repair may need to be completed anteriorly, since too much angulation of the esophagus may be created from excess posterior closure and posterior fixation of the GEJ to the preaortic fascia.

The Hill sutures are placed through the collar sling musculature of the GEJ. This lies immediately beneath the phrenoesophageal fat pad/ligament (Hill's phrenoesophageal bundles), commencing just to the patient's left/anterior of the anterior vagus nerve, extending over the angle of His, and ending just to the patient's right/posterior of the posterior vagus nerve. Thus the vagus nerves are important landmarks and must be identified. The anterior vagus nerve is found under tension by pulling down on the lesser curvature tissue.

The posterior vagus nerve is found by lifting the posterior fat pad upward/to the patient's right, as it consistently lies in the groove created by this maneuver.

Following hiatal closure, four Hill sutures of multicolored 48 inch 0-Ethibond (Ethicon Endosurgery multipack, Cat. #22970D8684) are placed through the tissue and left untied and clamped externally. The first two sutures are introduced through the surgeon's right-hand working port, while the third and fourth are introduced through the assistant port in the left upper quadrant. This is the most critical part of the repair, and exact placement is important (Fig. 13.3). There are three separate and distinct bites of tissue with each suture, the first being placement through the anterior bundle/collar sling musculature from inferior to superior; the second being placement through the posterior bundle/collar sling musculature from superior to inferior; and the third being transverse placement through the inferior aspect of the preaortic fascia.

The first bite of the first suture is placed immediately to the patient's left of the anterior vagus nerve. Grasping the bundle with the left hand and maneuvering the tissue over the needle facilitates this. This bite must go deeply enough to grab the collar sling musculature. It is usually necessary to trim away part of the anterior fat pad to expose this anatomy (Fig. 13.4).

The second bite is placement through the posterior bundle. The assistant retracts the lesser curvature tissue between the vagus nerves anteriorly and to the left, exposing

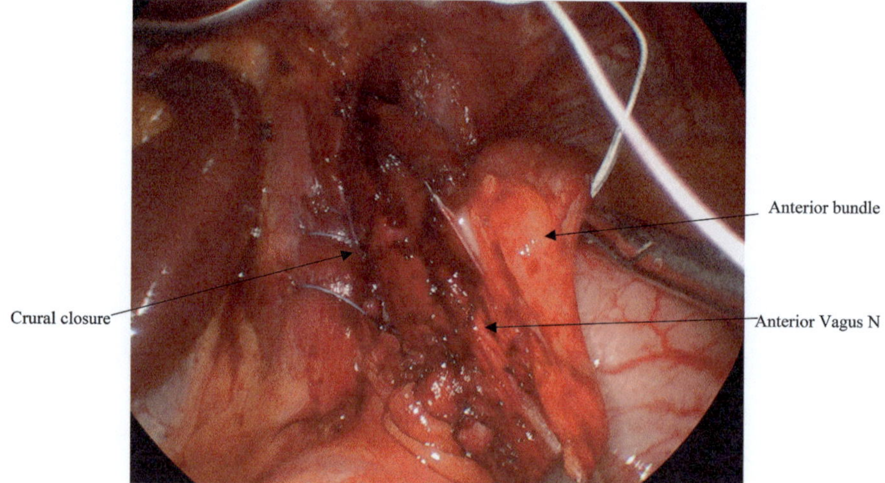

Fig. 13.4 First Hill suture, first bite: intra-operative view

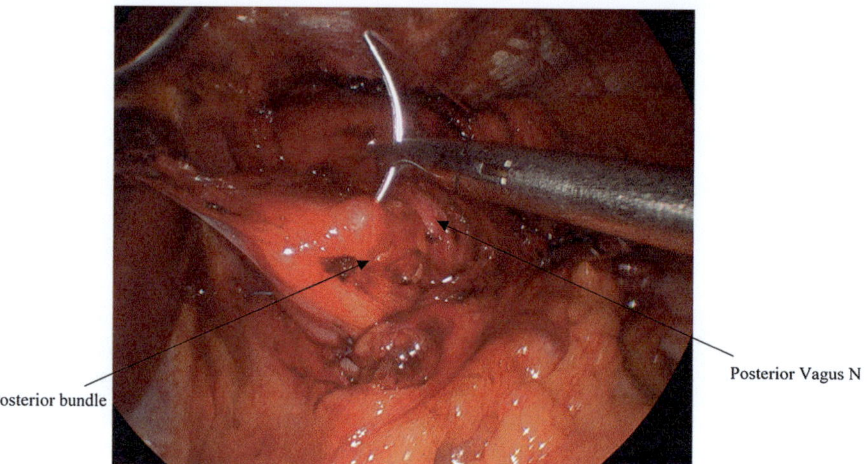

Fig. 13.5 First Hill suture, second bite: intra-operative view

the posterior vagus nerve. The surgeon grasps and manipulates the posterior bundle with the left hand. Beginning just posterior to the posterior vagus, the suture is passed through the bundle in a superior to inferior direction, including the underlying collar sling musculature. To do this successfully the needle will frequently need to be nearly upside down at the time of entry. Again, exposure is usually facilitated by trimming excess adipose tissue overlying the anatomy (Fig. 13.5). Posterior bundle suture placement may be aided by preliminarily fixing the superior aspect of the posterior fundus to the left crus and left aspect of the preaortic fascia with 1 or 2 sutures.

The third bite is transverse placement through the preaortic fascia. The assistant retracts the GEJ to the left and inferiorly for exposure. The suture is passed through the preaortic tissue inferiorly, immediately superior to the fatty tissue overlying the celiac axis. The location of this suture determines the final length of intra-abdominal esophagus, so it is important to be sufficiently inferior. The aorta lies 5–10 mm

deep, and may be avoided by lifting the tissue upward with a grasper and driving the needle transversely from left to right, rather than too deeply (Fig. 13.6). Finally the suture is brought out again through the right-hand port, taking care to buttress it with a grasper where it exits the tissue to avoid excess tissue trauma, and is clamped to itself with a hemostat (Fig. 13.7).

This same process is repeated with three more sutures, advancing each suture 2–3 mm further up the two bundles (e.g., in the direction of the angle of His) and the preaortic fascia. With excess advance the repair will be too snug, whereas with inadequate advance the repair may be too loose. The uppermost suture should enter the anterior bundle at approximately the left lateral border of the esophagus. It should enter the posterior bundle at its upper extent without going behind the esophagus. The third and fourth sutures are introduced and withdrawn through the assistant port. Colors should alternate to aid in preventing tangling. Care should be given to the angle of entry of the sutures through the ports, to

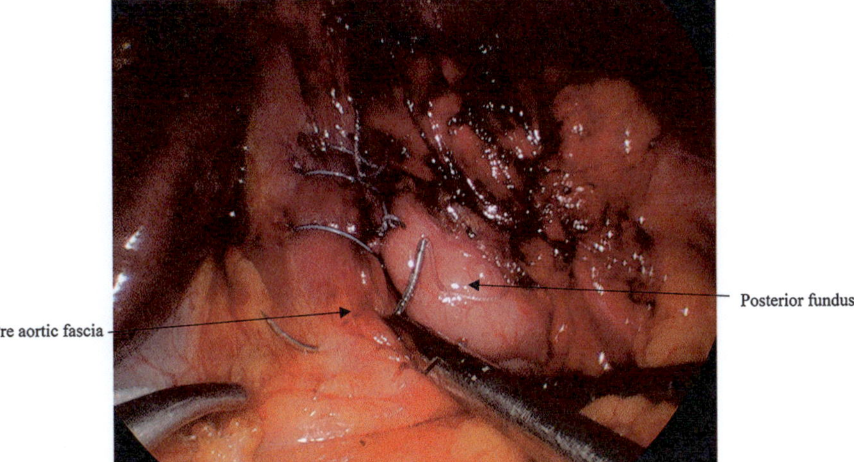

Fig. 13.6 First Hill suture, third bite: intra-operative view

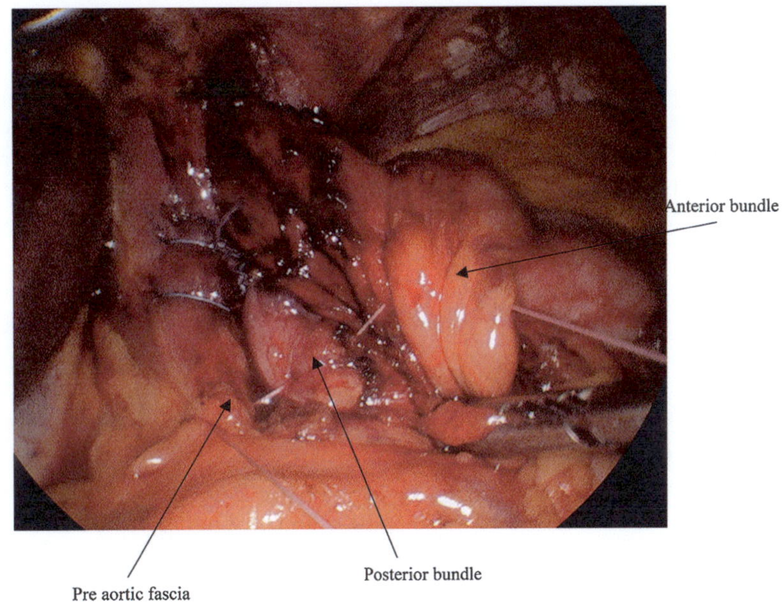

Fig. 13.7 First Hill suture, completed but not tied: intra-operative view

also prevent crossing. Three-eighths inch Teflon pledgets may be added to either end of the sutures; it has been our standard to add pledgets to the second and fourth sutures.

With all repair sutures placed but not tied, the 48 Fr dilator/manometry catheter is carefully advanced and positioned across the GEJ, and the top 2 sutures, i.e. those through the assistant port, are tied sequentially with a single half-hitch and clamped internally just above the knot with needle holders. The left hand instrument clamps the upper knot, while the right-hand instrument clamps the lower knot. Manometric measurements are taken by withdrawing the system until the pressure port is 5 cm below the repair, zeroing out background pressure, and withdrawing at a rate of 1 cm/s. This should be done more slowly if an arterial monitor is used, especially during crossing of the high-pressure zone, in order to capture the highest peak. The ideal pressure is 30–40 mmHg. The first increase in pressure encountered during pull-through is the repair, whereas an additional spike representing the diaphragm may be seen just above this. Sutures may be tightened or loosened at this time as needed. If the pressure is clearly too low an additional higher suture may be placed as deemed appropriate. When satisfactory pressure has been obtained, the dilator is again positioned across the GEJ again and all sutures are tied permanently at the established tension before taking a final manometric reading. Figure 13.8 shows the completed Hill repair.

The anterior hiatus is often reinforced with one or two sutures to prevent further attenuation and to avoid excess posterior closure. Mesh may be used at the discretion of the surgeon but excess posterior bulk should be avoided.

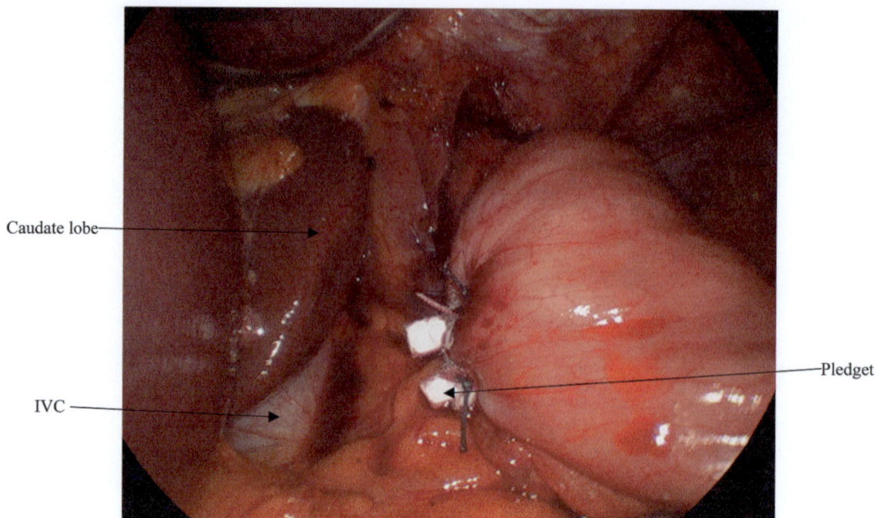

Fig. 13.8 Completed Hill repair: intra-operative view

The fundus is sutured to the anterior rim of the hiatus along both right and left crura, to prevent herniation and accentuate the valve. We routinely perform flexible upper endoscopy to assess calibration of the repair and the valve configuration. This is a helpful tool to aid the surgeon in refining technique, and will occasionally prevent a disastrous outcome.

Postoperative care is standard. Nasogastric suction is not routinely utilized. The patient is kept on full liquids for 2 weeks, and then advanced slowly to a normal diet by 6 weeks.

Results of the Hill Repair

The Hill repair is highly effective and durable. The durability of the Hill repair was shown in a large multi-institution study of over 1,000 patients followed for up to 25 years (mean follow-up of 10 years) demonstrating a 93 % long-term clinical success rate and only a 3 % reoperation rate [2].

The Hill repair has been successfully translated into laparoscopic technique, with over 2,500 laparoscopic repairs having been performed. Clinical results have been nearly identical to the open repair.

In a recent randomized controlled multi-institution trial comparing the laparoscopic Nissen and Hill repairs, the Hill was equivalent to the Nissen in every parameter of clinical success and repair failure, including symptomatic and physiologic control of reflux, except that, in contrast to the Nissen repair it did not raise lower esophageal sphincter pressure significantly above baseline. This may be an advantage in cases of ineffective esophageal motility. There was also a trend toward less gas bloating [3]. The results of this updated study supersede the only other randomized comparison of the two operations, done in the 1970s [8] in which the Nissen was deemed superior; however, the description of the Hill technique in this study raises concerns about the quality of the repair that was performed.

The effectiveness and safety of the Hill repair have been shown for patients with diminished esophageal peristalsis [4], and for those with para-esophageal hernia and short esophagus, without the need for an esophageal lengthening procedure [5].

The Nissen–Hill Hybrid Repair

The most common failure of the Nissen fundoplication is mediastinal herniation of the wrap; the second most common failure is a slipped Nissen, resulting from cephalad herniation of the GEJ and cardia through the wrap, which remains intra-abdominal [3, 9]. Both of these failures reflect inadequate fixation of the GEJ within the abdomen. Contrarily, the most common failure of the Hill repair is loosening from attenuation of the anterior repair sutures due to radial forces, with herniation of the GEJ being uncommon [3, 9]. In a recent randomized trial comparing 46 Nissen fundoplications to 56 Hill repairs, the two reoperations in the Nissen group were for mediastinal herniation of the wrap, whereas the two reoperations in the Hill group were for loosening of the repair [3].

The hybrid Nissen–Hill repair incorporates the structural features of both repairs, offsetting the weakness of one repair with the integrity of the other. Two Hill sutures securely anchor the GEJ within the abdomen to maintain axial integrity, while a full 360-degree Nissen wrap maintains radial integrity. This is not simply an anchored Nissen, in that it is the GEJ, rather than the wrap, which is anchored.

Nissen–Hill Hybrid Technique

Positioning and dissection are as described for the Hill repair, except that the port placement is the same as for a Nissen repair, with the surgeon's right-hand work port higher beneath the left costal margin and the 5 mm. assistant port placed left lateral, just below the costal margin. The dissection is similar except that the short gastric vessels are routinely taken and a Penrose drain is placed around the GEJ for downward traction during dissection and construction of the Nissen wrap. The gastroesophageal fat pad and associated hernia sac are routinely removed except along the lesser curvature, taking care to protect both vagus nerves. The hiatus is closed posteriorly with zero-gauge non-absorbable sutures.

There are four components to the Nissen–Hill hybrid repair:

Nissen Configuration

A marking suture is placed on the posterior fundus by traveling 6 cm below the GE junction along the greater curvature and one-third of the distance from greater to lesser curvature. A mirror-image mark is made on the anterior fundus. The posterior fundus is brought behind the esophagus and a "shoe-shine" maneuver is then performed to ensure full mobility of the fundus and a 1:1 relationship between anterior and posterior fundus. No fundoplication sutures are placed at this time.

Placement of Hill Sutures

The two lower of the four standard Hill sutures are then placed through the collar sling musculature and preaortic fascia as previously described (Fig. 13.1) [10]. The ends of each suture are brought out through the trocar, clipped together and returned into the abdomen and placed inferiorly and laterally out of the field until the Nissen is completed.

Nissen Construction

The Nissen repair is then completed in a standardized fashion [11, 12] over a 58 Fr dilator utilizing a horizontal mattress 2-0 double-armed prolene suture with double-mounted 5/8" Teflon pledgets on either side, suturing anterior to posterior fundus and incorporating the wall of the esophagus along its lesser curvature aspect (9:00 position) (Fig. 13.8). The sutures are tied using a Ti-Knot device (LSI Solutions, device; catalog # 030404, knots; catalog# 030510). Two

additional fundus-to-fundus sutures are then placed and tied, 5 mm above and 5 mm below the horizontal mattress suture, to create a 2 cm "floppy" Nissen wrap.

Completion of the Hill Sutures

With the dilator still in place, the Hill sutures are retrieved in reverse order, redundant tissue along the lesser curvature is retracted inferiorly, and the sutures are tied down with the Tie-knot (Fig. 13.9). Intra-operative manometry is not done as the repair is performed over a large dilator. The laxity of the anterior hiatus is assessed before and after removing the dilator, and is typically reinforced and/or further closed with 1 or more sutures to prevent subsequent widening and herniation. Biologic absorbable mesh is used routinely in cases of para-esophageal hernia. The corresponding intra-operative pictures of the Hybrid repair, with the Nissen already in place, and placement of mesh toward the end, can be seen in Figs. 13.10, 13.11, 13.12, and 13.13.

Results of the Hybrid Repair

With short-term follow-up in over 150 hybrid repairs, the results continue to exceed our initial expectations. After an initial feasibility and safety trial on patients with para-esophageal hernia and Barrett's metaplasia, the procedure has now been extended to patients with uncomplicated reflux. Gratifyingly there has been no noticeable increase in complications or short to mid-term side effects, and the recurrence rate has been lower than predicted with traditional repair.

In the first 50 patients with para-esophageal hernia undergoing hybrid repair, there was only 1 clinical recurrence at 13-month follow-up; there were 3 small asymptomatic fundic herniations with the GE junction intact and no reflux on pH testing; only two patients had resumed antisecretory medication, and preoperative symptoms were controlled in 98 %. There were significant improvements in all parameters of quality of life metrics, including dysphagia. Similar success has been achieved in a smaller group of patients with Barrett's metaplasia.

Summary

The Hill repair is at least equivalent in short-term clinical outcomes to the Nissen fundoplication in the surgical management of uncomplicated gastroesophageal reflux, and it may have advantages in the management of short esophagus and ineffective esophageal motility. In addition, as it is based

Fig. 13.9 Illustration of the
hybrid Hill–Nissen sutures in
place (Untied)

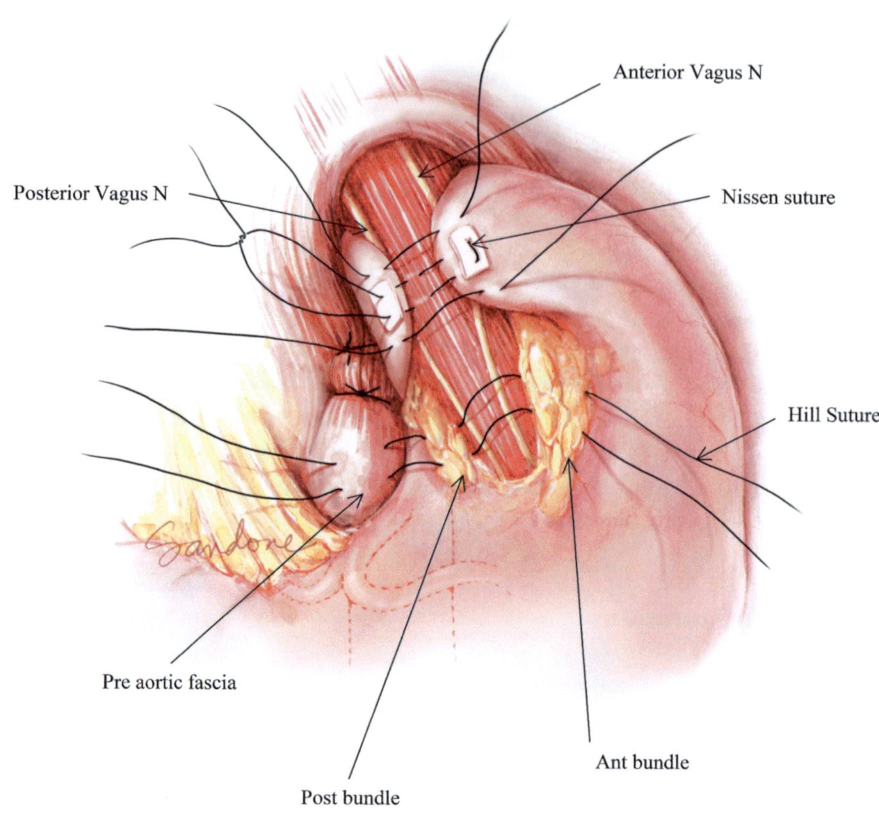

Fig. 13.10 Illustration of a
completed hybrid Hill–Nissen
repair

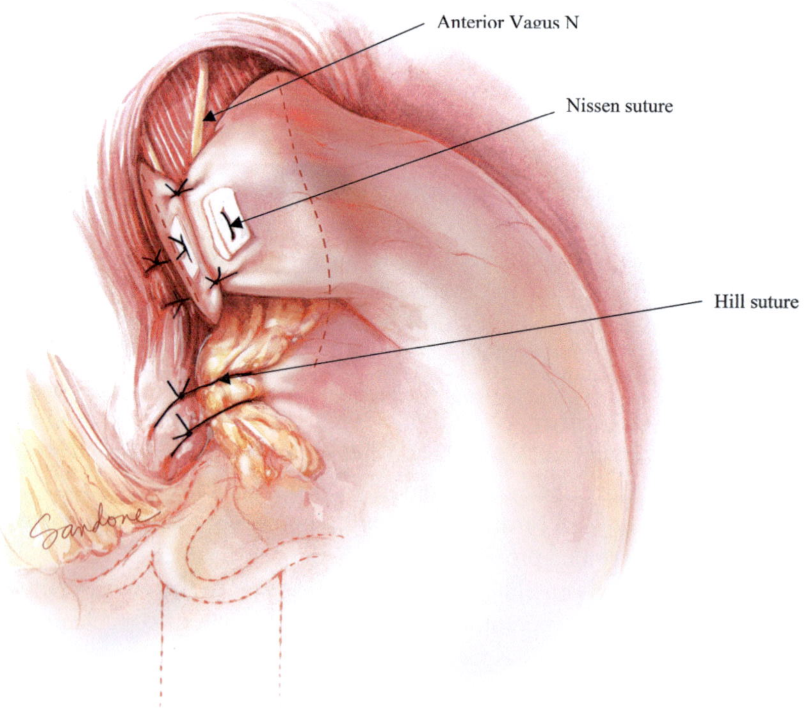

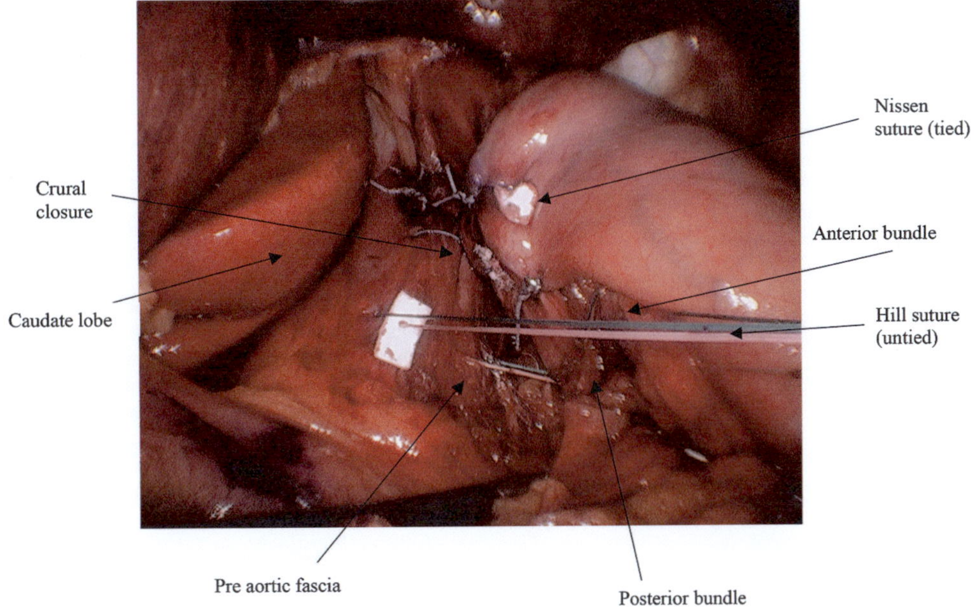

Fig. 13.11 Intra-operative view of the hybrid sutures in place, with the Nissen wrap completed

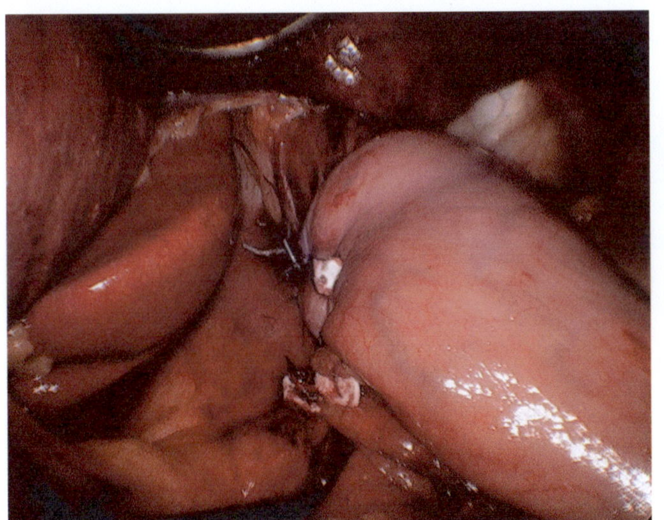

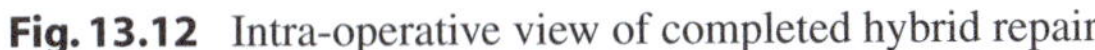

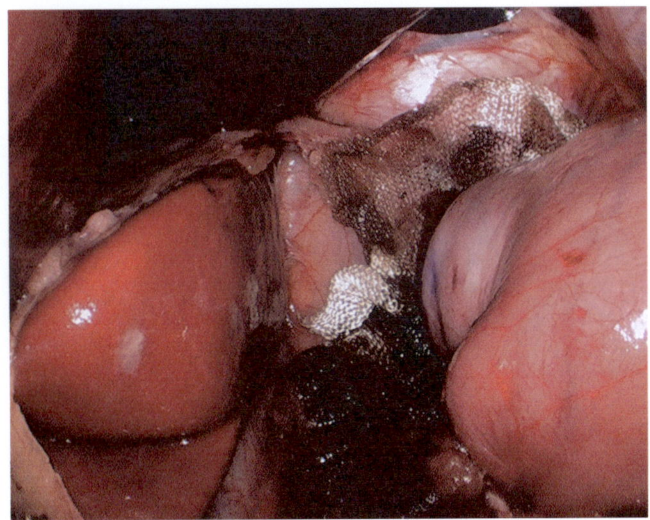

Fig. 13.12 Intra-operative view of completed hybrid repair

Fig. 13.13 Mesh placement in cases of para-esophageal hernia: intra-operative view

on different anatomic and functional concepts than the Nissen, it gives additional insight into the critical aspects of a successful antireflux operation. The open repair has been shown to be highly durable over at least a 10-year follow-up, and the operation has been successfully translated into a laparoscopic approach, with clinical results that match the open approach. Its technical performance is well within the scope of any qualified esophageal surgeon, and the technical details of manometric calibration and precise suture placement have been standardized and simplified.

The Hybrid Hill–Nissen repair incorporates features of both the techniques mentioned and acts in a synergistic manner, offsetting the weakness of one with the advantages of the other. Like the Hill repair, it is also useful particularly in cases of short esophagus, as it anchors the GE junction intra abdominally and obviates the need for an esophageal lengthening procedure. Short-term results suggest that this approach may be superior to either the Nissen or the Hill in cases of para-esophageal hernia or short esophagus, without an increase in side effects or complications.

References

1. Hill LD. An effective operation for hiatal hernia: an eight year appraisal. Ann Surg. 1967;166(4):681–92.
2. Aye RW, et al. The Hill antireflux repair at 5 institutions over 25 years. Am J Surg. 2011;201(5):599–604.
3. Aye RW, et al. A randomized multiinstitution comparison of the laparoscopic Nissen and hill repairs. Ann Thorac Surg. 2012;94(3): 951–8.
4. Aye RW, Mazza DE, Hill LD. Laparoscopic Hill repair in patients with abnormal motility. Am J Surg. 1997;173(5):379–82.
5. Jobe BA, et al. Laparoscopic management of giant type III hiatal hernia and short esophagus. Objective follow-up at three years. J Gastrointest Surg. 2002;6(2):181–8. discussion 188.
6. Low DE, et al. Fifteen- to twenty-year results after the Hill antireflux operation. J Thorac Cardiovasc Surg. 1989;98(3):444–9. discussion 449–50.
7. Korn O, et al. Gastroesophageal sphincter: a model. Dis Esophagus. 1997;10(2):105–9.
8. Demeester TR, Johnson LF, Kent AH. Evaluation of current operations for the prevention of gastroesophageal reflux. Ann Surg. 1974;180(4):511–25.
9. Horgan S, et al. Failed antireflux surgery: what have we learned from reoperations? Arch Surg. 1999;134(8):809–15. discussion 815–7.
10. Aye, RW. Current Therapy in Thoracic and Cardiovascular Surgery. The Hill Procedure for Gastroesophageal Reflux. 1st ed. Harcourt Health Sciences 2001.
11. DeMeester TR, Bonavina L, Albertucci M. Nissen fundoplication for gastroesophageal reflux disease. Evaluation of primary repair in 100 consecutive patients. Ann Surg. 1986;204(1):9–20.
12. Attwood SE, et al. Standardization of surgical technique in antireflux surgery: the LOTUS trial experience. World J Surg. 2008; 32(6):995–8.

Endoscopic Therapies for Reflux Disease

Toshitaka Hoppo, Astha J. Bhatt, and Blair A. Jobe

Introduction

Gastroesophageal reflux disease (GERD) is the most common esophageal disorder related to the retrograde flow of gastroduodenal contents into the esophagus, resulting in a spectrum of symptoms with or without tissue damage. Most patients with GERD have been treated with acid suppression therapy using antisecretory medications such as proton pump inhibitors (PPI) and/or H2 blockade but approximately 40 % of patients have recurrent or persistent symptoms despite a maximal dose of antisecretory medications [1]. Surgical fundoplication to anatomically restore an incompetent barrier function at the gastroesophageal junction (GEJ) has been recommended for patients with complicated and/or refractory GERD and has a long history of success. With the advancement of minimally invasive surgical techniques and instrumentations, laparoscopic fundoplication has become the standard surgical treatment option with an excellent long-term ability to control GERD symptoms in a minimally invasive fashion. However, many clinicians are still reluctant to refer their patients for surgical treatment because of possible surgical complications and postoperative side-effects such as dysphagia and gas bloat syndrome [2]. Since neither antisecretory medications nor surgical fundoplication can provide complete satisfaction, there is certainly a place for new options to treat GERD. In this context, transoral (endoscopic) incisionless approaches to restore the impaired barrier function has emerged as an alternative to medical and surgical treatment for GERD.

Endoscopic antireflux repairs (EAR), which use specialized devices to restore the competency of the LES, have been introduced and investigated over the last decade as a possible less invasive alternative between medical and surgical treatments to treat patients with GERD. Accumulated data have demonstrated the ability of endoluminal approaches to achieve short-term symptomatic improvement; but unfortunately, without dramatic improvement in objective measurements such as pH testing. This has definitely slowed the wide acceptance of EAR as a routine treatment option for GERD. In this chapter, we describe the concepts, procedures, and current status of EAR.

Indications

Currently, EAR is still in evolution and should be performed on highly selected patients; and probably only within a clinical trial. In most studies which have evaluated the efficacy and safety of EAR, patients were highly selected based on strict criteria including PPI-responsive typical GERD symptoms such as heartburn and/or regurgitation, small hiatal hernia (<2 cm), mild mucosal inflammation (Los Angeles classification grade A and B), normal esophageal motility, absence of Barrett's esophagus, and presence of pathological GERD confirmed by pH testing, all of which indicate a likely response to surgical fundoplication. Patients with lower BMI have also been found to have more favorable outcomes to EAR [3]. Patients who are unwilling to continue taking antisecretory medications, but who also fear or refuse surgical treatment, or who have failed previous surgical treatment, could potentially be good candidates for EAR procedures. By contrast, patients with hiatal hernia >2 cm, severely impaired esophageal motility, morbid obesity, and moderate to severe esophagitis (Los Angeles classification grade C and D)

T. Hoppo, MD, PhD • B.A. Jobe, MD (✉)
Department of Surgery, West Penn Hospital Part of Allegheny Health Network, Institute for the Treatment of Esophageal and Thoracic Disease, 4800 Friendship Avenue, Suite 4600 North Tower, Pittsburgh, PA 15224, USA
e-mail: thoppo@wpahs.org; bjobe1@wpahs.org

A.J. Bhatt, MD
Department of Surgery, St. Agnes Hospital, 900 S Caton Ave, Baltimore, MD 21075, USA
e-mail: drasthabhatt@gmail.com

L.L. Swanstrom and C.M. Dunst (eds.), *Antireflux Surgery*, DOI 10.1007/978-1-4939-1749-5_14, © Springer New York 2015

Table 14.1 Potential indications and contraindications for endoscopic antireflux repairs

Indications	Potential indications
Abnormal pH testing (positive DeMeester score)	Refractory GERD to surgical therapy (failed surgical treatment)
PPI-responsive typical GERD symptoms	Atypical GERD symptoms
Small hiatal hernia (<2 cm)	
Mild esophagitis (LA grade A or B)	
Normal esophageal motility	Contraindications
Absence of Barrett's esophagus	Large hiatal hernia (>2 cm)
Willingness to discontinue antisecretory medications	Severe esophagitis (LA grade C or D) or Barrett's esophagus
Inoperable due to severe co-morbidities	Severely impaired esophageal motility
Unwillingness to undergo surgery	Absence of PPI dependence

and/or Barrett's esophagus are not proper candidates for EAR (Table 14.1). Patients with worsening or non-improvement of GERD symptoms after a minimum of 8-weeks of PPI therapy are difficult clinical cases and probably should not be considered for EAR since they are at high risk of failing any GER treatment.

EAR Approaches

The principle goal of antireflux surgery (ARS) is to restore the structurally defective lower esophageal sphincter (LES) and return it to a subdiaphragmatic position in order to prevent the backflow of gastroduodenal contents into the esophagus, while maintaining egress of esophageal contents into the stomach. All antireflux procedures should achieve adequate pressure and length of the LES, while preserving receptive relaxation. Most recent EAR techniques such as transoral plication attempt a full-thickness serosa-to-serosa plication to restore the impaired LES. Another mechanism is to decrease the compliance of the LES in order to prevent transient sphincter relaxations (TSRL)—which have been proposed as an early phase of GERD.

For feasibility studies of EAR, the primary endpoints usually include symptomatic improvement and reduction and/or discontinuation of antisecretory medications in conjunction with objective measurements such as pH testing (distal esophageal acid exposure). Since EAR is associated with a high placebo effect, sham-controlled trials are often considered as the gold-standard trial design. Selection bias in EAR trials might occur because of unclear definitions of GERD particularly when based on subjective evaluation of response to medical therapy [4].

EAR Techniques

There have been a variety of endoluminal approaches to GERD such as implantation of synthetic bulking agents, thermal treatment of the LES, and endoscopic suturing and plication of the cardia. These approaches and their current status are summarized in Table 14.2, and their reported complications are summarized in Table 14.3.

Implantation of Synthetic Bulking Agents at the LES

The earliest endoscopic approach involved the injection of bovine dermal collagen into the LES in an attempt to reinforce the barrier function by enhancing the LES thickness both from a "bulking effect and also due to an inflammatory reaction" [5, 6]. Since then, several devices including Enteryx™ (Boston Scientific Corporate, Natick, MA) and Gatekeeper™ Reflux Repair System (Medtronic, Minneapolis, MN) had been introduced in the market and investigated.

Enteryx™ used a radio-opaque copolymer (Ethylene vinyl alcohol), which is an embolization agent, and which was injected into the distal esophageal wall under endoscopic and fluoroscopic guidance to create a permanent implant and a chronic foreign body reaction in the LES muscle layer (Fig. 14.1). An initial open-label, multicenter, international trial of Enteryx demonstrated sustained efficacy in the reduction of PPI use and esophageal acid exposure compared to baseline up to 2 years [7, 8]. This promising data led to a randomized sham-controlled multicenter trial involving 64 patients (Enteryx, $n=32$; control, $n=32$), which demonstrated that PPI cessation was achieved in 70 % of the Enteryx group compared to 40 % in the control group at a follow-up of 6 months. Interestingly enough, there was no significant difference in objective measurements of pH testing or LES pressure compared to baseline in both groups [9]. Because of reports of severe complications involving the mediastinum due to transmural injection or nearby inflammatory reaction that occurred after early large-scale commercialization, Enteryx was withdrawn from the market in 2005 [10–12].

Gatekeeper™ Reflux Repair System uses small hydrogel cylindrical prostheses, which are implanted into the submucosa at the level of GEJ. Similar to Enteryx, initial data was excellent, leading to a sham-controlled randomized study (Gatekeeper, $n=96$; sham, $n=48$), which resulted in an early termination due to lack of compelling efficacy with symptomatic control and objective measures of pH testing such as distal esophageal acid exposure [11]. Because of serious complications including esophageal

Table 14.2 Mechanisms and current status of EAR procedures

Mechanism of device	Product name	RCT	Current status in USA	History
Synthetic implant injection techniques – Prevents LES hypotension – Reduces Transient LES relaxation associated to acid reflux	Enteryx (Boston Scientific Corporate, Natick, MA) Gatekeeper (Medtronic, Minneapolis, MN)	Y Y	Not in use Not in use	Introduced in 2003 in USA Discontinued in 2005 due to severe complication Introduced in 2000 (in Netherlands), in 2003 (in USA) Discontinued in 2009 as no significant efficacy was shown
Radiofrequency ablation – Reduces the frequency of Transient LES relaxation episodes – Reduces LES hypersensitivity	Stretta (Mederi Therapeutics Inc., Greenwich, CT)	Y	In use	Introduced in 2000 (USA) Reintroduced by Mederi Therapeutics Inc. (Greenwich, CT) in April 2010
Plicating, suturing, stapling devices – Repairs the esophago-gastric flap valve – Correction of the angle of His – Shortening of the LES	EndoCinch (Bard Endoscopic technologies, Billerica, MA subsidiary of C.R Bard, Murray Hill, NJ)	Y	In use	Introduced in 1994 (in UK) and in 1998 (in USA)
	Endoscopic Suturing Device (ESD; Wilson-Cook Medical Inc, Winston-Salem, NC)	N	In use as a device for MIS	FDA approved in 2003
	NDO plicator (NDO Surgical, Inc., Mansfield, MA)	Y	Not in use	Introduced in 2003, Not being manufactured since 2008
	EsophyX (Endogastric Solutions, Redmond, WA)	N	In use	Introduced in 2005 (in Belgium) and 2007 (in USA)
	ARD Syntheon (Syntheon, Miami, FL)	N	Not in use	Not approved by FDA
	SRS device (Medigus, Omer, Israel)	N	Not in use	Tested in Europe, Australia, India, and early trials in US

Table 14.3 Reported adverse effects and complications of EAR procedures

Synthetic implant injection	Dysphagia Esophageal perforation (Gatekeeper) Pharyngeal perforation Pulmonary complications; chest pain, pneumothorax, pneumonitis, pneumomediastinum *Death*: severe bleeding due to esophago-aorta fistula (Enteryx)
Radiofrequency ablation	Fever Dysphagia Odynophagia Gastroparesis Perforation (Boerhaave syndrome, pneumoperitoneum) Ulcerative esophagitis Bleeding requiring blood transfusion Pleural effusion, atrial fibrillation, pancreatitis *Death case*: Leak-aspiration pneumonia-sepsis, bradycardia-asystole
Suturing devices	Gastric/esophageal perforation Pneumothorax, pneumomediastinum Retrosternal/pharyngeal pain Bleeding
Plicators	Esophageal perforation Pneumomediastinum Bleeding requiring blood transfusion Pleural effusion Permanent tongue numbness Persistent pain due to adhesion *Death*: ARDS due to aspiration

perforation ($n = 2$), pulmonary fistula related to perforation ($n = 1$), and severe chest pain ($n = 1$) [6, 13], the Gatekeeper™ Reflux Repair System was withdrawn from the market in 2009.

Radiofrequency Burns oft the LES

The application of radiofrequency to the GEJ creates a controlled thermal injury and possibly nerve ablation at the muscular layer of GEJ, producing fibrosis that decreases the compliance of the GEJ and has been shown to decrease the occurrence of transient LES relaxation [14, 15]. The Stretta System (Mederi Therapeutics, Greenwich, CT), which was reintroduced in the United States in April 2010 and is currently available for clinical use, is a transoral device used to deliver radiofrequency energy at the GEJ to treat GERD. This device uses a single-use, flexible catheter along with a balloon basket assembly with electrode needle sheaths. The catheter is inserted transorally proximal to the squamocolumnar junction, and the balloon is then inflated. Nickel–titanium electrodes are deployed into the muscular layer of the GEJ. Radiofrequency energy at 465 kHz and 2–5 W is delivered while microcircuitry monitors the mucosal temperature [16]. Serial thermal ablations are applied to the muscular layer every 0.5 cm extending from 1.5 cm distal to 2 cm proximal to the squamocolumnar junction. The consequent

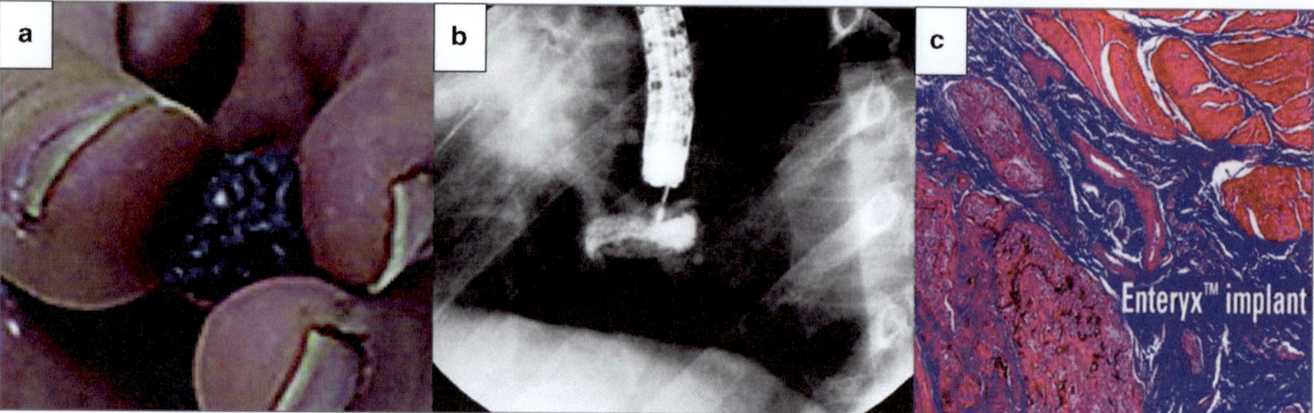

Fig. 14.1 Implantation of synthetic bulking agents. (**a**) Foamy particles of biopolymer after solidification in water. (**b**) Ring-like aspect of biopolymer after injection at the gastroesophageal junction. (**c**) Histological feature of the reaction induced by biopolymer injection

fibrotic tissue, and perhaps collagen contraction, reactions that can be seen for up to 12 month, result in a reinforcement of the LES [17]. Aberrant nerve pathways may also be ablated, as observed in cardiac arrhythmia ablation. It is possible that radiofrequency treatments may delay gastric emptying due to accidental thermal damage of the vagal nerves [18–20].

Although previous studies have demonstrated the safety and potential efficacy of the Stretta system, the therapeutic outcomes have been somewhat conflicting. A case series of 109 patients who had undergone the Stretta procedure demonstrated a significant improvement of GERD-HRQL score and reduction in the need for daily antisecretory medications at a follow-up period of 4 years. Furthermore, a second session of ablation was proposed for those with GERD-HRQL scores that did not improve by 75 % at the end of 4 months and showed additional response [21]. A randomized controlled study involving 64 patients with GERD (Stretta, $n=32$; control, $n=32$) demonstrated that the Stretta procedure improved clinical symptoms such as heartburn and GERD-HRQL score at 6 months after intervention compared to the placebo group; however there was no significant difference in antisecretory medication use or esophageal acid exposure at 6 months [22]. Another randomized controlled study involving 40 patients (Stretta, $n=20$; control, $n=20$) demonstrated that PPIs were discontinued in 3 patients and reduced in 15 patients at 12 months after intervention in the Stretta group, whereas none in the control group reduced their dose of PPIs [23]. However, there was no difference in objective measurements of acid exposure by pH testing. In the most recent prospective, sham-controlled randomized trial, 36 patients with chronic GERD were randomly assigned to single-dose Stretta group ($n=12$), double-dose Stretta group ($n=12$), or sham group ($n=12$). The Stretta procedure significantly reduced GERD-HRQL scores, PPI use, distal esophageal acid exposure, and grade of esophagitis compared to the sham procedure at a 12-month follow-up. Double-dose Stretta appeared to have superior outcomes to single-dose Stretta, although this was not a significant difference [24].

Overall, the Stretta system appears to improve GERD symptoms and quality of life, and potentially reduces the need for PPIs during intermediate follow-up; however the impact of Stretta on objective measurements of GERD such as distal esophageal acid exposure remains unpredictable.

Transoral Suturing and Plication

Devices that are applied transorally and attempt tissue approximation by deploying nonabsorbable sutures, staples, or plastic fasteners through the gastric and/or esophageal wall have a long history. Some devices such as the EndoCinch use a suctioning chamber for mucosa-to-mucosa approximation, whereas the NDO System and EsophyX use a grasping tool (e.g., a screw-shaped needle) to retract the tissue for subsequent serosa-to-serosa full-thickness plication. The primary goal of these suturing and plication devices is to restore the impaired gastroesophageal flap valve by recreating the acute angle of His with either stitches or fasteners, thus leading to the reduction of esophageal acid exposure [25–29]. In addition an attempt is made with some approaches to envelop the distal esophagus with the proximal stomach so as to replicate the nipple valve seen with a Nissen.

Bard EndoCinch Gastroplication Device (Bard Endoscopic Technologies, Billerica, MA)

The EndoCinch (Bard Endoscopic technologies, Billerica, MA subsidiary of C.R Bard, Murray Hill, NJ) was the first device to be approved for clinical use to treat GERD by endoluminal gastroplication. This device was a transoral suturing device that was attached onto a standard endoscope

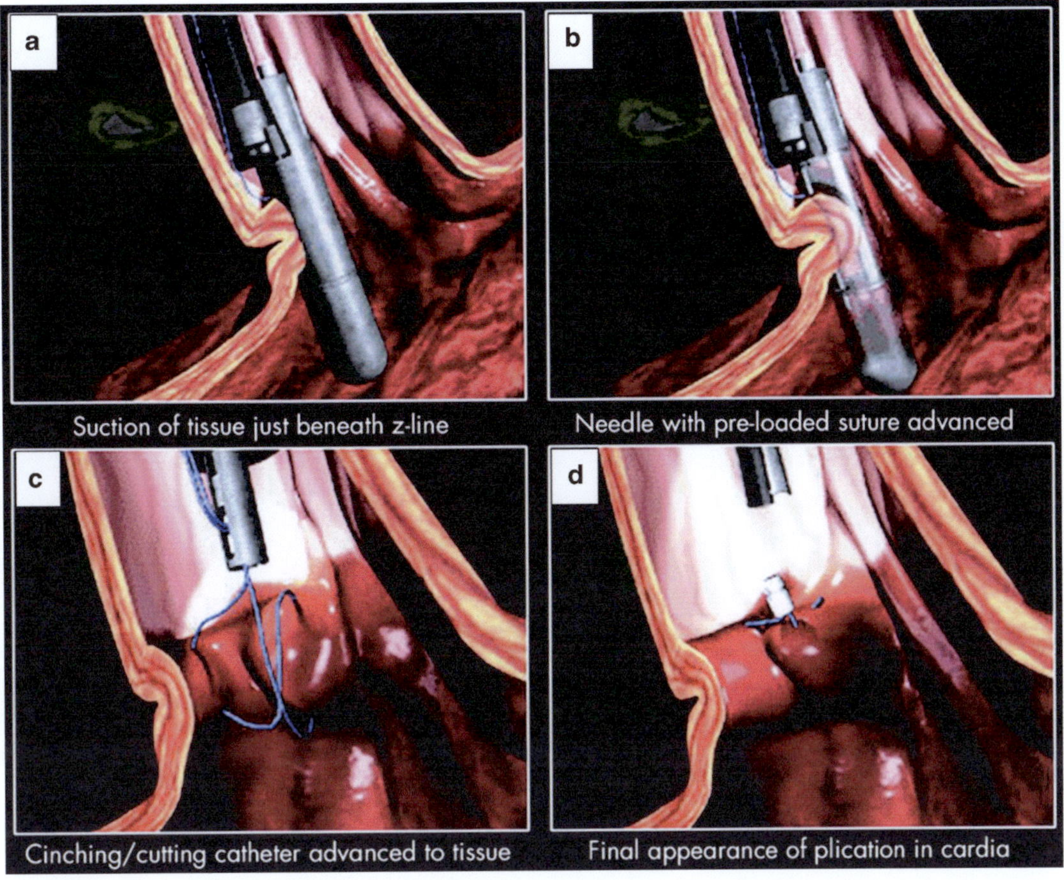

Fig. 14.2 Bard EndoCinch device. (**a**) The sewing chamber located 1–2 cm below the esophago-gastric junction and the tissue is brought into a lateral opening using suction. (**b**) A push wire is advanced through the hollow needle, pushing tag, and suture through the tissue to place first stitch through the suctioned tissue. (**c**) A second tag is also loaded and placed 1 cm adjacent the first suture. (**d**) The plication is completed by locking the two existing threads together and cutting extra thread. (Reproduced from Arts, J et al. Gut 2004;53:1207–14)

and created mucosa-to-mucosa gastroplication immediately distal to or at the level of GEJ. The device was inserted transorally and advanced to the level of GEJ where mucosa to be sutured was identified and could be captured into the suction and sewing chamber attached to the distal tip of endoscope. Subsequently, two adjoining stitches are placed through the captured mucosa and are tied together to create a figure-of-eight pleat that tightened the impaired valve and increased its ability to serve as an antireflux barrier (Fig. 14.2) [30]. This device was originally hoped to be able to perform a full-thickness plication; however the suction chamber was unable to incorporate the entire thickness of the stomach or esophageal wall before deploying the suture, thus leading to mucosa only sutures and probably explaining subsequent failure. Despite modifications of this procedure, including additional interventions to provide more sutures and supplemental use of electrocautery to enhance tissue adhesion, none of the studies demonstrated a long-term sustained efficacy in terms of improvement of clinical symptoms, reduction of PPI use, or normalization of acid exposure [27, 31]. In addition, this procedure is associated with complications including phar-

yngitis, vomiting, abdominal pain, mucosal tears, and perforation [29, 30, 32]. It was therefore withdrawn from the market in 2009.

In a double-blind, randomized, sham-controlled trial to evaluate the efficacy of EndoCinch, 60 patients with pH-proven GERD were randomly assigned to either EndoCinch ($n=20$), sham procedure ($n=20$), or observation ($n=20$). At 3 months, 65 % of patients in the EndoCinch group had a 50 % reduction in PPI use compared to 25 % in the sham group ($p=0.01$); however this effect was lost at 6 and 12 months. In the EndoCinch group, 29 % of patients were retreated with a mean of 1.4 extra plications after a median follow-up period of 4 months, and functional sutures were found in only 19 % of all sutures placed [30]. Another randomized placebo-controlled study involving 46 patients with documented GERD, who were randomly assigned to either the EndoCinch group with 2–4 plications ($n=22$) or a sham (placebo) group ($n=24$), demonstrated that on the short-term EndoCinch was able to control clinical symptoms and reduce PPI use; however there was no difference in objective measurements such as endoscopic findings and distal esophageal acid exposure [33].

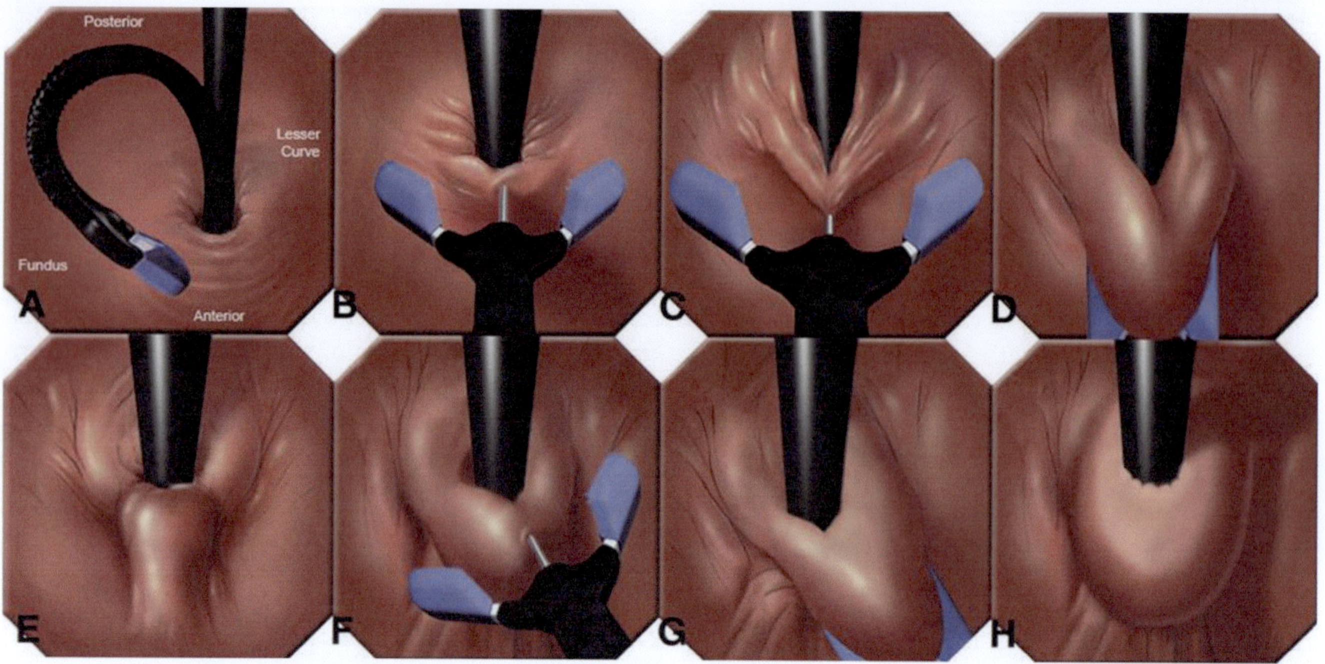

Fig. 14.3 NDO plicator. (**a**) Plicator and gastroscope retroflexed to the GEJ in the anterior position. (**b**) Plicator arms are opened and the tissue retractor pulls a full-thickness wall of anterior gastric cardia. (**c**) Gastric wall is retracted into the plicator arms. (**d**) The first pre-tied implant is deployed. (**e**) Full-thickness serosa-to-serosa plication after the first implant is restructuring the GEJ. (**f**) For serial plication, the instrument arms are opened, and the tissue retractor again pulls a full-thickness gastric wall. (**g**) Gastric wall is again retracted into the Plicator arms, and the second suture is deployed. (**h**) The serial placation technique restructures the antireflux barrier. (Reproduced from Renteln D, et al. Gastrointest Endosc. 2008;68(5):833–44)

Wilson-Cook Endoscopic Suturing Device (ESD; Wilson-Cook Medical Inc, Winston-Salem, NC)

This endoluminal suturing device was first approved for clinical use in 2003. The device works on the same principle as the Endocinch with the main difference being that it uses an external working channel to avoid repeated endoscope insertions and withdrawals for suture passing, locking, and cutting. However, this technique had the same deficits as the EndoCinch, including superficial bites and a high rate of suture failure. In a small study involving 20 patients who had undergone the ESD procedure, there were no significant changes in the LES pressure, PPI use, or objective measurements of pH testing at 6 months, and only 5 % of all sutures remained in situ [34]. No further evaluation was performed. Currently, this device has been introduced in the market as the Sew-Right suturing device for laparoscopic surgery by LSI solutions® (Victor, NY) but is no longer available for endoscopic use.

NDO Surgical Endoscopic Plication System (NDO Surgical, Inc., Mansfield, MA)

This device was designed to create a full-thickness serosa-to-serosa plication of anterior gastric cardia using a pledgeted T-shaped implant. Endoscopic visualization was provided by retroflexion of a slim gastroscopy inserted through a working channel of this device. Once visualized, the GEJ is identified and a corkscrew-shaped tissue retractor is used to aggressively grasp the lip of the valve and pull it toward the device. The large jaws are closed, capturing full thickness of the GEJ and a pre-tied pledgeted suture is deployed to create a full-thickness plication (Fig. 14.3). The procedure was approved to create a single plication between the anterior gastric wall and fundus 1 cm distal to the GEJ to avoid damage to major branches of left gastric artery and vagus nerve trunks.

A multicenter, single-blind, randomized prospective trial comparing the NDO Plicator ($n=78$) with a sham procedure ($n=82$) demonstrated that the NDO Plicator significantly improved GERD-HRQL score and reduced PPI use and distal esophageal acid exposure compared to the sham group at a follow-up of 3 months, indicating that the short-term outcome of NDO Plicator is superior to that of the sham procedure. There was no mortality or severe complications such as esophageal perforation [35]. Following this randomized trial, a multicenter, prospective study with 5-year follow-up demonstrated that cessation of daily PPI therapy was achieved in 67 % of patients who had undergone a single full-thickness placation by using the NDO plicator, and GERD-HRQL scores remained significantly improved

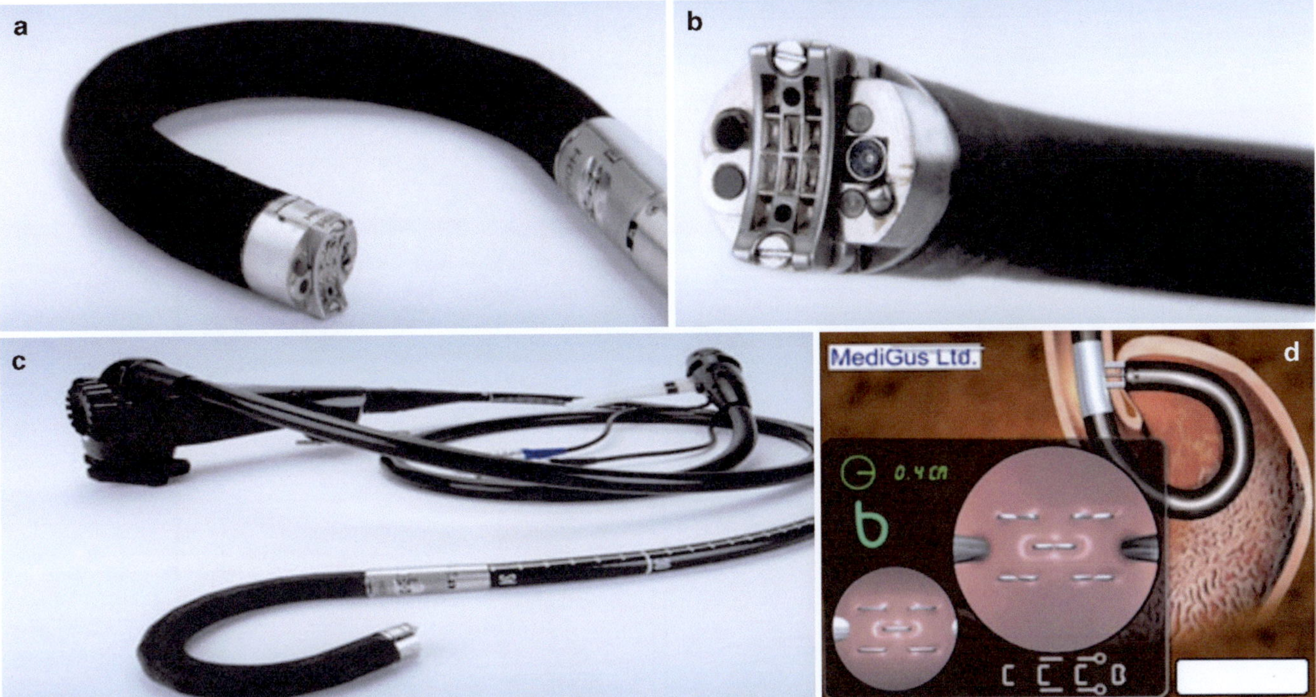

Fig. 14.4 *Medigus SRS device*: (**a–c**) The device has two stapler components; the anvil is at the tip and the cartridge at the shaft. The accurate alignment is performed using ultrasonic guidance. (**d**) The endoscope is inserted transorally and top of fundus is caught by the anvil and brought against the shaft that contains stapler cartridges fired with standard 4.8-mm staples. The device is partially withdrawn, then rotated 120°, and the procedure is repeated. (Obtained with permission from www.medigus.com/AboutGerd/GERD.aspx) MUSE™ System by Medigus

compared to baseline (pre-intervention), indicating that symptomatic control and reduction in the need for PPIs are maintained up to 5 years. The device was FDA approved for application of a single suture, but many surgeons found that additional firings resulted in even better results. A European multicenter, prospective study with 12-month follow-up supported the safety and efficacy of multiple plicator implants to improve clinical symptoms and reduce antisecretory medication use [36]. Despite these promising results, the device was withdrawn in 2008 due to financial difficulties.

ARD Syntheon (Syntheon, Miami, FL)

The Syntheon Anti-Reflux Device (ARD) used a titanium compression implant that creates a full-thickness serosa-to-serosa plication in the gastric cardia anteriorly and along the lesser curve. This plication was performed with a standard endoscope and was removable in the first 48 h after placement.

A multicenter pilot feasibility study involving 70 patients demonstrated that, of 57 patients who completed a 6-month follow-up, 79 % of patients showed a 50 % or more improvement in GERD-HRQL scores and 63 % discontinued antisecretory medications. Ambulatory pH testing showed that there was a median decrease of 27 % in the proportion of pH < 4, and abnormal pH was normalized in 26 % of patients [37]. Since this study, this device has not been further evaluated and never reached the market.

MUSE Device (Medigus, Omer, Israel)

The MUSE device uses a flexible gastroscopy containing a specialized stapling system and an ultrasound unit to attempt to create an anterior fundoplication via the transoral approach. The stapling system consists of an anvil located at the tip of the device and the stapler cartridge (4.8-mm staples) mounted on the shaft, and these components come together under a combination of visual and ultrasonic guidance. Once contact between the gastric and esophageal walls is confirmed, staples are fired to create a full-thickness plication, thus recreating the angle of His. The device is then partially withdrawn, rotated 120°, and the procedure is repeated (Fig. 14.4). A preclinical study using a swine model demonstrated the feasibility and safety of this device, however a clinical trial has not yet been published [38]. The original SRS device was withdrawn from the market due to technical issues but has been reintroduced as the MUSE in 2014 and is currently FDA approved and available for use. At the SAGES meeting in April, 2014, results of a clinical trial on 69 patients were presented and showed that 85 % of patients

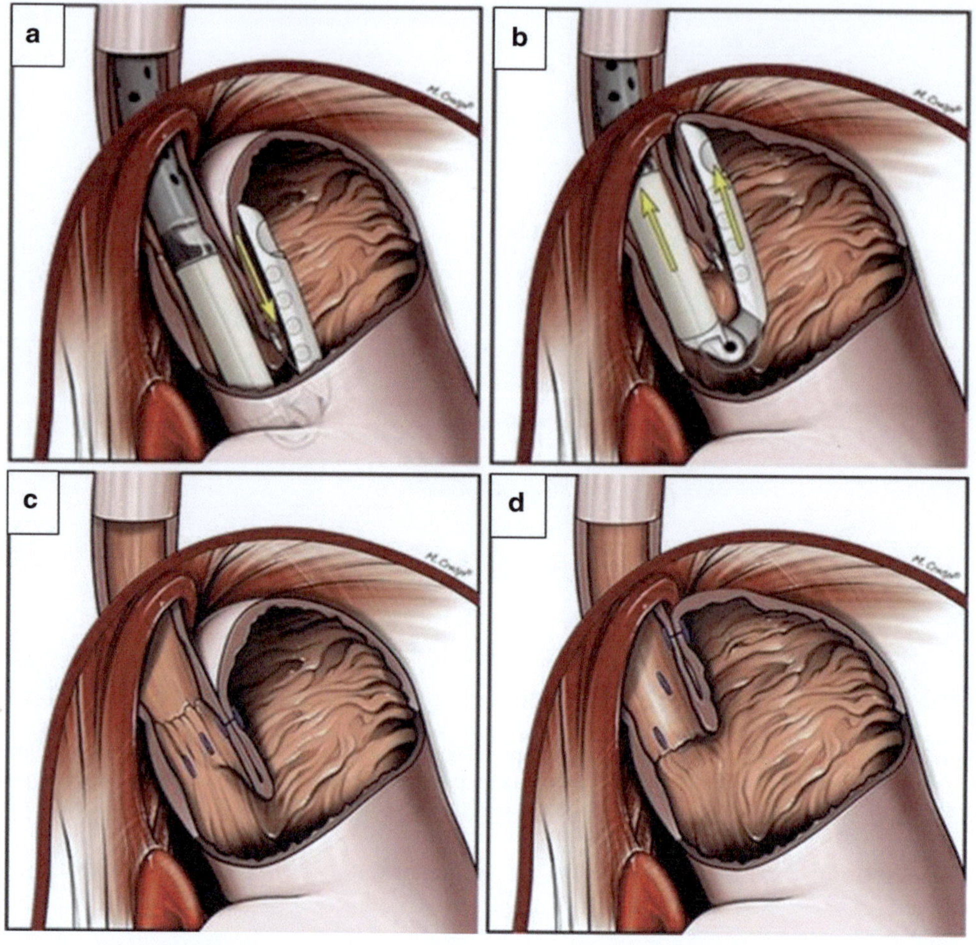

Fig. 14.5 *Illustration of endoluminal fundoplication (EsophyX device).*
(**a**) The device is inserted up to gastric cardia and a screw-shaped retractor is applied to the squamocolumnar junction. (**b**) The squamocolumnar junction is retracted, and the device is closed and H-shaped fasteners are deployed to create full-thickness serosa-to-serosa plication. (**c**) Scheme of TIF 1.0 procedure (gastro-gastric plications). (**d**) Scheme of TIF 2.0 procedure (Gastroesophageal placation). (Reproduced from Bell RCW, et al. Surg Endosc. 2011;25:2387–99)

reduced GERD medication use by ≥50 % with 65 % of subjects eliminating GERD medication entirely after 6 months. The study also found that 73 % of subjects improved quality of life scores by ≥50 %. This has not been published yet.

Transoral Incisionless Fundoplication

The EsophyX™ device (Endogastric Solutions, Redmond, WA, USA) is another FDA-approved device to perform transoral incisionless fundoplication (TIF), which attempts to wrap the gastric cardia around the distal esophagus to recreate a fundoplication-like nipple valve at the GEJ. The safety and efficacy of EsophyX™ has been intensively investigated and seems to be the most promising endoluminal device that creates a full-thickness serosa-to-serosa plication. The wrap is then fixed in place by deployment of plastic H-shaped fasteners (Fig. 14.5). The TIF procedure has evolved through clinical experience. TIF 1.0 was a gastro-gastric plication that created an omega-shaped valve. Efficacy of the TIF 1 was not Bourne out by clinical studies. Currently, the TIF 2.0

procedure is performed which uses extra fasteners to create an esophago-gastric plication attempting to wrap the esophagus 270–310° in circumference and lengthen the valve 3–4 cm (Fig. 14.6) [39].

In a canine model to evaluate the feasibility of the TIF procedure, serosa-to-serosa fusion was histologically observed on the newly created valve at 4 weeks (Fig. 14.6), and TIF 2.0 procedure normalized distal esophageal acid exposure and increased LES pressure over a 2-week period [39]. Following this, a company-sponsored, European multicenter, prospective study involving 86 patients with chronic GERD evaluating the safety and efficacy of TIF 1.0 procedure demonstrated that 68 % of patients discontinued PPIs at a 12-month follow-up. A clinically significant improvement in GERD-HRQL scores was achieved in 73 % of patients, and distal esophageal acid exposure was reduced in 61 % of patients but normalized in only 37 % of patients. In a 2-year follow-up of this study, the effectiveness of TIF 1.0 procedure to eliminate heartburn was sustained in 93 % of patients

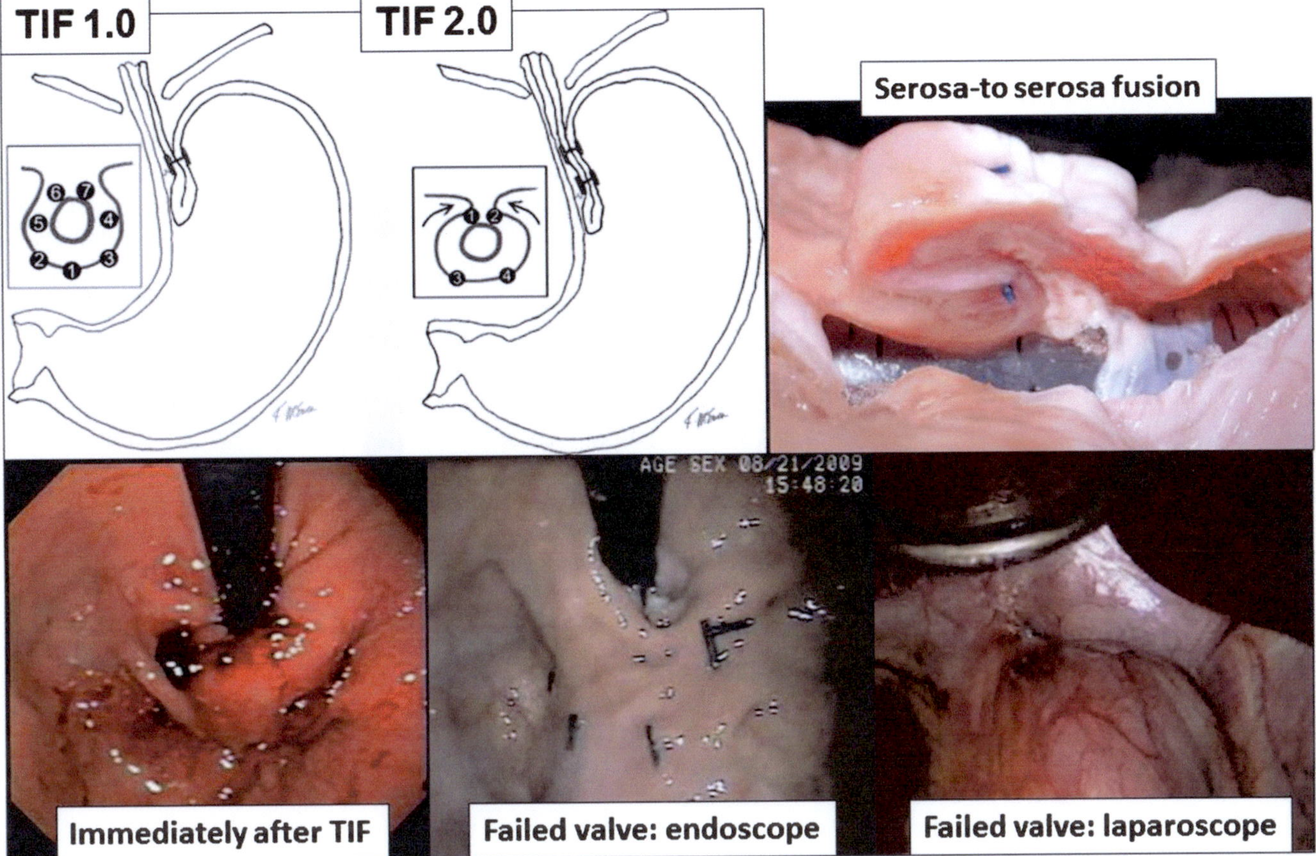

Fig. 14.6 TIF procedure (*left upper panel*) illustrations of TIF 1.0 and TIF 2.0 procedures. (*Right upper panel*) Serosa-to-serosa fusion was found at 4 weeks after TIF procedure. (*Lower panel*) Endoscopic appearance of gastroesophageal valve immediately after TIF 2.0 procedure (*left*) and failed valve (*middle*) and laparoscopic appearance of failed valve (*right*). (Reproduced from Jobe BA, et al. Ann Surg. 2008;248(1):69–76)

who completed a 2-year follow-up, and 71 % had no need for PPIs [39, 40]. These encouraging data led to several clinical studies; however the outcomes have been conflicting. Furthermore, the TIF 2.0 procedure was expected to be superior to the TIF 1.0 procedure; however our series of 19 highly selected patients who had undergone the TIF 2.0 procedure demonstrated that 53 % (10/19) of patients required re-intervention for recurrent symptoms within the first 12 months and 68 % (13/19) were considered to be unsuccessful, indicating that even TIF 2.0 procedure is associated with high rates of early symptomatic failure and the need for surgical re-intervention [40]. These results led to additional modifications of the procedure with more aggressive attempts to create a "wrap" and more fasteners being deployed. Anecdotal reports suggest that results may be better with the latest technique modifications [41]. A randomized, sham-controlled study (RESPECT trial) was recently completed and early reports suggest moderately good results for the most recent TIF procedure. Complete results of the RESPECT

trial have not been published as of mid 2014. Early reports are required to evaluate the true efficacy and durability of TIF procedure.

Further modifications of the device are being made by the company and may further improve the outcomes of this procedure.

Current Status and Future Prospective for EAR

Accumulating evidence has suggested that the most challenging aspect of EAR is to achieve long-term sustained improvements in objective measurements such as distal esophageal acid exposure, although most of EAR techniques appear to be safe, and effective at least to the point of improved clinical symptoms and quality of life, and reduction of PPI use for a short period of time. Many EAR devices have disappeared primarily due to inadequate or poor long-term clinical data and resulting lack of financial support, and only three FDA-approved devices are currently available on the market; the Stretta radiofrequency system, the EsophyX device, and most recently the MUSE device. However, none of these can be considered standards of care and are not widely performed outside of a few specialist centers. A systematic review of EAR techniques for the treatment of GERD advised that none of the currently available randomized controlled trials have supported their routine use for the treatment of GERD [42]. It can be expected though, that further refinement of devices and techniques will improve outcomes.

GERD is caused by an anatomically impaired gastroesophageal flap valve, which allows retrograde flow of gastric contents into the esophagus. Acid suppression therapy eliminates heartburn by reducing the acid production and turning off the acidity of gastric contents but never address the incompetent valve at the GEJ. The important components of surgical repair are to adequately mobilize the stomach and to achieve a 2–3 cm tension-free intra-abdominal esophagus in order to avoid a persistent downward forcing tension onto the fundoplication, which causes recurrent hernia or disruption of the fundoplication. None of the current EAR techniques can fully achieve this principle of surgical valve repair, though the Esophyx procedure at least makes an attempt to do. It may be that a totally different approach or combination with some additional technology may be required to achieve the optimal long-term outcomes. As one of such approaches, an endoscopic implantation technique combined with tissue engineering has been investigated, in which skeletal muscle-derived cells are transplanted into the muscular layer at the GEJ for attempting to restore the LES function [43].

Although there is lack of long-term sustained efficacy, the EAR procedures may continue to be an alternative option, somewhere between surgical and medical therapies, especially for patients having refractory GERD to medical therapy, who are not candidates for surgery due to severe co-morbidities or are unwilling to take medications or undergo surgery. Since the surgical fundoplication for patients with massive obesity has been challenging due to high rate of recurrence, the EAR procedures could also be a good option to treat GERD in this population [44]. A recent retrospective study demonstrated that seven patients with massive obesity, who had undergone Roux-en-Y gastric bypass with documented GERD, underwent the Stretta procedure to treat GERD, and 5 of 7 patients had complete symptomatic resolution and normalization of pH testing at a follow-up of 20 ± 2 months. Additionally, reversibility is an important component of the EAR procedures. Some studies have demonstrated that the EAR procedures can be repeated or converted to surgical fundoplication in case of recurrence or unsatisfied outcome of the initial treatment. However, it is noted that a prior or repeated EAR procedures potentially make the following surgical fundoplication more difficult due to severe adhesion at the level of GEJ [40].

Guidelines recently published by SAGES [46] (http://www.sages.org/publications/guidelines/endoluminal-treatments-for-gastroesophageal-reflux-disease-gerd/) collated the most recent published data on EAR [44]. For Esophyx, they concluded that: "Long term data is not yet available for EsophyX. In short term follow-up, from 6 months to 2 years, EsophyX may be effective in patients with a hiatal hernia ≤ 2 cm with typical and atypical GERD. Further studies are required to define optimal techniques and most appropriate patient selection criteria, and to further evaluate device and technique safety. [Quality of Evidence: (++). GRADE Recommendation: Weak]". For Stretta their conclusions were: " Stretta is considered appropriate therapy for patients being treated for GERD who are 18 years of age or older, who have had symptoms of heartburn, regurgitation, or both for 6 months or more, who have been partially or completely responsive to antisecretory pharmacologic therapy, and who have declined laparoscopic fundoplication. [Quality of Evidence: (++++). GRADE Recommendation: Strong]." There were insufficient publications to support any comment about the MUSE device.

Conclusion

EAR so far has consisted of three major endoluminal techniques; radiofrequency energy, synthetic implants, and plication techniques. It is evident that EAR procedures should be performed on highly selected patients with documented GERD, who have small or no hiatal hernia (<2 cm), normal esophageal motility, are not obese, and do not have severe esophagitis or Barrett's esophagus. None of the EAR procedures has been widely adopted as a routine treatment of GERD due to skepticism of their sustained long-term efficacy, and failure of the companies to achieve a reimbursement pathway. Further modification of the devices and/or combination with additional technology will continue to improve outcomes, and further randomized, sham-controlled studies with long-term follow-up are required to assess the true benefit of EAR.

References

1. Inadomi JM, McIntyre L, Bernard L, Fendrick AM. Step-down from multiple- to single-dose proton pump inhibitors (PPIs): a prospective study of patients with heartburn or acid regurgitation completely relieved with PPIs. Am J Gastroenterol. 2003;98(9):1940–4.
2. Hogan WJ. Clinical trials evaluating endoscopic GERD treatments: is it time for a moratorium on the clinical use of these procedures? Am J Gastroenterol. 2006;101(3):437–9.

3. Khajanchee YS, Ujiki M, Dunst CM, Swanstrom LL. Patient factors predictive of 24-h pH normalization following endoluminal gastroplication for GERD. Surg Endosc. 2009;23(11):2525–30.

4. O'Connor KW, Lehman GA. Endoscopic placement of collagen at the lower esophageal sphincter to inhibit gastroesophageal reflux: a pilot study of 10 medically intractable patients. Gastrointest Endosc. 1988;34(2):106–12.

5. Deviere J, Pastorelli A, Louis H, et al. Endoscopic implantation of a biopolymer in the lower esophageal sphincter for gastroesophageal reflux: a pilot study. Gastrointest Endosc. 2002;55(3):335–41.

6. Fockens P, Cohen L, Edmundowicz SA, et al. Prospective randomized controlled trial of an injectable esophageal prosthesis versus a sham procedure for endoscopic treatment of gastroesophageal reflux disease. Surg Endosc. 2010;24(6):1387–97.

7. Johnson DA, Ganz R, Aisenberg J, et al. Endoscopic, deep mural implantation of Enteryx for the treatment of GERD: 6-month follow-up of a multicenter trial. Am J Gastroenterol. 2003; 98(2):250–8.

8. Cohen LB, Johnson DA, Ganz RA, et al. Enteryx implantation for GERD: expanded multicenter trial results and interim postapproval follow-up to 24 months. Gastrointest Endosc. 2005;61(6):650–8.

9. Deviere J, Costamagna G, Neuhaus H, et al. Nonresorbable copolymer implantation for gastroesophageal reflux disease: a randomized sham-controlled multicenter trial. Gastroenterology. 2005; 128(3):532–40.

10. Wong RF, Davis TV, Peterson KA. Complications involving the mediastinum after injection of Enteryx for GERD. Gastrointest Endosc. 2005;61(6):753–6.

11. Tintillier M, Chaput A, Kirch L, Martinet JP, Pochet JM, Cuvelier C. Esophageal abscess complicating endoscopic treatment of refractory gastroesophageal reflux disease by Enteryx injection: a first case report. Am J Gastroenterol. 2004;99(9):1856–8.

12. Veerappan GR, Koff JM, Smith MT. Enteryx polymer migration to lymph nodes and beyond. Endoscopy. 2008;40 Suppl 2:E10–1.

13. Fockens P, Bruno MJ, Gabbrielli A, et al. Endoscopic augmentation of the lower esophageal sphincter for the treatment of gastroesophageal reflux disease: multicenter study of the Gatekeeper Reflux Repair System. Endoscopy. 2004;36(8):682–9.

14. Utley DS. The Stretta procedure: device, technique, and pre-clinical study data. Gastrointest Endosc Clin N Am. 2003;13(1):135–45.

15. Tam WC, Schoeman MN, Zhang Q, et al. Delivery of radiofrequency energy to the lower oesophageal sphincter and gastric cardia inhibits transient lower oesophageal sphincter relaxations and gastro-oesophageal reflux in patients with reflux disease. Gut. 2003;52(4):479–85.

16. Triadafilopoulos G, Utley DS. Temperature-controlled radiofrequency energy delivery for gastroesophageal reflux disease: the Stretta procedure. J Laparoendosc Adv Surg Tech A. 2001; 11(6):333–9.

17. Kim MS, Holloway RH, Dent J, Utley DS. Radiofrequency energy delivery to the gastric cardia inhibits triggering of transient lower esophageal sphincter relaxation and gastroesophageal reflux in dogs. Gastrointest Endosc. 2003;57(1):17–22.

18. Arts J, Sifrim D, Rutgeerts P, Lerut A, Janssens J, Tack J. Influence of radiofrequency energy delivery at the gastroesophageal junction (the Stretta procedure) on symptoms, acid exposure, and esophageal sensitivity to acid perfusion in gastroesophageal reflux disease. Dig Dis Sci. 2007;52(9):2170–7.

19. Triadafilopoulos G. Changes in GERD symptom scores correlate with improvement in esophageal acid exposure after the Stretta procedure. Surg Endosc. 2004;18(7):1038–44.

20. Triadafilopoulos G. Clinical experience with the Stretta procedure. Gastrointest Endosc Clin N Am. 2003;13(1):147–55.

21. Coron E, Sebille V, Cadiot G, et al. Clinical trial: radiofrequency energy delivery in proton pump inhibitor-dependent gastro-oesophageal reflux disease patients. Aliment Pharmacol Ther. 2008;28(9):1147–58.

22. Noar MD, Noar E. Gastroparesis associated with gastroesophageal reflux disease and corresponding reflux symptoms may be corrected by radiofrequency ablation of the cardia and esophagogastric junction. Surg Endosc. 2008;22(11):2440–4.

23. Corley DA, Katz P, Wo JM, et al. Improvement of gastroesophageal reflux symptoms after radiofrequency energy: a randomized, sham-controlled trial. Gastroenterology. 2003;125(3):668–76.

24. Aziz AM, El-Khayat HR, Sadek A, et al. A prospective randomized trial of sham, single-dose Stretta, and double-dose Stretta for the treatment of gastroesophageal reflux disease. Surg Endosc. 2010;24(4):818–25.

25. Hill LD, Kozarek RA, Kraemer SJ, et al. The gastroesophageal flap valve: in vitro and in vivo observations. Gastrointest Endosc. 1996;44(5):541–7.

26. Kadirkamanathan SS, Yazaki E, Evans DF, Hepworth CC, Gong F, Swain CP. An ambulant porcine model of acid reflux used to evaluate endoscopic gastroplasty. Gut. 1999;44(6):782–8.

27. Lin BR, Wong JM, Chang MC, et al. Abnormal gastroesophageal flap valve is highly associated with gastroesophageal reflux disease among subjects undergoing routine endoscopy in Taiwan. J Gastroenterol Hepatol. 2006;21(3):556–62.

28. Liu JJ, Glickman JN, Li X, et al. Smooth muscle remodeling of the gastroesophageal junction after endoluminal gastroplication. Gastrointest Endosc. 2007;65(7):1023–7.

29. Schiefke I, Zabel-Langhennig A, Neumann S, Feisthammel J, Moessner J, Caca K. Long term failure of endoscopic gastroplication (EndoCinch). Gut. 2005;54(6):752–8.

30. Schwartz MP, Wellink H, Gooszen HG, Conchillo JM, Samsom M, Smout AJ. Endoscopic gastroplication for the treatment of gastro-oesophageal reflux disease: a randomised, sham-controlled trial. Gut. 2007;56(1):20–8.

31. Schiefke I, Neumann S, Zabel-Langhennig A, Moessner J, Caca K. Use of an endoscopic suturing device (the "ESD") to treat patients with gastroesophageal reflux disease, after unsuccessful EndoCinch endoluminal gastroplication: another failure. Endoscopy. 2005;37(8):700–5.

32. Chen YK, Raijman I, Ben-Menachem T, et al. Long-term outcomes of endoluminal gastroplication: a U.S. multicenter trial. Gastrointest Endosc. 2005;61(6):659–67.

33. Montgomery M, Hakanson B, Ljungqvist O, Ahlman B, Thorell A. Twelve months' follow-up after treatment with the EndoCinch endoscopic technique for gastro-oesophageal reflux disease: a randomized, placebo-controlled study. Scand J Gastroenterol. 2006;41(12):1382–9.

34. Chuttani R, Sud R, Sachdev G, et al. A novel endoscopic full-thickness plicator for the treatment of GERD: a pilot study. Gastrointest Endosc. 2003;58(5):770–6.

35. Rothstein R, Filipi C, Caca K, et al. Endoscopic full-thickness plication for the treatment of gastroesophageal reflux disease: a randomized, sham-controlled trial. Gastroenterology. 2006; 131(3):704–12.

36. von Renteln D, Schiefke I, Fuchs KH, et al. Endoscopic full-thickness plication for the treatment of gastroesophageal reflux disease using multiple plicator implants: 12-month multicenter study results. Surg Endosc. 2009;23(8):1866–75.

37. Ramage JI, Rothstein RI, Edmundowicz SA, et al. Endoscopically placed titanium plicator for GERD: pivotal phase – preliminary 6-month results. Gastrointest Endosc. 2006;63(5):AB126.

38. Kauer WK, Roy-Shapira A, Watson D, et al. Preclinical trial of a modified gastroscope that performs a true anterior fundoplication for the endoluminal treatment of gastroesophageal reflux disease. Surg Endosc. 2009;23(12):2728–31.

39. Jobe BA, O'Rourke RW, McMahon BP, et al. Transoral endoscopic fundoplication in the treatment of gastroesophageal reflux disease: the anatomic and physiologic basis for reconstruction of the esophagogastric junction using a novel device. Ann Surg. 2008; 248(1):69–76.

40. Hoppo T, Immanuel A, Schuchert M, et al. Transoral incisionless fundoplication 2.0 procedure using EsophyX for gastroesophageal reflux disease. J Gastrointest Surg. 2010;14(12):1895–901.

41. Wendling MR, Melvin WS, Perry KA. Impact of transoral incisionless fundoplication (TIF) on subjective and objective GERD indices: a systematic review of the published literature. Surg Endosc. 2013;27(10):3754–61.

42. Chen D, Barber C, McLoughlin P, Thavaneswaran P, Jamieson GG, Maddern GJ. Systematic review of endoscopic treatments for gastro-oesophageal reflux disease. Br J Surg. 2009;96(2):128–36.

43. Pasricha PJ, Ahmed I, Jankowski RJ, Micci MA. Endoscopic injection of skeletal muscle-derived cells augments gut smooth muscle sphincter function: implications for a novel therapeutic approach. Gastrointest Endosc. 2009;70(6):1231–7.

44. Mattar SG, Qureshi F, Taylor D, Schauer PR. Treatment of refractory gastroesophageal reflux disease with radiofrequency energy (Stretta) in patients after Roux-en-Y gastric bypass. Surg Endosc. 2006;20(6):850–4. Auyang ED[1], Carter P, Rauth T, Fanelli RD; SAGES Guidelines Committee. SAGES clinical spotlight review: endoluminal treatments for gastroesophageal reflux disease (GERD).

Magnetic LES Augmentation: The LINX Procedure

Luigi Bonavina, Greta Saino, Stephanie G. Worrell, and Tom R. DeMeester

Background

Gastroesophageal reflux disease (GERD), as recently redefined and classified by the Montreal consensus conference, is a chronic foregut disorder in which the barrier function of the lower esophageal sphincter (LES) fails and gastroduodenal contents are allowed to reflux into the esophagus causing troublesome symptoms and/or anatomical lesions [1]. Chronic GERD represents a significant cost burden on the healthcare economy, with nearly $10 billion of annual direct costs in the United States alone, the highest cost of any digestive disorder [2].

The two primary treatment options for GERD patients are long-term medical acid suppression therapy or a surgical reconstruction of the LES. Currently, approximately one third of patients are resistant or only partial responders to daily acid suppression therapy with proton-pump inhibitors (PPI) [3, 4], and even high dose pharmacological therapy is often inadequate to maintain a symptom-free state in individuals with a mechanically defective LES [5]. Additionally, there are growing concerns over the long-term effects of chronic acid suppression. Many patients suffer from persis-

L. Bonavina, MD (✉)
Division of General Surgery, Department of Biomedical Sciences for Health, IRCCS Policlinico San Donato, University of Milano, Via Decembrio 19a, Milan 20137, Italy
e-mail: luigi.bonavina@unimi.it

G. Saino, MD
IRCCS Policlinico San Donato, University of Milano Medical School, Piazza Malan, San Donato Milanese, Milan 20092, Italy
e-mail: greta.saino@grupposandonato.it

S.G. Worrell, MD
Department of Surgery, Keck Medical Center of USC, 1510 San Pablo St, Los Angeles, CA 90033, USA
e-mail: stephanie.worrell@med.usc.edu

T.R. DeMeester, MD
Department of Surgery, Keck Medical Center of USC, 892 Huntington Garden Drive, Los Angeles, CA 91108, USA
e-mail: Tom.DeMeester@med.usc.edu

tent non-acid reflux and nocturnal acid breakthrough, and may progress to serious complications of the disease, such as volume regurgitation with pulmonary aspiration and Barrett's metaplasia, the leading risk factor for esophageal adenocarcinoma. A large European open cohort multicenter study (ProGERD) showed that 9.7 % of patients under routine medical care progressed to Barrett's esophagus in 5 years of follow-up [6]. Recent literature also indicates that chronic acid suppression with PPI may reduce the effectiveness of medications such as clopidogrel, reduce the absorption of vitamin B12 and magnesium, and increase the risk of Clostridium difficile infection [7]. There is some evidence suggesting chronic acid suppression may even be associated with an increased incidence of gastric cancer [8]. Other consequences of prolonged PPI therapy include hypergastrinemia, enterochromaffin-like cell hyperplasia, and parietal cell hypertrophy, leading to rebound acid hypersecretion [9].

The laparoscopic Nissen fundoplication is a safe, effective, and durable therapy for GERD when performed in specialized and high-volume centers. However, despite a remarkably low 30-day morbidity and mortality rates, the operation is underused due to the high incidence of short-term side effects and fear of failure, which impacts referral patterns [10]. Also, wide variability in clinical outcomes due to the subtleties of expert surgical results has limited the adoption of this procedure [11]. Patients undergoing a Nissen fundoplication are especially at risk for potential side effects of the procedure such as bloating, the inability to belch and vomit, and the occurrence of persistent dysphagia that may occasionally require revisional surgery [12]. These are the main reasons why gastroenterologists tend to limit their referrals for fundoplication only to patients with long-lasting severe disease and large hiatal hernias. Currently, fewer than 30,000 Nissen fundoplication procedures are performed annually in the US, corresponding to less than 1 % of the GERD population [13]. This is dramatically less than the number in the first decade following introduction of laparoscopic fundoplication. The decline in surgical volume has been attributed to the perceived risk of fundoplication failure,

L.L. Swanstrom and C.M. Dunst (eds.), *Antireflux Surgery*,
DOI 10.1007/978-1-4939-1749-5_15, © Springer New York 2015

Table 15.1 Side effects of the Nissen fundoplication ($n > 100$ patients with long-term follow-up)

	Open 1986[a] (%)	Lap 1998[b] (%)	Lap 2006[c] (%)	Lap 2011[d] (%)
Inability to belch	36	20	–	–
Inability to vomit (if tried)	63	25	–	–
Increased flatus	38	47	40	57
Symptomatic gas bloat	15	44	31	40
Persistent dysphagia	3	2	2	11

Adapted from: [a]DeMeester T, et al. Ann Surg. 1986;204:9–20 (Open series, median follow-up 5 years)
[b]Peters J, et al. Ann Surg. 1998;228:40–50 (Lap series, mean follow-up 21 months.)
[c]Dallemagne B, et al. Surg Endosc. 2006;20:159–65 (Lap series, follow-up 10 years)
[d]Galmiche JP, Lundell L, et al. JAMA 2011;305:1969–77 (Lap series, follow-up 5 years)

to the availability of over-the-counter PPIs and endoscopic therapies, and to the rise of bariatric surgery [14].

The limitations of both pharmacologic therapy and fundoplication leave many patients and clinicians in the equivocal position to either tolerate a lifetime drug dependence with incomplete symptom relief or to undertake the risk of a surgical procedure that alters gastric anatomy and may have considerable side effects. This large population of patients suffer from such a "therapy gap" in effective GERD treatment. The result is a large population of patients with incomplete relief of symptoms who could benefit from a simple sphincter augmentation procedure rather than choosing life-long medical therapy or an anatomic altering fundoplication.

Consequently, it is reasonable that patients with progressive disease who get incomplete relief of their symptoms, develop new symptoms, or require higher doses of PPIs are frustrated by the ineffectiveness of the medical therapy and the lack of a dependable and durable surgical solution to their problem that is free of side effects. The specific issues they are anxious about are the persistence of symptoms while on PPI therapy, life-long dependency on medication, disease progression while on medication, the side effects of medication, and the finality and side effects of a surgical fundoplication. They are asking themselves, what does this mean for me in the long-term? The limitations of both medical therapy and laparoscopic fundoplication leave this group of patients in the equivocal position of either tolerating a lifetime of drug dependence with incomplete symptom relief and the risk of progressive disease or accepting the risk of a surgical procedure that alters gastric anatomy, has significant side effects and is not easily reversible (Table 15.1).

Improved understanding of the LES has led to the development of procedures that augment the sphincter without causing side effects. The procedures are applicable to patients who have earlier evidence of progressive disease manifested by incomplete relief of their symptoms with PPI therapy. On clinical testing, these patients have increased esophageal acid exposure, adequate esophageal body function, and a normal or near normal LES. Such patients have a transient failure of the LES due to excessive shortening of its overall length when challenged by gastric distension or dilation. A promising surgical therapy for these patients is the implantation of a new device that focused on augmenting the function of the existing LES. The anatomy of the hiatus is not altered and unlike a fundoplication the procedure does not attempt to improve the exposure of the abdominal length of the LES to the positive environmental pressure of the abdomen. There are three such operations; augmentation of the LES with radio-frequency [15], with electrical stimulation [16], and with magnetic beads [17]. Of these, the most extensive clinical experience has been with magnetic sphincter augmentation using a device known as the LINX.

The LINX™ Reflux Management System

The LINX procedure was developed to address the existing "therapy gap" in the treatment of GERD. The LINX is a simple mechanical device designed to augment the physiologic barrier to reflux by magnetic force. It remedies transient failure of the LES by preventing shortening of its overall length when challenged by gastric distension or dilation [17]. The procedure requires only limited dissection, does not alter the anatomy of the esophageal hiatus, has minimal side effects, and is reversible (Table 15.2).

The device consists of a series of titanium beads with magnetic cores hermetically sealed inside. The beads are interlinked with independent titanium wires to form a flexible and expandable ring. Interestingly, each bead can move independent of the adjacent beads, creating a dynamic implant that mimics the physiological movement of the esophagus without limiting its range of motion (Fig. 15.1). The strength of the magnetic core contained in each bead is calibrated by mass to provide a resisting force that precisely augments the sphincter's function. For reflux to occur, the intragastric pressure must overcome the resistance to opening of both the patient's native LES pressure and the magnetic bonds of the device. The device is manufactured in different sizes and is capable of nearly doubling its diameter when all beads are separated. The magnetic attraction force to be counteracted to allow beads separation is independent of the number of beads contained in the device. The LINX device, while augmenting the LES, allows for expansion to accommodate a swallowed bolus or the escape of elevated gastric pressure associated with belching or vomiting. This provides control of reflux without compromising the physiologic function of the LES [18]. The LINX device can be easily removed if necessary, thereby preserving the option for a subsequent fundoplication if necessary. More importantly the LINX device produces little to no persistent side effects and was designed to limit the technical variability that occurs with fundoplication.

Surgical Procedure

The goal was to develop a more standardized and gentler antireflux procedure that is applicable and acceptable to patients with early progressive disease with reproducible outcomes. The principles of implanting the LINX device are proper sizing of the device, proper positioning of the device, and constructing, with limited dissection, a tunnel behind the esophagus and between its posterior wall and the posterior vagus nerve through which the LINX device is passed. The phrenoesophageal ligament is not dissected and the esophageal hiatus is not explored. Guarding the integrity of the phrenoesophageal ligament during LINX implantation is

imperative as the ligament functions to maintain the abdominal length of the LES. This is counter to doing a fundoplication where the hiatus is completely dissected out and the LES is enveloped with the gastric fundus to provide a conduit to transmit intra-abdominal pressure around the LES.

The critical benchmark steps of the procedure are listed in Table 15.3. The steps of the procedure are illustrated in Fig. 15.2. Briefly, surgical dissection begins by dividing the peritoneum on the anterior surface of the gastroesophageal junction (GEJ) below the insertion of the inferior leaf of the phrenoesophageal ligament and above the junction of the hepatic branch to the anterior vagus nerve. The lateral surface of the left crus is freed from the posterior fundic wall without dividing any short gastric vessel. The gastro-hepatic ligament is opened above and below the hepatic branch to facilitate the preparation of the retro-esophageal window. Gentle dissection from the right side is made toward the left crus just above the crural decussation to identify the posterior vagus nerve. A tunnel is then created between the vagus and the posterior esophageal wall, and a penrose drain is passed in a left to right direction. The circumference of the esophagus is measured with a proprietary sizer to determine the proper size of the LINX device to be implanted. The sizing tool is a laparoscopic instrument with a soft, circular curved tip actuated by coaxial tubes through a handset. The handset contains a numerical indicator that corresponds with the size range of the LINX device. Alternatively, the original sizing device mimics the LINX implant with special color-coding of each bead to measure the circumference of the esophagus. The sizing tool is placed around the esophagus in the dissected space between the posterior esophageal wall and the posterior vagus nerve bundle. Once the appropriate LINX device has been selected, it is introduced through the posterior tunnel. The opposing ends are then brought to the anterior surface of the esophagus and connected together; this completes the implant procedure.

Table 15.2 Side effects following the LINX

	Surg. Endosc. [17]	NEJM [23]	JACS [25]
Follow-up time (months)	48	36	36
Dysphagia-moderate or severe (%)	0[a]	0[a]	0[b]
Ability to belch (%)	95	98	99
Ability to vomit (%)	95	98	99

[a]Per adverse reporting event
[b]Per GERD–HRQL score >3

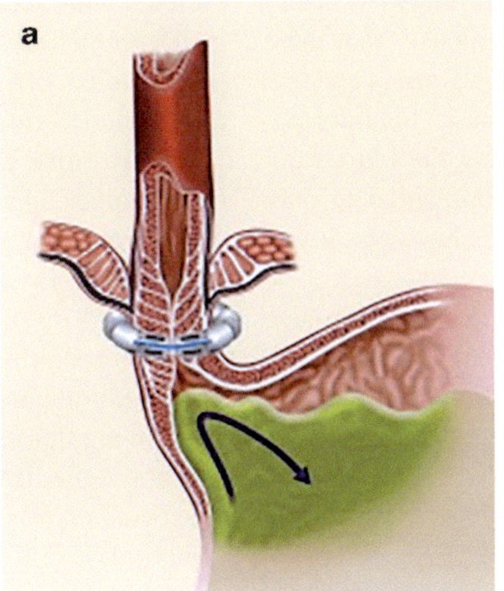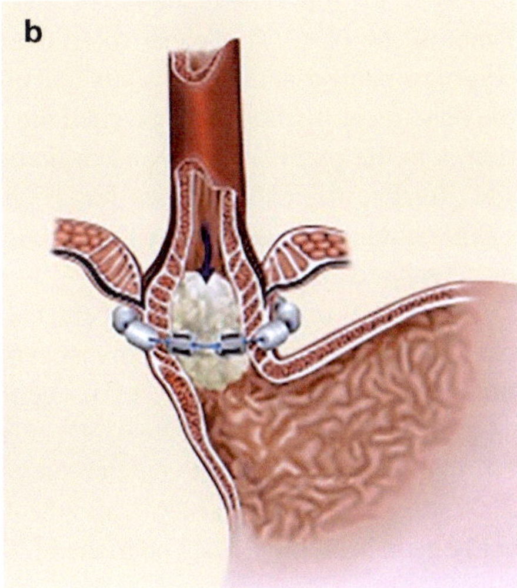

Fig. 15.1 The LINX reflux management system encircling the distal esophagus in the closed position (**a**) and in the open position (**b**)

Table 15.3 Critical benchmarks in performing the LINX

1. Mobilization of the fundus of the stomach from the diaphragm and surface of the left crus
2. Open the fascia for 1–2 cm along the inferior–anterior margin of the left crus just above the crural decussation
3. Initiate the dissection of a tunnel from the left through the fascial incision and posterior to the esophagus for about 1 cm
4. Open the gastro-hepatic ligament above and below the hepatic branch of the anterior vagal nerve
5. Open the fascia along the inferior–anterior margin of the right crus for 1–2 cm just above the crural   decussation
6. Identify the posterior vagal nerve by slow and gentle dissection while retracting the stomach in an anterior–inferior direction
7. Dissect a tunnel posterior to the esophagus just above the GEJ and between the posterior vagus nerve and the posterior wall of the esophagus
8. Pull a 1/4 inch penrose drain through the tunnel
9. If necessary, mobilize the anterior gastroesophageal fat pad inferiorly or trench across the fat pad on the anterior surface of the esophagus above the level of the posterior tunnel
10. Measure the circumference of the esophagus at the level of the GEJ
11. Implant the appropriate sized LINX device through the tunnel and around the esophagus
12. Endoscope the patient if appropriate to check the position of the LINX device

Preliminary observations suggest that patients with minimal to no hiatal hernia achieve the best results with the LINX augmentation. However, sliding hernias, up to 3 cm in size, can be effectively repaired by approximating the crura with interrupted posterior stitches and then the device can safely be implanted. The decision to proceed with a posterior crural repair depends on the size of the hernia that is found intra-operatively.

Operative time is about half-an-hour. Patients are discharged the same day of surgery or on the first postoperative day under direction to return to a normal diet as quickly as possible and to discontinue use of acid suppression medication immediately. Patients typically return to normal physical activity in less than a week. The most common complaint following the LINX procedure is mild dysphagia that is usually easily tolerated and requires only temporary diet adjustments.

Clinical Experience

The LINX Reflux Management System has been recently reviewed by the Gastroenterology and Urology Advisory Panel of the FDA. This panel voted unanimously that there was reasonable assurance of safety and effectiveness and that the benefits of treatment outweighed the risks. This information is in the public domain and available at the FDA website. To date the LINX device has been implanted in over 1,000 patients worldwide and the outcomes have confirmed its safety and efficacy [19].

Two initial prospective, multicenter, clinical studies have been conducted under an FDA investigational device exemption to evaluate the LINX System. The first study evaluated 44 patients implanted with the LINX at four study centers in USA and in Europe between February 2007 and October 2008; the short-term, mid-term, and the 4-year results of this study have been previously published [20–22].

The second study evaluated 100 patients implanted in USA between January and September 2009 [23]. No significant differences were seen between the studies in terms of safety and efficacy. A registry of antireflux surgery is currently enrolling patients in Europe to include treatment with either the LINX System or the Nissen fundoplication.

The feasibility study was a prospective, multicenter, single-arm, controlled clinical trial. Patients served as their own control to assess the effect of treatment on esophageal acid exposure, symptoms, and use of PPI. The trial protocol was approved by the institutional review board at each of the four study centers. The primary criteria for inclusion in the feasibility trial were the following: age >18 and <85 years, typical reflux symptoms at least partially responsive to PPI therapy, abnormal esophageal acid exposure, and normal contractile amplitude and wave form in the esophageal body. The primary criteria for exclusion from the trial were the following: history of dysphagia, previous upper abdominal surgery, previous endoluminal antireflux procedures, sliding hiatal hernia >3 cm, esophagitis > grade A, and/or the presence of histologically documented Barrett's esophagus. Patients with abnormal manometric findings (distal esophageal contraction amplitude of less than 35 mmHg on wet swallows or <70 % propulsive peristaltic sequences) were also excluded from the study.

Preoperative evaluation consisted of symptom questionnaire, upper gastrointestinal endoscopy, barium swallow, esophageal manometry, and 24-h esophageal pH monitoring. The Gastro-Esophageal Reflux Disease–Health Related Quality of Life (GERD–HRQL) validated questionnaire was administered prior to any diagnostic test and off PPI therapy. The questionnaire consists of six heartburn questions, two swallowing questions, one gas bloat question, and one question about medication use. The responses to these questions are scored on a scale of 0 (no symptoms) to 5 (incapacitating symptom).

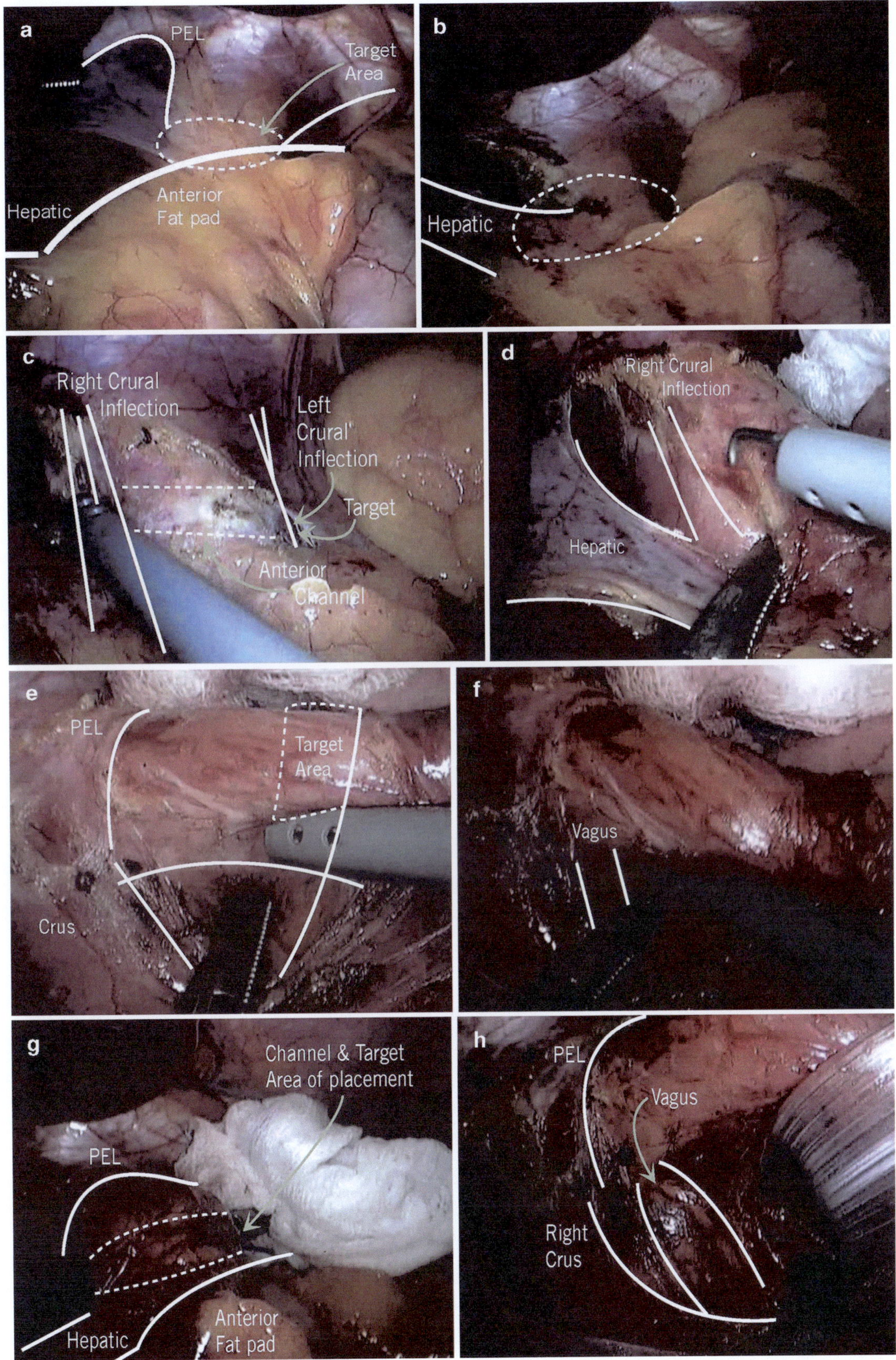

Fig. 15.2 Surgical steps of the LINX procedure. (**a**) Establish area for device placement; (**b**) if no or small hernia, preserve phrenoesophageal ligament (PEL)—if large hernia make routine dissection; (**c**) identify depression between left crus and esophagus. Create left "target" dissection and anterior channel (being careful to preserve PEL and anterior vagus); (**d**) identify inflection between right crus and esophagus; (**e**) dissect to separate right crus from esophagus; (**f**) identify and exclude posterior vagus; (**g**) complete "tunnel" through to "target" on left lateral side of esophagus; (**h**) place penrose drain for traction; (**i**) place distal end of sizer past mid-point of posterior esophagus and release traction on stomach;

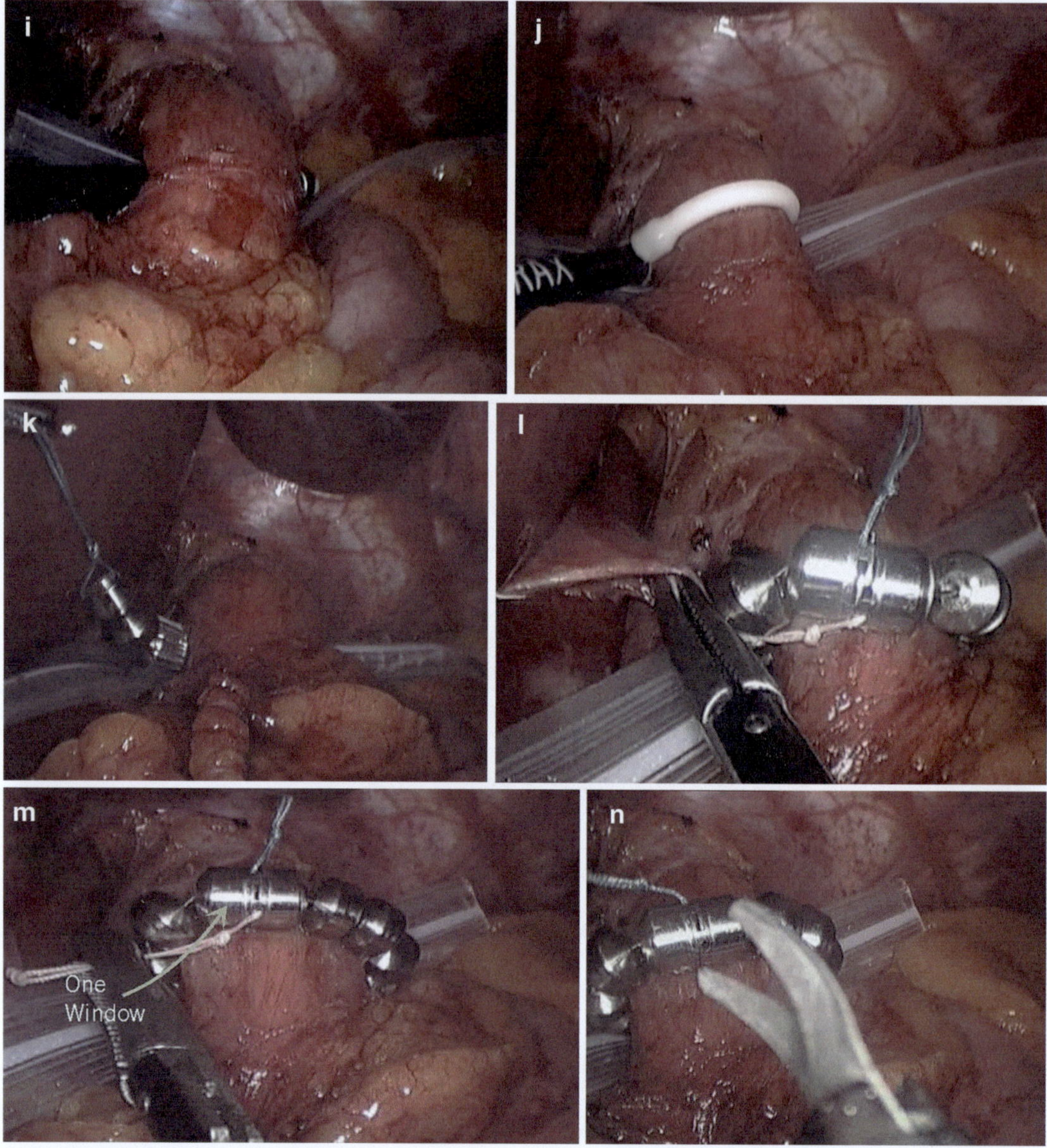

Fig. 15.2 (continued) (**j**) make certain that esophagus is clear of nasogastric tube or endoscope and no excess tissue is between sizer and esophagus. Leave any traction on stomach; (**k**) place LINX inside penrose drain and position in tunnel behind esophagus, then remove penrose drain; (**l**) grasping sutures, place one clasp end up on the esophagus, hold in position while maneuvering second clasp into alignment with open clasp. Do not clasp wires, make certain clasps are free of tissue; (**m**) once clasps are engaged confirm that device is locked. Make certain there is a single window visible between clasps. *Tug green* and *white sutures* at 180° opposition; (**n**) Confirm (*1*) no excess or connective tissue remains between device and esophagus (*2*) no beads are separated—without traction (*3*) no space exists between device and esophagus

The presence of esophagitis was assessed by upper gastrointestinal endoscopy using the Los Angeles or Savary–Miller classification. The size of hiatal hernia, if present, was measured as the distance between the GEJ, defined by the proximal limit of the gastric folds, and the crural impression. The LES resting pressure and length were measured by esophageal manometry using a station pull-through technique. The percent of LES relaxation and the LES residual pressure were assessed with five wet swallows. The amplitude of esophageal contractions was measured by averaging ten wet swallows of 5 ml each, taken 30 s apart. Abnormal motility was defined as a mean amplitude of less than 35 mmHg and/or a greater than 30 % prevalence of simultaneous, dropped, or interrupted waves. Prolonged (24–48 h) esophageal pH monitoring was used to confirm abnormal esophageal acid exposure off PPI therapy. The pH-probe or Bravo capsule was placed 5 cm above the manometric upper border of the LES as determined by manometry or 6 cm above the Z-line determined by endoscopy.

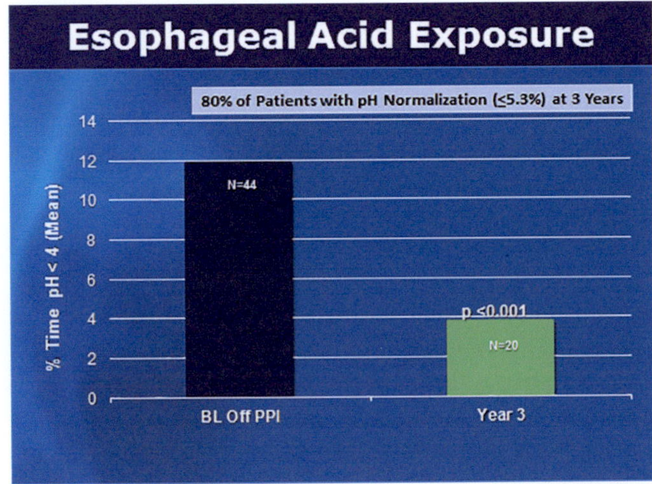

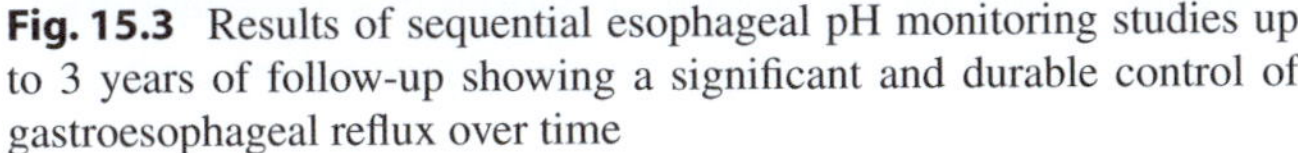

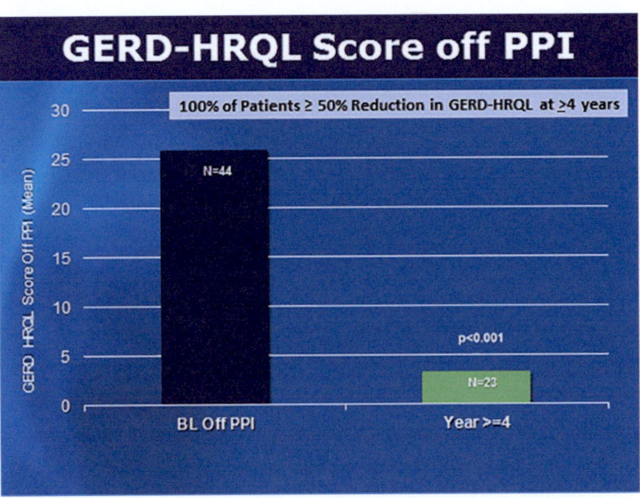

Fig. 15.3 Results of sequential esophageal pH monitoring studies up to 3 years of follow-up showing a significant and durable control of gastroesophageal reflux over time

Fig. 15.4 The GERD–HRQL total score significantly decreased and remained stable after the implant

All LINX devices were successfully implanted via a standard 5 port laparoscopic approach. The median operative time was 40 min (range 19–104). No intraoperative complications occurred. Patients were instructed to resume a regular diet after a chest film and radiological assessment of the esophageal transit were performed. All patients except one were discharged within 48 h.

The impression of the device was observed at the level of the z-line. The passage of a standard 9 mm endoscope through the GEJ was smooth and no increased resistance was felt at the GEJ. Mucosal erosions of the device, the most feared complication is very rare, with only 0.1 % being reported in the literature [24].

Thirty-two patients had both baseline and one-year postoperative manometric testing. The LES resting pressure increased from 6.5 to 14.6 mmHg ($p<.005$) in the nine patients with a hypotensive LES pressure. No significant changes in pressure occurred in the 23 patients with normal LES pressure at baseline. There were no statistically significant changes in the length of the LES nor in the amplitude of esophageal contractions.

Esophageal pH testing was completed in 20 patients at 3 years after surgery. The mean total % time pH was <4 decreased from a preoperative baseline of 11.9–3.8 % ($p<0.001$). All the other components of the 24-h pH test and the DeMeester composite score were significantly reduced compared to baseline. The esophageal acid exposure was normalized in 80 % of patients (Fig. 15.3).

At 4 years, the mean total GERD–HRQL score at 4 years or more was 3.3 compared to the baseline score of 25.7 ($p<.0001$); all patients had at least a 50 % reduction in the total GERD–HRQL score (Fig. 15.4). Interestingly, 87.5 % of patients were satisfied with their present condition, and

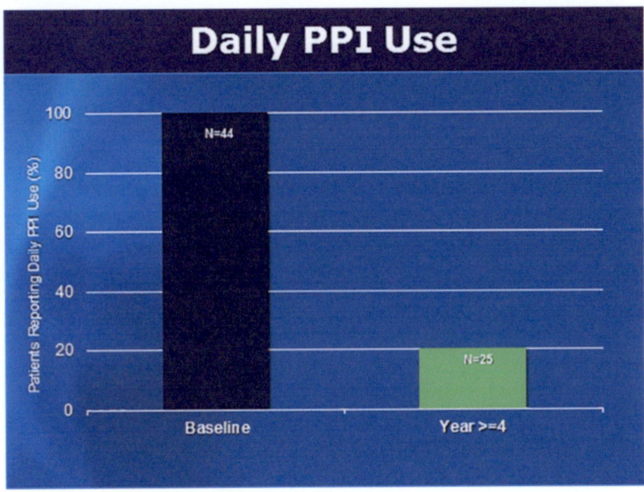

Fig. 15.5 The proportion of patients requiring daily use of proton-pump inhibitors significantly decreased and remained stable after the implant

80 % of patients were free from daily dependence on PPI (Fig. 15.5).

Forty-three percent of patients complained of mild dysphagia during the postoperative period; in all individuals the symptom resolved by 90 days without treatment. Three patients were explanted: one because of persistent dysphagia, one because of the need to undergo a MRI study, and the last one who elected to have a Nissen fundoplication for persisting GERD symptoms. Inability to belch or vomit was reported by less than 5 % of patients.

Similar rigorous inclusion criteria and perioperative subjective and objective evaluations were used in the larger second study involving 100 patients at 13 centers in the United States and one in the Netherlands. Dramatic improvements were seen in GERD related quality of life, regurgitation, and esophageal acid exposure. Proton-pump inhibitor use dropped to 13 % at 3 years and patient satisfaction with their reflux control increased from 13 to 94 % after implantation. Importantly, these positive results are stable showing no degradation over the study time period. Although 14 % of patients reported some bloating after implantation, no patients rated this symptom as severe. Patients retained their ability to belch and vomit. Dysphagia proved to be quite common—present to some extent in 68 % of patients but decreasing to 4 % by 3 years. Five percent rated the dysphagia as severe and the device was removed in three of these patients with complete resolution.

Two single-center studies have further validated the efficacy of the LINX procedure. In Milan, Italy, 100 consecutive patients underwent Linx implantation between 2007 and 2012. The median implant duration was 3 years, ranging from 378 days to 6 years. There was a significant reduction of acid exposure time and improvement of GERD Health Related Quality of Life score; freedom from daily dependence on PPI was achieved in 85 % of the patients [25]. Another study from USA, including 66 patients with an average follow-up of 5.8 months, showed similar satisfactory results [26].

Finally, a study of the Linx safety profile has been performed on the first 1,000 patients implanted worldwide in 82 hospitals [24]. The median implant duration was 274 days. The reoperation rate was 3.4 %. The primary reason for device removal was dysphagia, and erosion of the device occurred in one patient (0.1 %).

Why a New Antireflux Procedure?

The limitations of current therapeutic strategies have left a large proportion of patients with GERD dissatisfied and in an equivocal position, i.e., to continue with a lifetime dependence on a medication that does not provide complete relief of symptoms or to undergo a surgical procedure that requires significant alteration of gastric anatomy and may deteriorate over time. Laparoscopic fundoplication has been plagued with well described side effects, variable outcomes when done by less experienced surgeons and high recurrence rates. Consequently there is a reluctance for physicians to refer patients with symptoms and signs of progressive disease for surgery early in the course of their progression. Studies on the perception patients have about laparoscopic fundoplication show that 90 % are concerned about long-term failure of the procedure, 75 % are concerned about the possibility of dysphagia after the procedure, and 41 % are concerned about reversing the fundoplication if necessary [25]. Further, patients are concerned about developing new symptoms after fundoplication such as bloating in 31–44 % of patients,

increased flatus in 47–57 % of patients, and the inability to belch or vomit [27–30].

Based upon the clinical experience to date, the LINX System represents a new therapeutic option that addresses the limitations of existing therapies and provides a permanent and more physiologic solution to GERD with what appears to be a more favorable side effect profile.

The LINX does not alter gastric anatomy and can be easily reversed if necessary thereby preserving the option of fundoplication or other therapies in the future. As a matter of fact, once healing is complete after the implant, the device is encapsulated in fibrous tissue but is not incorporated in the esophageal wall; this makes possible to remove the device without damage to the esophagus. Importantly, the LINX procedure is designed to limit technical variability which will hopefully result in more standardization of antireflux surgery and more consistent clinical outcomes—a recognized shortcoming of other available surgical antireflux therapies.

The potential limitations of the new technique are the untested efficacy in the presence of sliding or paraesophageal herniation, short esophagus and Barrett's esophagus, the current contraindication to undergo magnetic resonance imaging, and the potential long-term consequences of a permanent foreign body implant. It is also uncertain if the LINX device will be effective in patients with a completely destroyed LES. Consequently, at present, patients with a hiatal hernia >3 cm, endoscopic grade C or D esophagitis, or endoscopic Barrett's esophagus, are not considered candidates for sphincter augmentation and should be treated with a fundoplication. Future studies will compare reflux control and side effects with the LINX device to varying degrees of fundoplications. It should be understood that the device is not intended to be a substitute for the Nissen and is intended to be used earlier in the disease process in patients with normal or early deterioration of their LES to prevent the progression of GERD. Despite these limitations and the lack of long-term results, the LINX system remains a promising new method that might overcome the current limitations in the GERD treatment in the future.

In addition, the LINX procedure has the potential to be broadly and successfully adopted by the surgical community due to the simple and standardized laparoscopic procedure required for the implant. Patients should still be counseled regarding the presence of dysphagia which is to be expected with any treatment aimed at restoring the gastroesophageal reflux barrier.

How to Identify the Patient for Sphincter Augmentation

The two primary treatment options for patients with GERD are long-term acid suppressive therapy or surgery. Acid suppression therapy with PPIs is the first line therapy. Medical therapy is focused on reducing the acidity of the gastric juice while accepting that reflux continues to occur unabated [31]. Consequently, patients experience breakthrough symptoms with daily PPI use, making medical therapy often inadequate to maintain a symptom-free state [32]. Consequently, 13 % of patients will have progression of their disease over 5 years while on acid suppression therapy [6]. Clinical flags of progression are evidence that PPIs are becoming less effective over time. The ineffectiveness of PPIs can be identified by the emergence of incomplete symptom relief, the onset of new symptoms, the need to escalate the dose of PPIs to achieve symptomatic relief, the development of nocturnal symptoms, and the onset of regurgitation and/or extra-esophageal symptoms [6, 33]. The clinical signs of progression are related to the deterioration of the LES and include *bi-positional*. LB reflux on 24 h esophageal pH monitoring, abnormal esophageal acid exposure on both days of a 48 h pH monitoring study, a motility study showing a defective LES, and/or persistent esophagitis despite therapy [33].

Summary

Over the last five decades surgical therapy for GERD has gone through an evolution. More so now than ever, antireflux surgery requires proper patient selection, proper procedure selection, and proper performance of the surgical procedure. Fundoplications are safe, provide substantial symptomatic improvement, and reduce esophageal acid exposure to super normal levels. However, it alters gastric and hiatal anatomy which can lead to herniation, slippage, or breakdown of the repair and induces side effects that annoy patients. It is too much surgery for patient with early progressive disease. New surgical procedures have been developed for patients with early progressive disease and a normal or near normal LES that transiently fails when challenged by gastric distention or dilation. Of these procedures the most extensively studied is the LINX device. It is safe, provides substantial symptom improvement, reduces esophageal acid exposure, preserves gastric and hiatal anatomy, and has minimal side effects. The modern approach to antireflux surgery is moving toward utilizing a form of fundoplication for patients with end stage advanced disease with uncontrolled symptoms from a partial or completely damaged LES and utilizing sphincter augmentation for patients who, despite PPI therapy, have symptoms and signs of early progressive disease.

References

1. Vakil N, van Zanten SV, Kahrilas P, Dent J, Jones R. The Montreal definition and classification of gastroesophageal reflux disease: a global evidence-based consensus. Am J Gastroenterol. 2006;101: 1900–20.
2. Shaheen NJ, Hansen RA, Morgan DR, Gangarosa L, Ringel Y, Thiny M, et al. The burden of gastrointestinal and liver diseases, 2006. Am J Gastroenterol. 2006;101:2128–38.
3. Dean BB, Gano AD, Knight K, et al. Effectiveness of proton pump inhibitors in nonerosive reflux disease. Clin Gastroenterol Hepatol. 2004;2:656–64.
4. AGA Institute: GERD patient study – patients and their medications. Harris Interactive; 2008.
5. Lord R, DeMeester S, Peters J, Hagen J, Elyssnia D, Sheth C, DeMeester T. Hiatal hernia, lower esophageal sphincter incompetence, and effectiveness of Nissen fundoplication in the spectrum of gastroesophageal reflux disease. J Gastrointest Surg. 2009;13: 602–10.
6. Malfertheiner P, Nocon M, Vieth M, Stolte M, Jaspersen D, Koelz HR, et al. Evolution of gastro-oesophageal reflux disease over 5 years under routine medical care – the ProGERD study. Aliment Pharmacol Ther. 2012;35:154–64.
7. Heidelbaugh JJ, Kim AH, Chang R, Walker PC. Overutilization of proton-pump inhibitors: what the clinician needs to know. Therap Adv Gastroenterol. 2012;5(4):219–32.
8. Poulsen AH, Christensen S, McLaughlin JK, Thomsen RW, Sorensen HT, Olsen JH, et al. Proton pump inhibitors and risk of gastric cancer: a population-based cohort study. Br J Cancer. 2009;100:1503–7.
9. McColl K, Gillen D. Evidence that proton-pump inhibitor therapy induces the symptoms it is used to treat. Gastroenterology. 2009;137:20–2.
10. Niebisch S, Fleming FJ, Galey KM, Wilshire CL, Jones CE, Litle VR, et al. Perioperative risk of laparoscopic fundoplication: safer than previously reported – analysis of the American College of Surgeons National Surgical Quality Improvement Program 2005 to 2009. J Am Coll Surg. 2012;215:61–9.
11. Richter JE, Dempsey DT. Laparoscopic antireflux surgery: key to success in the community setting. Am J Gastroenterol. 2008;103: 289–91.
12. Khajanchee YS, O'Rourke R, Cassera MA, Gatta P, Hansen PD, Swanstrom LL. Laparoscopic reintervention for failed antireflux surgery: subjective and objective outcomes in 176 consecutive patients. Arch Surg. 2007;142:785–91.
13. Finks JF, Wei Y, Birkmeyer JD. The rise and fall of antireflux surgery in the United States. Surg Endosc. 2006;20:1698–701.
14. Colavita PD, Belyansky I, Walters AL, Tsirline VB, Zemlyak AY, Lincourt AE, Heniford BT. Nationwide inpatient sample: have antireflux procedures undergone regionalization? J Gastrointest Surg. 2013;17(1):6–13. doi:10.1007/s11605-012-1997-0.
15. Perry KA, Banerjee A, Melvin WS. Radiofrequency energy delivery to the lower esophageal sphincter reduces esophageal acid exposure and improved GERD symptoms: a systemic review and meta-analysis. Surg Laparosc Endosc Percutan Tech. 2012;22:283–8.
16. Rodriguez L, Rodriguex P, Gomez B, et al. Long-term results of electrical stimulation of the lower esophageal sphincter for the treatment of gastroesophageal reflux disease. Endoscopy. 2013; 45:595–604.
17. Lipham JC, DeMeester TR, Ganz RA, et al. The LINX reflux management system: confirmed safety and efficacy now at 4 years. Surg Endosc. 2012;26(10):2944–9.
18. Ganz R, Gostout C, Grudem J, Swanson W, Berg T, DeMeester TR. Use of a magnetic sphincter for the treatment of GERD: a feasibility study. Gastrointest Endosc. 2008;67:287–94.
19. Lipham JC, Louie BE, Smith CD, et al. Safety analysis of the first 1000 patients treated with magnetic sphincter augmentation for gastroesophageal reflux disease. Diseases Esophagus. 2014; Epub ahead of print. doi:10.1111/dote.12199
20. Bonavina L, Saino G, Bona D, Lipham J, Ganz RA, Dunn D, et al. Magnetic augmentation of the lower esophageal sphincter: results of a feasibility clinical trial. J Gastrointest Surg. 2008;12: 2133–40.

21. Bonavina L, DeMeester TR, Fockens P, Dunn D, Saino G, Bona D, et al. Laparoscopic sphincter augmentation device eliminates reflux symptoms and normalizes esophageal acid exposure. Ann Surg. 2010;252:857–62.

22. Lipham JC, DeMeester TR, Ganz RA, Bonavina L, Saino G, Dunn D, et al. The Linx reflux management system: confirmed safety and efficacy now at 4 years. Surg Endosc. 2012; doi:10.1007/s00464-012-2289-1.

23. Ganz RA, Peters JH, Horgan S, Bemelman WA, Dunst CM, et al. Esophageal sphincter device for gastroesophageal reflux disease. NEJM. 2013;368(8):719–27.

24. Lipham JC, Taiganides PA, Louie BE, Ganz RA, DeMeester TR. Safety analysis of first 1000 patients treated with magnetic sphincter augmentation for gastroesophageal reflux disease. Dis Esophagus 2014; doi:10.1111/dote.12199.

25. Bonavina L, Saino G, Bona D, Sironi A, Lazzari V. One hundred consecutive patients treated with magnetic sphincter augmentation for gastroesophageal reflux disease: 6 years of clinical experience from a single center. J Am Coll Surg. 2013;217:577–85.

26. Smith CD, Devault KR, Buchanan M. Introduction of mechanical sphincter augmentation for gastroesophageal reflux disease into practice: early clinical outcomes and keys to successful adoption. J Am Coll Surg. 2014;218:776–81.

27. Richter JE. Gastroesophageal reflux disease treatment: side effects and complications of fundoplication. Clin Gastroenterol Hepatol. 2013;11(5):465–71.

28. Peters JH, DeMeester TR, Crookes P, et al. The treatment of gastroesophageal reflux disease with laparoscopic Nissen fundoplication: prospective evaluation of 100 patients with "typical" symptoms. Ann Surg. 1998;228(1):40–50.

29. Dallemagne B, Weerts J, Markiewicz S. Clinical results of laparoscopic fundoplication at ten years after surgery. Surg Endosc. 2006;20:159–65.

30. Galmiche JP, Hatlebakk J, Attwood S, et al. Laparoscopic antireflux surgery vs esomeprazole treatment for chronic GERD: the LOTUS randomized clinical trial. JAMA. 2011;305:1969–77.

31. Hemmick GJM, Bredenoord AJ, Weusten BLAM, et al. Esophageal pH-impedance monitoring in patients with therapy-resistant reflux symptoms: on or off proton pump inhibitor? Am J Gastroenterol. 2008;103:2446–53.

32. Fass R. Alternative therapeutic approaches to chronic proton pump inhibitor treatment. Clin Gastroenterol Hepatol. 2012;10:338–45.

33. Falkenback D, Oberg S, Johnsson F, et al. Is the course of gastroesophageal reflux disease progressive? A 21-year follow-up. Scand J Gastroenterol. 2009;44(11):1277–87.

GERD Treatment in the Bariatric Population

Ashwin Anthony Kurian and Kevin M. Reavis

Background

The prevalence of both obesity and gastroesophageal reflux disease (GERD) has increased in parallel to one another over the last few decades. More than 25 % of the population of the United States is affected by GERD and its incidence is increasing every year [1, 2]. Similar trends are seen in obesity with 50 % of the United States population now either overweight or obese, with 5 % of the population meeting criteria for weight loss surgery. The prevalence of GERD is higher in morbidly obese patients with up to 70 % of morbidly obese patients report some degree of GERD symptoms, making it one of the most common comorbidities in the obese patient [3].

There is a direct correlation between increasing body mass index (BMI; calculated in kg/m^2) and the prevalence of GERD. Patients with a BMI greater than 35 kg/m^2 are six times more likely to have symptoms of reflux as compared with normal weight patients [4]. Markers of visceral adiposity and central obesity such as waist circumference and waist-to-hip ratios demonstrate an even stronger correlation with GERD [5]. Morbid obesity is associated with an increased incidence of mechanically defective flower esophageal sphincter (LES) as well as with hiatal hernias [6]. Obesity has also been shown to be associated with an increased frequency and duration of transient LES relaxations [7]. Finally, the morbidly obese not only have more

GERD symptoms, they are also at increased risk for the sequelae of reflux such as esophagitis and adenocarcinoma as compared with patients with normal weight [8].

Morbid obesity is a systemic disorder, resulting in a profound reduction in life expectancy. Along with GERD, these patients have associated conditions including diabetes, hypertension, osteoarthritis, dyslipidemia, and others affecting every major organ system in the body [9]. It is estimated that a 25-year-old morbidly obese man has a 22 % reduction in life expectancy compared to a normal-weight individual, relating to a calculated loss of life of 12 years [10]. Unfortunately reductions in weight by nonsurgical methods fail in the vast majority of patients and bariatric surgery is currently the only method that results in consistent, significant, durable weight loss [11].

GERD and the Obese Patient

As with normal weight patients, the first level of therapy for the management of mild to moderate degrees of GERD in obese patients is nonsurgical. In addition to a trial of antacid medications, conservative measures that aim at weight loss are often effective. A physician supervised diet and exercise regimen, or medical intervention in the form of appetite suppression and metabolic enhancement for mild to moderate obesity, typically results in a 10–15 % loss of excess body weight, which can also mitigate GERD symptoms. However it remains challenging to lose greater amounts of weight and effectively keep it from returning in the long-term using nonsurgical means. Lifestyle modifications such as avoiding certain refluxogenic foods, cessation of eating 2–3 h after dinner prior to sleeping, and using favorable sleeping positions are often recommended for GERD patients and can also help with mild weight loss. Although agents like antacids, histamine$_2$ blockers, and proton pump inhibitors (PPI) are quite successful in managing GERD symptoms, about 30–40 % of patients are incompletely responsive to PPIs and 50–75 % of patients have recurrence of symptoms when they stop using

Disclosure: The senior author serves as a consultant for Endogastric Solutions.

A.A. Kurian, MBBS, MD
SurgOne Foregut Institute, 401 West Hampden Place,
Suite 230, Englewood, CO 80110, USA
e-mail: ashwinkurian@hotmail.com

K.M. Reavis, MD (✉)
Division of Gastrointestinal and Minimally Invasive Surgery,
The Oregon Clinic, 4805 NE Glisan St., Ste. 6N60,
Portland, OR 97213, USA
e-mail: kreavis@orclinic.com

L.L. Swanstrom and C.M. Dunst (eds.), *Antireflux Surgery*,
DOI 10.1007/978-1-4939-1749-5_16, © Springer New York 2015

these medications [12]. These numbers are magnified in the obese population. Long-term use of antisecretory agents is increasingly associated with side effects such as loss of bone mineral density leading to increased fracture risk, which has resulted in the U.S. Food and Drug Administration issuing a warning regarding their prolonged use [13]. Morbidly obese GERD patients who fail life style modifications and medical therapy, or who do not wish to be on long-term antisecretory medications, should be considered for surgical intervention to potentially improve their quality of life.

Patient Selection

In order to confirm a diagnosis of GERD in the morbidly obese patient population, symptom severity and frequency, especially dysphagia, should be carefully recorded as it may influence the type of operative intervention employed. A typical GERD workup includes contrast esophagography, upper endoscopy, pH testing, and esophageal manometry with impedance [14].

If a patient presenting with a chief complaint of GERD is also morbidly obese (BMI>40), a discussion of the impact the excess weight has on not only their GERD but also on their general health is mandatory. Consideration of bariatric surgery as a dual treatment for GERD and morbid obesity is reasonable for patients who have exceeded specific weight and comorbidity thresholds. It is important to note however, that not all obese patients with GERD are interested in bariatric surgery despite the overall health benefits it may afford. To date, there is insufficient evidence to suggest that antireflux surgery alone is contraindicated in the obese patient although the risks may be higher than in the normal weight individual. Patients should be carefully educated on the potential risks and benefits of their choice to have a bariatric procedure versus isolated antireflux surgery in order to make an informed decision about their healthcare.

If a patient is interested in pursuing bariatric surgery as a treatment for their GERD, their preoperative evaluation needs to involve evaluation of the patient's clinical background including duration of obesity, previous attempts at weight loss, and psychosocial factors. Consultation using a team approach including a psychologist, a physical therapist, and a dietician is typical in most programs. Patients who might be candidates for bariatric surgery should meet the recommendations set forth in 1991 by the National Institutes of Health of a BMI ≥ 35 kg/m^2 with at least one significant comorbidity such as diabetes, hypertension, or dyslipidemia, or if they have a BMI ≥ 40 kg/m^2 with or without comorbidities [15]. To more accurately stratify these patients obesity was further classified in the 1998 National Institutes of Health Clinical Guidelines on the Identification, Evaluation, and Treatment of Overweight and Obesity in Adults into

Class I (BMI 30.0–34.9 kg/m^2), Class II (BMI 35.0–39.9 kg/m^2), and Class III (BMI ≥ 40 kg/m^2) [16].

Surgical Options

Surgical interventions for GERD in the obese patient can be either antireflux procedures that augment the LES or bariatric procedures which counteract reflux by a number of different mechanisms including the promotion of weight loss and the decrease in the volume of refluxate. It is not known what amount of weight loss is necessary or the critical amount of refluxate diversion necessary to achieve symptomatic relief. Of the bariatric procedures available there is a large variation in improvement for both obesity and GERD. This is illustrated by the fact that the biliopancreatic diversion with duodenal which (BPD-DS) is associated with less GERD symptom resolution as compared with the roux-en-y gastric bypass even though the BPD-DS is associated with more postoperative weight loss compared to the gastric bypass. Some other bariatric procedures such as the sleeve gastrectomy have been shown to reduce or in some studies induce GERD in different patients and therefore is probably not an ideal surgery for someone presenting for GERD treatment (Table 16.1) [17].

Antireflux Surgery

Laparoscopic fundoplication, either complete (Nissen) or partial (Toupet) has well-documented efficacy for GERD. Other less popular procedures include the Hill repair and various endoluminal procedures. The Nissen fundoplication is associated with 90–94 % postoperative patient satisfaction and overall outcomes during long-term follow-up when employed to treat medically refractory GERD [18–21]. At 5-year and 10-year follow-up of laparoscopic Nissen and Toupet fundoplications revealed that 93 % of

Table 16.1 Antireflux and bariatric operations with comparative effects

Operation	Antireflux barrier	Decreased acid secretion	Bile diversion	Weight loss
Fundoplication	Yes	No	No	No
Gastric banding	Yes	No	No	Yes
Sleeve gastrectomy	No	Yes	No	Yes
Roux-en-Y gastric bypass	No	Yes	Yes	Yes
Biliopancreatic diversion with duodenal switch	No	No	Yes	Yes

Data partially from Schauer P, Hamad G, Ikramuddin S. Surgical management of gastroesophageal reflux disease in obese patients. Semin Laparosc Surg. 2001;8(4):256–64

the patients were free of significant reflux symptoms at 5 years after surgery and 89.5 % of the patients were still free of significant reflux at 10 years of clinical follow-up. The symptom-free status was higher following Nissen (93.3 %) than Toupet (81.8 %). However, both procedures resulted in respectable levels of GERD amelioration compared with similar patients being treated with medication (proton pump inhibitors) alone [22].

Concerns exist regarding the long-term durability of the fundoplication in the morbidly obese population. Evidence regarding the impact of obesity on surgical outcomes and recurrence of GERD is however variable. In a study following 224 patients for 3 years after fundoplication, Perez et al. noted a higher recurrence rate following surgery in obese patients. The increasing recurrence rates corresponded with increasing BMI. Recurrent GERD was noted in 4.5 % of patients with BMI less than 25 kg/m^2, 8 % recurrence for BMI 25–30 kg/m^2, and 27 % recurrence for BMI greater than 30 kg/m^2 [23]. In contrast another study following 194 patients for a mean of 3.2 years after Nissen fundoplication found that there was no correlation between increasing BMI and a poorer overall outcome regarding recurrence of GERD after dividing the patients into 3 groups: normal weight (BMI < 25 kg/m^2), overweight (BMI 25–29.9 kg/m^2), and obese (BMI > 30 kg/m^2) [24]. A multivariate analysis assessing symptomatic outcomes after laparoscopic antireflux surgery in 199 consecutive patients undergoing complete fundoplication revealed that obesity was not predictive of worse outcomes during a mean follow-up of 15 months [25]. Likewise Winslow and colleagues identified no association between BMI and complications or anatomic failure three years following surgery. The majority of 505 patients (84 %) in the study were either overweight or obese, yet the complication and failure rates were comparable to those reported for individuals of normal weight [26]. There have been longer follow-up reports supporting these findings as well. In one study 481 patients were studied. One hundred three (21 %) had a normal BMI, 208 (43 %) were class I obese, 115 (24 %) were class II obese, and 55 (12 %) were class III–IV obese. Mean follow-up was 7.5 years. Conversion to an open operation and requirement for revision surgery were not influenced by preoperative weight. Operating time was longer in the obese patients (mean 86 vs 75 min) yet clinical outcomes improved following surgery regardless of BMI [27]. Yet another pattern has been reported from the group at Emory University in which initial data from a large cohort suggested that obesity did not initially adversely affect postoperative GERD recurrence rates [28]. However during 11-year follow-up analysis of the cohort, durability issues emerged. Although patients with class I obesity remained similar to normal habitus patients in regards to GERD recurrence, those with class II–III obesity demonstrated an odds ratio of failure nearly 5 times that of their normal weight

counterparts [29]. Overall, the preponderance of data supports that a standard antireflux surgery in the obese and morbidly obese is very effective but is probably more difficult to perform and probably is slightly less effective and/or long lived than when performed in normal weight patients. What is certain is that fundoplication improves only the function of the LES without addressing other health concerns and comorbid conditions of the morbidly obese. With that in mind, an operation that addresses GERD as well as weight associated comorbid conditions in the obese patient would be the optimal solution.

Bariatric Surgery Options

As opposed to standard antireflux surgery, which reconstructs the gastroesophageal valve, bariatric procedures affect reflux through other mechanisms. These include the reduction in gastric acid production, reduced gastric refluxate volume, diversion of biliopancreatic juices, and the induction of weight loss. Of the laparoscopic procedures commonly used for weight loss, only Roux-en-Y gastric bypass has a consistent impact on GERD other than the general benefit of weight reduction. Laparoscopic malabsorptive operations such as biliopancreatic diversion with duodenal switch have no effect on GERD and therefore would be a contraindicated procedure for a primary GERD treatment [30] (Table 16.1).

Roux-En-Y Gastric Bypass

The Roux-en-Y Gastric bypass is the most commonly performed bariatric procedure in the United States and is the only bariatric procedure with a consistently beneficial effect on GERD. It consists of three components. The proximal stomach is divided to create an approximately 30–50 cm^3 pouch. A Roux limb is then created 40–100 cm beyond the ligament of Treitz and anastomosed to the gastric pouch. The proximal jejunal limb (biliopancreatic limb) is then anastomosed to the Roux limb 100–150 cm distal to the gastrojejunostomy (Fig. 16.1). The restrictive gastric pouch and malabsorptive bypass of the gastric remnant and proximal small bowel combine to induce significant weight loss (less than that seen with BPD-DS and more than that seen with adjustable gastric banding and sleeve gastrectomy). The gastroesophageal junction however is not augmented. Acid exposure to the distal esophagus is markedly reduced since the gastric pouch contains fewer parietal cells resulting in reduced acid production in the gastric remnant and potential refluxate volumes are less. Biliopancreatic juices are also diverted which may also be a benefit particularly in patients with Barrett's esophagus (Table 16.1). Overall, the Roux-en-Y

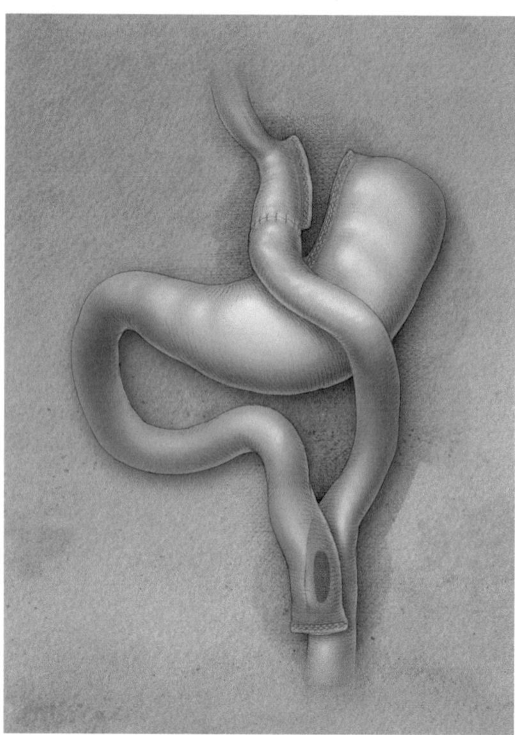

Fig. 16.1 Roux-en-Y gastric bypass

gastric bypass has been shown to be the most reliable operation to treat severe GERD in the obese patient population.

Frezza et al. followed 152 morbidly obese patients with GERD for 12 months following Roux-en-Y gastric bypass and reported a significant decrease in GERD symptoms: heartburn (from 87 to 22 %), water brash (from 18 to 7 %), wheezing (from 40 to 5 %), laryngitis (from 17 to 7 %), and aspiration (from 19 to 2 %). It is also associated with significant reduction of antisecretory medication use from between 40 and 60 % preoperatively to 10 % postprocedure and a concurrent improvement in quality-of-life measures [31]. Perry and colleagues reported similar findings in 57 patients with a mean BMI of 47 who underwent gastric bypass with 18 month follow-up. Specifically all patients reported improvement or no symptoms of GERD, there was a mean weight loss of 40 kg, and quality-of-life scores (SF-36) were above national norms for physical and mental components [32]. Another study enrolled 12 morbidly obese patients with six undergoing laparoscopic complete fundoplication (mean BMI 40 kg/m^2) and six undergoing laparoscopic gastric bypass (mean BMI 55 kg/m^2). Postoperative symptom scores and 24-h pH scores were normal in both groups after surgery. While outcomes focused on GERD physiology were similar between the two operations, gastric bypass carried the additional benefit of comorbidity resolution [33].

Gastric bypass is also comparable to laparoscopic fundoplication in its safety profile. Varela and colleagues analyzed the University Health System Consortium database for patients who underwent laparoscopic fundoplication or laparoscopic gastric bypass from 2004 to 2007 ($n=27{,}264$). Gastric bypass was associated with significantly lower overall in-hospital complications and comparable mean length of stay, observed mortality, risk-adjusted mortality, and hospital cost as compared with laparoscopic fundoplication [34].

In addition to the level of safety observed with gastric bypass in the treatment of GERD and comorbid conditions due to obesity, impressive prescription medication use and costs are also reduced. Nguyen et al. followed 77 morbidly obese patients for one year following gastric bypass. The mean excess body weight loss was 67+/−14 % one year after surgery. The mean number of prescription medications per patient was reduced from 2.4 preoperatively to 0.2 one year after surgery. The mean monthly medication cost decreased from $196 preoperatively to $54 one month after surgery, representing a 72 % cost savings. One month postoperatively, medication cost saving for GERD was 81 %; for diabetes it was 69 %; for dyslipidemia it was 53 %; and for hypertension it was 43 %. The mean monthly medication cost savings for the first year after surgery was $168 with a yearly savings of $2,016 per patient [35]. Gastric bypass has also been associated with a 40 % decrease in all-cause mortality, a 56 % decrease in mortality from coronary artery disease, 60 % decrease in mortality from cancer, and a 92 % decrease in mortality from diabetes as compared with age, sex, and BMI-matched control subjects in large population studies [36].

The additional benefit of bariatric procedures, particularly gastric bypass in the treatment of GERD and concomitant illnesses in the morbidly obese population has led some surgeons to avoid offering fundoplication in higher BMI patients. In a recent survey of foregut surgeons with expertise in bariatrics the majority of respondents felt that laparoscopic Roux-en-Y gastric bypass was the best option (91 %), distantly followed by laparoscopic sleeve gastrectomy (6 %). Many reported having morbidly obese patients with a primary surgical indication of GERD who were denied a bariatric procedure by a third-party payer (57 %), and some (35 %) of those surgeons would choose to do nothing rather than proceed with fundoplication alone, which they felt was suboptimal as it did not address all of the obesity related comorbidities. The majority of respondents felt that bariatric surgery should be recognized as a standard surgical option for treating GERD in the obese (96 %). Currently however, third-party payers in the US often decline to provide benefits for a bariatric procedure for this indication [37].

Evidence that gastric bypass not only resolves GERD symptoms as an index procedure but also does so when employed following failed fundoplication in obese patients was demonstrated in a study by Stefanidis et al. in which 25 patients with class I obesity who suffered recurrent GERD following fundoplication were converted to Roux-en-Y gastric bypass with resultant substantial improvement in quality-of-life scores and gastrointestinal symptoms rating scale scores after a mean of 14 months following conversion [38].

The concerns echoed above regarding long-term durability of fundoplication when exposed to increased intra-abdominal pressures in the obese population are magnified when these patients who suffer from GERD have an associated hiatal or paraesophageal hernia. While treating this particularly challenging patient population foregut surgeons have reported the combination of hiatal and paraesophageal hernia repair with gastric bypass or sleeve gastrectomy with minimal recurrence of GERD or hernia symptoms [39–42].

Adjustable Gastric Band

The laparoscopic adjustable gastric band is performed less and less worldwide due to efficacy questions and need for surgical reinterventions. It acts as a purely restrictive bariatric operation (Fig. 16.2). Its sole advantage is based on the minimally disruptive nature of the procedure. An adjustable silicone band is placed immediately distal to the gastroesophageal junction followed by imbrication of the gastric fundus over the band, to create an approximately 15 cm^3 proximal gastric pouch. A subcutaneous port is accessed percutaneously with a Huber needle to adjust band volume (0–12 mL) and control the degree of gastric restriction. There are conflicting reports to as to the improvements of GERD symptoms following adjustable gastric band placement. Some reports suggest a 90 % resolution or improvement in GERD symptoms, [43]. while others note that GERD is the most common complication requiring reoperation (4.7 %) after band placement [44]. The band may be particularly inducive of GERD if it slips distally or the proximal gastric pouch dilates. While this might be corrected by laparoscopically unbuckling the band and replacing it in the correct anatomical position, it seems like a bad idea to do such a revision for GERD. More recently, Brancatisano and colleagues followed 838 patients and showed moderate weight loss (54 % EBWL) but a fairly mediocre 66 % improvement in GERD symptoms. No objective testing was reported [45].

Another concern regarding the band for GERD surgeons is the occurrence of band-related esophageal dysmotility. Several animal and human studies report severe esophageal dysmotility secondary to gastric banding. O'Rourke and colleagues placed nonadjustable bands around the proximal stomach of opossums and followed them for 14 weeks. There was a 36 % decrease in both baseline mean resting LES pressure and in the distal esophageal peristaltic pressure in banded animals. Motility disorders developed during the study in more than one-third of the banded animals [46]. This problem has been reported in up to 70 % of patients, with 25 % of patients presenting with esophageal dilation

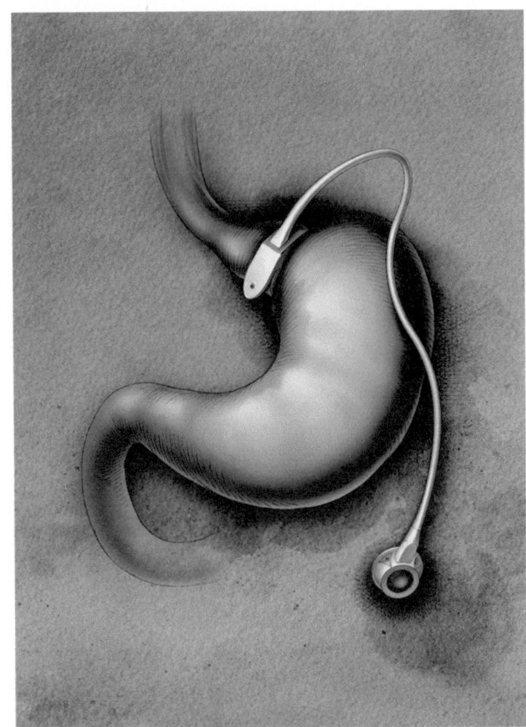

Fig. 16.2 Adjustable gastric band

[47]. Overall it is clear that the LAGB is a very poor choice for treating the obese patient seeking GERD treatment [48].

Sleeve Gastrectomy

The laparoscopic sleeve gastrectomy is the most recent bariatric procedure to gain acceptance by third-party payers. It consists of a stapled resection of the greater curve of the stomach initiated 2–6 cm proximal to the pylorus and proceeding cephalad to the angle of His. It is commonly performed over a 32–40 French bougie, placed along the lesser curvature resulting in gastric volumes of 50–80 cm^3 (Fig. 16.3). The lesser curvature is less compliant than the resected greater curvature resulting in a fairly stable restrictive endolumenal environment. This degree of gastric resection probably results in a reduction in gastric acid production, but also reduces the production of the hunger-inducing hormone Ghrelin (produced by the resected greater curvature gastric tissue) resulting in increased satiety. This metabolic component adds to the restrictive component of the procedure to cause significant weight loss which is typically less than that seen with gastric bypass and more than that seen with adjustable gastric band. GERD resolution after sleeve gastrectomy is very variable and in general suboptimal. Any benefit is probably related to the weight loss that results post procedure. Due to the resected parietal cell rich fundus and greater curvature during sleeve gastrectomy, acid secretion

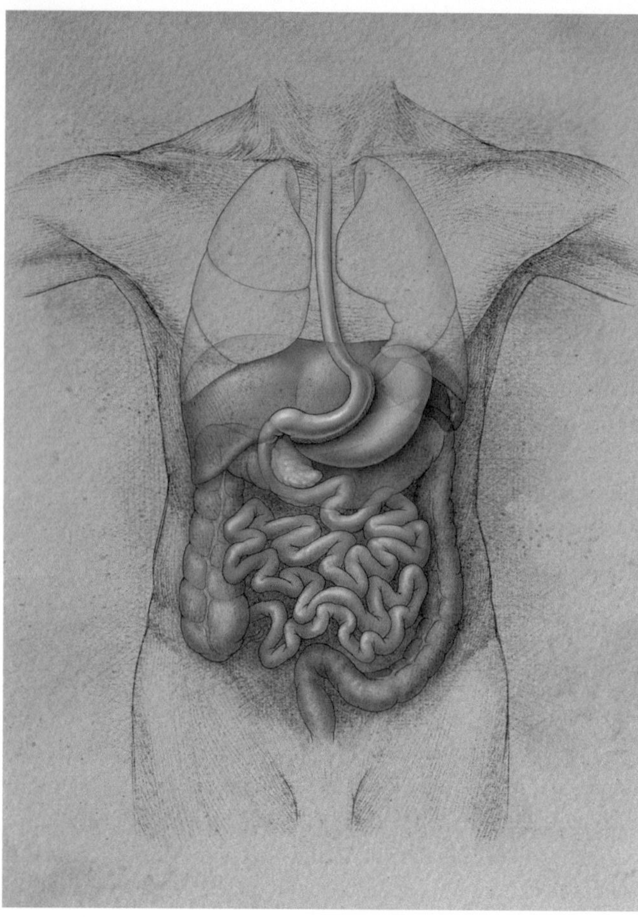

Fig. 16.3 Sleeve gastrectomy

within the tubularized stomach should be decreased, however biliopancreatic juices are not diverted.

Sleeve gastrectomy has been implicated with both the amelioration as well as the development of GERD. A few studies have shown improved GERD symptoms [49, 50]. Most studies however showed the same or worse incidence of GERD symptoms [51, 52]. One of the few studies performing objective pH testing after surgery showed an increase in upright pH exposure (5–12.6 %) and supine exposure (1.4–11 %). This study also showed a deterioration of the LES pressures post sleeve (18.3 mm/Hg to 11) [52].

A recent meta-analysis of 15 studies reporting postoperative GERD symptoms after sleeve gastrectomy found increased incidence of GERD in four studies and reduced GERD in seven studies [53]. Overall, the evidence points to sleeve resection as being a poor treatment option for the GERD patient and should probably be considered contraindicated for this indication.

To assess the impact of each of the bariatric procedures discussed so far on GERD, The Bariatric Outcomes Longitudinal Database (a prospective database of patients who undergo bariatric surgery by a participant in the American Society of Metabolic and Bariatric Surgery Center of Excellence program) recently assessed the results from 22,870 morbidly obese patients with GERD who were undergoing adjustable gastric banding, sleeve gastrectomy, and gastric bypass. The mean BMI was 46.3 kg/m². All three operations resulted in improved GERD symptom scores 6 months following surgery. GERD symptom score reduction was most pronounced in gastric bypass patients (56.5 %; 7,955 of 14,078) followed by adjustable gastric banding (46 %; 3,773 of 8,207) and sleeve gastrectomy patients (41 %; 240 of 585) [54]. Overall, this seems to indicate a rather poor effect of bariatric surgery on GERD making it clear that more well constructed studies based on objective test endpoints are needed.

Emerging Therapies

Innovative methods of GERD treatment in the obese patient are now being pursued via both laparoscopic and endoscopic approaches. Greater curvature gastric plication is being investigated as a potential alternative to sleeve gastrectomy for weight loss but would not be expected to be any better a treatment for GERD than standard sleeve resection [55].

A different technological approach to the treatment of GERD utilizes a magnetic bracelet made of titanium beads and magnetic core placed laparoscopically around the gastroesophageal junction to augment the antireflux function of the LES has received U.S. Food and Drug Administration approval [56, 57]. In non-obese patients there was a significant reduction in the mean esophageal acid exposure time with pH normalization achieved in 80 % of the patients 3 years following insertion. At >4 years there was a significant improvement in quality-of-life measures for GERD in all the patients with complete cessation in the use of PPIs in 80 % of the patients. Transient postoperative dysphagia was common but typically resolved by 12 weeks following surgery [58]. The use of this device in the obese population has not been completely evaluated. It may have a role in palliation of post bypass or sleeve induced GERD but this has not yet been defined or published (Fig. 16.4).

Treating Refractory GERD After Bariatric Surgery

While gastric bypass is often associated with amelioration or resolution of GERD in the morbidly obese patient, there are certainly circumstances where GERD persists, is induced, or recurs. In mild to moderate cases, such refractory GERD can be managed by life style adjustments and/or medication. Fundoplication via mobilization of the remnant stomach and radiofrequency treatment of the LES have been described with some success [59, 60]. In more severe cases, revisional surgery may be required. GERD persistence or development

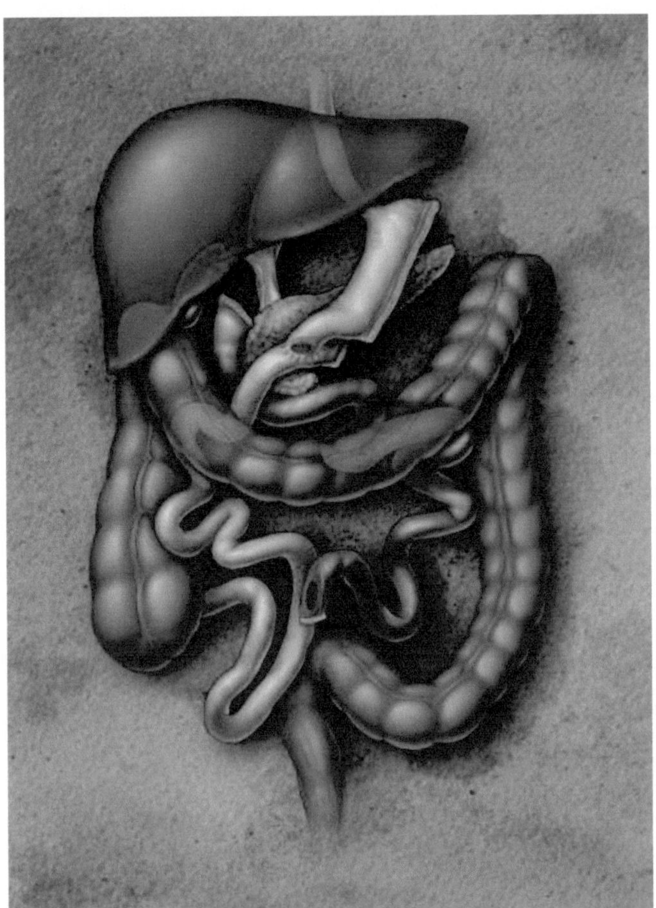

Fig. 16.4 Biliopancreatic diversion with duodenal switch

ment [62]. Gastric bypass has been identified as a relatively effective as treatment strategy for patients suffering from GERD following adjustable gastric banding, sleeve gastrectomy, and other procedures such as vertical banded [63].

Although gastric bypass functions as an effective exit strategy for GERD following other bariatric operations, there are also cases of recurrent GERD following gastric bypass. This can be caused by a technical error resulting in a large pouch created at the time of the initial operation, due to progressive pouch dilation or could be due to an underlying gastro-gastric fistula. If excessive acid exposure is present resulting in esophageal or marginal ulceration of the proximal jejunum within the Roux limb, revision of the gastro-jejunostomy (via resection and reanastomosis with a small or no gastric pouch) is warranted if medical management fails. An enlarged gastric pouch resulting in regurgitation or a pouch-remnant fistula resulting in increased acid in the pouch and regurgitation or development of marginal ulcer have been shown to be amenable to endoscopic suture repair [64]. If however the pouch is of adequate size and an underlying fistula is ruled out, then the situation becomes more challenging. Endolumenal strategies using radiofrequency energy to improve the robustness of the LES and antireflux mechanism may be indicated. This applies to both gastric bypass patients and sleeve patients suffering recalcitrant GERD without outflow obstructions. Mattar et al. treated seven patients a mean of 27 months following gastric bypass who had pH confirmed GERD. Of the seven patients, five patients had complete resolution of their symptoms, with normalization of pH studies. Follow-up was 20 +/− 2 months. One patient did not have adequate relief of symptoms after the treatment, and one patient was lost to follow-up [65]. Post bypass complete fundoplication has also been described using the adjacent bypassed remnant stomach with satisfactory short-term results [66]. Surgical augmentation of the LES following bypass or sleeve gastrectomy without the use of surrounding viscera can alternatively be completed with a Hill valvuloplasty [67]. New endolumenal devices are being evaluated that act to restrict or divert food intake while excluding the stomach or duodenum, or that overlay the distal esophagus to effectively shield the various components of the foregut from one another [68–71]. No conclusive evidence exists that these devices are successful in long-term resolution of either GERD or obesity; however it seems at this time that many investigative efforts are moving toward endolumenal treatments as an area of potential growth in this field.

following adjustable gastric banding can be related to technical issues secondary to band slippage or proximal pouch dilation or induced esophageal dysmotility. Slippage can be corrected laparoscopically as mentioned earlier. If this is not adequate, or if the underlying problem is esophageal dysfunction masquerading as GERD, then removing the band and conversion to gastric bypass is appropriate. Ardestani et al. followed 19 patients requiring conversion of adjustable gastric band to gastric bypass due to inadequate weight loss or band erosion. Perioperative complications were acceptable with 2 of 19 (10.5 %) having surgical site infections without major intracorporeal complications [60].

Sleeve gastrectomy has been associated with the resolution of GERD in a few studies and implicated in the development of GERD in many others. In patients who develop GERD secondary to distal stenosis near the angularis incisura, opening the affected area via endoscopic dilation, distal gastroplasty (similar to a Heineke-Mikulicz pyloroplasty), or antrectomy with primary anastomosis can be performed [61]. If this is not an effective option then patients presenting with recalcitrant GERD after sleeve gastrectomy should be treated by transecting the sleeve proximally in a similar fashion as that used for standard bypass pouch creation and reconstructing with a Roux limb to provide definitive treat-

Summary

GERD and obesity are two of the most common chronic illnesses afflicting our society. Although the etiology and manifestations of each are very different, they commonly co-exist and require coordinated treatment. Although patients may be presenting with a primary concern of GERD, if they have morbid obesity as well it stands to reason that this should be discussed with the patient as part of treatment counseling. The GERD surgeon can certainly advocate to the patient the benefits surgical weight loss would provide: improvements in diabetes, hypertension, and dyslipidemia will markedly improve the patient's quality of life, and even life expectancy. If the patient doesn't want or can't have obesity surgery, evidence would support providing the patient with a fundoplication to control their GERD symptoms in most cases. The caveat here should be that the patient must be warned that surgery may be more difficult and at low volume centers may have more complications, that subsequent bariatric surgery is more complicated and that long-term outcomes may be slightly worse for fundoplication in the face of morbid obesity. In fact, most GERD surgeons would agree that there is almost certainly morbidly obese patients who should not be offered a fundoplication—those with such severe comorbidities that anesthesia is a high risk or such a high BMI that fundoplication would be practically impossible. As far as which bariatric surgery is most suitable for the morbidly obese GERD patient, evidence would point to the gastric bypass as the only suitable option in most cases. Bypass results in relatively good reflux control and also a significant and sustained weight loss. For many patients who are referred to the surgeon for GERD, the discussion of bariatric surgery to treat his or her concomitant diseases may the first time that options regarding bariatric surgery have been introduced. Not uncommonly this discussion may require more than one office visit to complete due to the substantial psychosocial preparation needed for bariatric surgery. Additional specialists are also often typically involved in the preparation of these patients. Surgeons who are interested in offering bariatric surgical procedures themselves should either complete appropriate training or refer those patients to a qualified surgeon who can offer these options.

Several innovative laparoscopic and endolumenal technologies are being evaluated for the index and revisional management of both GERD and obesity. These and related technologies will likely transform the management of these chronic diseases in the future.

References

1. Center for Disease Control and Prevention. Overweight and Obesity. Available at: http://www.cdc.gov. Accessed 20 Sept 2005.
2. Friedenberg FK, Hanlon A, Vanar V, et al. Trends in gastroesophageal reflux disease as measured by the National Ambulatory Medical Care Survey. Dig Dis Sci. 2010;55:1911–7.
3. Fisher BL, Pennathur A, Mutnick JL, et al. Obesity correlates with gastroesophageal reflux. Dig Dis Sci. 1999;44:2290–4.
4. Eslick GD. Gastrointestinal symptoms and obesity: a meta-analysis. Obes Rev. 2012;13(5):469–79.
5. Tai CM, Lee YC, Tu HP, et al. The relationship between visceral adiposity and the risk of erosive esophagitis in severely obese Chinese patients. Obesity (Silver Spring). 2010;18(11):2165–9.
6. Ayazi S, Hagen JA, Chan LS, et al. Obesity and gastroesophageal reflux: quantifying the association between body mass index, esophageal acid exposure, and lower esophageal sphincter status in a large series of patients with reflux symptoms. J Gastrointest Surg. 2009;13(8):1440–7.
7. Schneider JH, Küper M, Königsrainer A, et al. Transient lower esophageal sphincter relaxation in morbid obesity. Obes Surg. 2009;19(5):595–600.
8. Hampel H, Abraham NS, El-Serag HB. Meta-analysis: obesity and the risk for gastroesophageal reflux disease and its complications. Ann Intern Med. 2005;143:199–211.
9. Calle EE, Thun MJ, Petrelli JM, et al. Body-mass index and mortality in a prospective cohort of US adults. N Engl J Med. 1999;341:1097–105.
10. Fontaine KR, Redden DT, Wang C, Westfall AO, Allison DB. Years of life lost due to obesity. JAMA. 2003;289:187–93.
11. National Institutes of Health Consensus Development Conference Statement. Gastrointestinal surgery for severe obesity. Am J Clin Nutr. 1992;55:487S–619S.
12. Cadière GB, Van Sante N, Graves JE, et al. Two-year results of a feasibility study on antireflux transoral incisionless fundoplication using EsophyX. Surg Endosc. 2009;23:957–64.
13. http://www.fda.gov/consumer.
14. Reavis KM. Management of the obese patient with gastroesophageal reflux disease. Thorac Surg Clin. 2011;21(4):489–98. doi:10.1016/j.thorsurg.2011.08.004. Epub 2011 Sep 16. Review.
15. Gastrointestinal surgery for severe obesity: National Institutes of Health Consensus Development Conference Statement. Am J Clin Nutr 1992;55(Suppl 2): 615S–9S.
16. Pi-Sunyer FX, Becker DM, Bouchard C, et al. Clinical guidelines on the identification, evaluation, and treatment of overweight and obesity in adults. The Evidence Report. NIH Publication No. 98-4083 National Institutes of Health. 1998
17. Schauer P, Hamad G, Ikramuddin S. Surgical management of gastroesophageal reflux disease in obese patients. Semin Laparosc Surg. 2001;8(4):256–64.
18. Dent J. Landmarks in the understanding and treatment of reflux disease. J Gastroenterol Hepatol. 2009;24 Suppl 3:S5–14.
19. Terry M, Smith CD, Branum GD, et al. Outcomes of laparoscopic fundoplication for gastroesophageal reflux disease and paraesophageal hernia. Surg Endosc. 2001;15:691–9.
20. Lafullarde T, Watson DI, Jamieson GG, et al. Laparoscopic Nissen fundoplication: five-year results and beyond. Arch Surg. 2001; 136:180–4.
21. Hunter JG, Trus TL, Branum GD, et al. A physiologic approach to laparoscopic fundoplication for gastroesophageal reflux disease. Ann Surg. 1996;223:673–87.
22. Dallemagne B, Weerts J, Markiewicz S, et al. Clinical results of laparoscopic fundoplication at ten years after surgery. Surg Endosc. 2006;20:159–65.
23. Perez AR, Moncure AC, Rattner DW. Obesity adversely affects the outcome of antireflux operations. Surg Endosc. 2001;15(9):986–9.
24. Fraser J, Watson DI, O'Boyle CJ, et al. Obesity and its effect on outcome of laparoscopic Nissen fundoplication. Dis Esophagus. 2001;14(1):50–3.
25. Campos GM, Peters JH, DeMeester TR, et al. Multivariate analysis of factors predicting outcome after laparoscopic Nissen fundoplication. J Gastrointest Surg. 1999;3:292–300.
26. Winslow ER, Frisella MM, Soper NJ, Klingensmith ME. Obesity does not adversely affect the outcome of laparoscopic antireflux surgery (LARS). Surg Endosc. 2003;17:2003–11.
27. Chisholm JA, Jamieson GG, Lally CJ, Devitt PG, Game PA, Watson DI. The effect of obesity on the outcome of laparoscopic

antireflux surgery. J Gastrointest Surg. 2009;13(6):1064–70. doi:10.1007/s11605-009-0837-3. Epub 2009 Mar 4.

28. McNatt SS, Smith CD, Hunter JG, Galloway JG. Morbid obesity does not predict a poor outcome after laparoscopic antireflux surgery. Gastroenterology. 2000;118:A1033.

29. Morgenthal CB, Shane MD, Stival A, et al. The durability of laparoscopic Nissen fundoplication: 11-year outcomes. J Gastrointest Surg. 2007;11(6):693–700.

30. Prachand VN, Ward M, Alverdy JC. Duodenal switch provides superior resolution of metabolic comorbidities independent of weight loss in the super-obese (BMI >or 5 50 kg/m^2) compared with gastric bypass. J Gastrointest Surg. 2010;14(2):211–20.

31. Frezza EE, Ikramuddin S, Gourash W, et al. Symptomatic improvement in gastroesophageal reflux disease (GERD) following laparoscopic Roux-en-Y gastric bypass. Surg Endosc. 2002;16(7): 1027–31.

32. Perry Y, Courcoulas AP, Fernando HC, Buenaventura PO, McCaughan JS, Luketich JD. Laparoscopic Roux-en-Y gastric bypass for recalcitrant gastroesophageal reflux disease in morbidly obese patients. JSLS. 2004;8(1):19–23.

33. Patterson EJ, Davis DG, Khajanchee Y, Swanstrom LL. Comparison of objective outcomes following laparoscopic Nissen fundoplication versus laparoscopic gastric bypass in the morbidly obese with heartburn. Surg Endosc. 2003;17(10):1561–5.

34. Varela JE, Hinojosa MW, Nguyen NT. Laparoscopic fundoplication compared with laparoscopic gastricbypass in morbidly obese patients with gastroesophageal reflux disease. Surg Obes Relat Dis. 2009;5(2):139–43.

35. Nguyen NT, Varela JE, Sabio A, et al. Reduction in prescription medication costs after laparoscopic gastric bypass. Am Surg. 2006;72(10):853–6.

36. Adams TD, Gress RE, Smith SC, Halverson RC, Simper SC, Rosamond WD, et al. Long-term mortality after gastric bypass surgery. N Engl J Med. 2007;357:753–61.

37. Pagé MP, Kastenmeier A, Goldblatt M, et al. Medically refractory gastroesophageal reflux disease in the obese: what is the best surgical approach? Surg Endosc. 2014;28(5):1500–4.

38. Stefanidis D, Navarro F, Augenstein VA, Gersin KS, Heniford BT. Laparoscopic fundoplication takedown with conversion to Roux-en-Y gastric bypass leads to excellent reflux control and quality of life after fundoplication failure. Surg Endosc. 2012;26(12):3521–7. doi:10.1007/s00464-012-2380-7. Epub 2012 Jun 13.

39. Kasotakis G, Mittal SK, Sudan R. Combined treatment of symptomatic massive paraesophageal hernia in the morbidly obese. JSLS. 2011;15(2):188–92. doi:10.4293/108680811X13022985132164.

40. Merchant AM, Cook MW, Srinivasan J, Davis SS, Sweeney JF, Lin E. Comparison between laparoscopic paraesophageal hernia repair with sleeve gastrectomy and paraesophageal hernia repair along in morbidly obese patients. Am Surg. 2009;75(7):620–5.

41. Rodriguez JH, Kroh M, El-Hayek K, Timratana P, Chand B. Combined paraesophageal hernia repair and partial longitudinal gastrectomy in obese patients with symptomatic paraesophageal hernias. Surg Endosc. 2012;26(12):3382–90. doi:10.1007/s00464-012-2347-8. Epub 2012 Jun 3.

42. Krpata DM, Criss CN, Gao Y, Sadava EE, Anderson JM, Novitsky YW, Rosen MJ. Effects of weight reduction surgery on the abdominal wall fascial wound healing process. J Surg Res. 2013;184(1): 78–83.

43. Dixon JB, O'Brien PE. Gastroesophageal reflux in obesity: the effect of lap-band placement. Obes Surg. 1999;9:527–31.

44. Forsell P, Hallerback B, Glise H, et al. Complications following Swedish adjustable gastric banding: a longterm follow-up. Obes Surg. 1999;9:11–6.

45. Brancatisano A, Wahlroos S, Brancatisano R. Improvement in comorbid illness after placement of the Swedish Adjustable Gastric Band. Surg Obes Relat Dis. 2008;4(3 Suppl):S39–46.

46. O'Rourke RW, Seltman AK, Chang EY, et al. A model for gastric banding in the treatment of morbid obesity: the effect of chronic partial gastric outlet obstruction on esophageal physiology. Ann Surg. 2006;244(5):723–33.

47. Naef M, Mouton WG, Naef U, et al. Esophageal dysmotility disorders after laparoscopic gastric banding–an underestimated complication. Ann Surg. 2011;253(2):285–90.

48. Merrouche M, Sabaté JM, Jouet P, Harnois F, Scaringi S, Coffin B, Msika S. Gastro-esophageal reflux and esophageal motility disorders in morbidly obese patients before and after bariatric surgery. Obes Surg. 2007;17(7):894–900.

49. Lazoura O, Zacharoulis D, Triantafyllidis G, et al. Symptoms of gastroesophageal reflux following laparoscopic sleeve gastrectomy are related to the final shape of the sleeve as depicted by radiology. Obes Surg. 2011;21(3):295–9.

50. Daes J, Jimenez ME, Said N, et al. Laparoscopic sleeve gastrectomy: symptoms of gastroesophageal reflux can be reduced by changes in surgical technique. Obes Surg. 2012;22(12):1874–9.

51. Carter PR, Leblanc KA, Hausmann MG, et al. Association between gastroesophageal reflux disease and laparoscopic sleeve gastrectomy. Surg Obes Relat Dis. 2011;7(5):569–72.

52. Burgerhart JS, Schotborgh CA, Schoon EJ et al. The Effect of Sleeve Gastrectomy on Gastroesophageal Reflux. Obes Surg. 2014. [Epub ahead of print].

53. Chiu S, Birch DW, Shi X, et al. Effect of sleeve gastrectomy on gastroesophageal reflux disease: a systematic review. Surg Obes Relat Dis. 2011;7(4):510–5.

54. Pallati PK, Shaligram A, Shostrom VK, Oleynikov D, McBride CL, Goede MR. Improvement in gastroesophageal reflux disease symptoms after various bariatric procedures: review of the Bariatric Outcomes Longitudinal Database. Obes Relat Dis. 2013; pii: S1550-7289(13)00259-1. doi: 10.1016/j.soard.2013.07.018. http://www.ncbi.nlm.nih.gov/pubmed/24238733Surg. [Epub ahead of print].

55. Lee WJ, Han ML, Ser KH, Tsou JJ, Chen JC, Lin CH. Laparoscopic Nissen fundoplication with gastric plication as a potential treatment of morbidly obese patients with gerd, first experience and results. Obes Surg. 2014; [Epub ahead of print].

56. Ganz RA, Gostout CJ, Grudem J, et al. Use of a magnetic sphincter for the treatment of GERD: a feasibility study. Gastrointest Endosc. 2008;67(2):287–94.

57. Bonavina L, DeMeester T, Fockens P, et al. Laparoscopic sphincter augmentation device eliminates reflux symptoms and normalizes esophageal acid exposure: one- and 2-year results of a feasibility trial. Ann Surg. 2010;252(5):857–62.

58. Lipham JC, Demeester TR, Ganz RA, et al. The LINX(®) reflux management system: confirmed safety and efficacy now at 4 years. Surg Endosc. 2012;26(19):2944–9.

59. Mattar SG1, Qureshi F, Taylor D, Schauer PR. Treatment of refractory gastroesophageal reflux disease with radiofrequency energy (Stretta) in patients after Roux-en-Y gastric bypass. Surg Endosc. 2006;20(6):850-4. Epub 2006 May 12.

60. Nilton T, Kawahara IC, Alster IF, Maluf-Filho IIW, Polara IIIG, Campos IV M. Luiz Francisco Poli-de-Figueiredo (in memoriam)I modified Nissen fundoplication: laparoscopic antireflux surgery after Roux-en-Y gastric bypass for obesity. Clinics. 2012; 67(5):531–3.

61. Ardestani A, Lautz DB, Tavakkolizadeh A. Band revision versus Roux-en-Y gastric bypass conversion as salvage operation after laparoscopic adjustable gastric banding. Surg Obes Relat Dis. 2011;7(1):33–7. Epub 2010 Oct 16.

62. Naef M, Mouton WG, Naef U, van der Weg B, Maddern GJ, Wagner HE. Esophageal dysmotility disorders after laparoscopic gastric banding – an underestimated complication. Ann Surg. 2011;253(2):285–90.

63. Langer FB, Bohdjalian A, Shakeri-Leidenmühler S, Schoppmann SF, Zacherl J, Prager G. Conversion from sleeve gastrectomy to

Roux-en-Y gastric bypass – indications and outcome. Obes Surg. 2010;20(7):835–40.

64. Ekelund M, Oberg S, Peterli R, et al. Gastroesophageal reflux after vertical banded gastroplasty is alleviated by conversion to gastric bypass. Obes Surg. 2012;22(6):851–4.

65. Jirapinyo P, Watson RR, Thompson CC. Use of a novel endoscopic suturing device to treat recalcitrant marginal ulceration (with video). Gastrointest Endosc. 2012;76(2):435–9. doi:10.1016/j.gie.2012.03.681. Epub 2012 May 31.

66. Mattar SG, Qureshi F, Taylor D, Schauer PR. Treatment of refractory gastroesophageal reflux disease with radiofrequency energy (Stretta) in patients after Roux-en-Y gastric bypass. Surg Endosc. 2006;20(6):850–4.

67. Kawahara NT, Alster C, Maluf-Filho F, Polara W, Campos GM, Poli-de-Figueiredo LF. Modified Nissen fundoplication: laparoscopic antireflux surgery after Roux-en-Y gastric bypass for obesity. Clinics (Sao Paulo). 2012;67(5):531–3.

68. Pescarus R, Sharata A, Shlomovich E, Reavis KM, Dunst CM, Swanstrom LS, Hill procedure for recurrent GERD post gastric bypass. submitted ASMBS2014.

69. Available at: http://www.usgimedical.com/news/releases/20100915.htm.

70. Available at: http://clinicaltrials.gov/ct2/show/NCT01207804.

71. Available at: http://www.endogastricsolutions.com/esophyx_overview.htm.

Perioperative Complications and Their Management

Silvana Perretta

Introduction

Early in the era of laparoscopic antireflux surgery, the significance of the learning curve was recognized to be highly dependent on the volume of operations performed at the institution. In fact, while high-volume centers of excellence report long-term success rates greater than 90 %, general population-based LF outcomes are reported to be markedly worse, indicating that the operation is highly dependent on the learning curve phenomenon [5]. The lack of standardization of the technique and the lack of tools to calibrate objectively the repairs are probably the primary reasons for the variability in the outcomes [6]. In 1999, Rantanen et al. reported the morbidity and mortality rates extracted from official data of the National Research and Development Center for Welfare and Health, which collected data on all operations performed in Finland. Between 1987 and 1996, 5,502 antireflux operations were performed, 72.6 % of which open and 21.1 % laparoscopically [4]. Fatal and life-threatening complications were observed in 0.6 % of patients after open procedures (mortality: 0.2 %) and in 1.3 % of patients after laparoscopic procedures (mortality: 0.1 %) ($P<0.05$) [4]. At that time, the authors posited that these results might compromise the advantages of the laparoscopic technique. Ten years later, the same group conducted exactly the same study on patients undergoing operation between 1992 and 2001 [7]. There was an inversion of the trend, with the laparoscopic approach (63 %) prevailing over the open procedure (37 %) in a total of 10,841 fundoplications performed. Although morbidity rate was comparable, the mortality rate was significantly lower in the laparoscopic group (0.04 vs. 0.2 % in the open group).

S. Perretta, MD (✉)
Department of Digestive and Endocrine Surgery,
NHC Strasbourg, hopitaux universitaires Strasbourg,
1 place de l'hopital, 67000 Strasbourg, France
e-mail: silvana.perretta@ircad.fr

Visceral perforation was still the leading cause of severe complications in both groups. The authors concluded that the first 10-year experience of laparoscopic fundoplication reduced the rate of serious complications, which are mainly associated with technical failures related to the lack of a standardized surgical technique. Richter confirmed this data in 2013 reporting a decrease in the inpatient mortality rate after LAF from 0.82 % in 1993 to 0.26 % in 2000, but then a sudden increase in 2006 to 0.54 % [8]. This latter rise in mortality was related to a different patient population, older and with more comorbidity. Another review covering 10 years (1990–2001) was a review of the database from the department of Veterans Affairs that showed 0.8 % mortality for a cohort of 3,145 patients [9]. The main causes of death were gastrointestinal bleeding, gastric necrosis, gastric or esophageal perforation, cardiac arrest, respiratory complication, and pulmonary embolism.

Perforations and Leaks

Perforations are rare (<1 %) in the fundoplication literature. They are more common in redo surgery but not higher than in open surgery [7, 10, 11]. Perforations usually occur at the level of the esophagus or the proximal stomach. The underlying mechanism can be improper dissection, rough tissue manipulation, improper use of electrocautery devices, or faulty transoral introduction of a calibration bougie or nasogastric tube. Perforations can also be secondary to the pull-through of gastroesophageal sutures. In the case of Collis gastroplasty, performed in patients presenting with a "short esophagus," a leak from the gastric staple line can occur in a "not insignificant" percent of cases. This is presumably more likely to happen when previous antireflux or other gastroesophageal surgery has taken place, as multiple dissections interfere with the blood supply to this area. In a series of 210 patients Schauer reported 17 perforations, 10 related to improper retro-esophageal window dissection, 5 to bougie introduction, and 2 occurring at the site of gastric sutures

L.L. Swanstrom and C.M. Dunst (eds.), *Antireflux Surgery*,
DOI 10.1007/978-1-4939-1749-5_17, © Springer New York 2015

"pullthrough" [10]. It should be noted that, independently of the location, (esophageal or gastric), most perforation occur posteriorly. Since the most frequent site of injury is the posterior GEJ, it follows that the creation of the retro-esophageal window requires optimal exposure and adequate identification of the main anatomical landmarks: such the right and left diaphragmatic crura, the aorta and the posterior esophagus, and stomach (Fig. 17.1). This is particularly true in redo cases and the morbidly obese where the anatomical planes are usually distorted and obscured.

Incorrect traction on the stomach and esophagus during passage of a bougie for sizing the fundoplication can result in severe angulation of the distal esophagus or proximal stomach and possible subsequent perforation (Fig. 17.2). Bougies and nasogastric tubes should be placed always under laparoscopic view, by experienced medical personnel and with direct communication by the surgery team.

If the perforation is recognized and repaired the post-operative course should be uneventful with an unchanged functional outcome. When the perforation is detected intra-operatively the repair can and should be easily performed by primary closure, which is then incorporated in the fundoplication wrap.

The greatest threat to the patient is an unrecognized perforation. The presenting signs and symptoms may differ from classical teachings about the acute abdomen. Postoperative upper gastrointestinal series may also be misleading. Even in the absence of obvious radiological, biological, and peritoneal signs of sepsis, a high level of suspicion should be there for patients presenting with persistent, and

relatively increased, post-operative pain, tachycardia and/or respiratory distress; since these symptoms are better indicator of a potential complication than history, labs, or examination. In these patients a diagnostic laparoscopy should be a first approach and should include a systematic exploration of

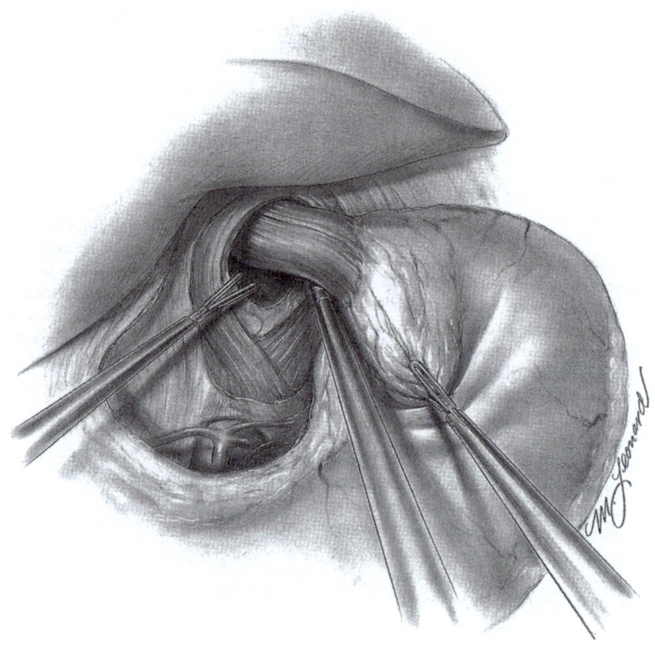

Fig. 17.1 Avoidance of dissection injury of the gastroesophageal junction requires careful retraction, identification of critical structures, precise dissection, and careful use of energy. An angled laparoscope allows dissection behind the GEJ to be performed under direct vision

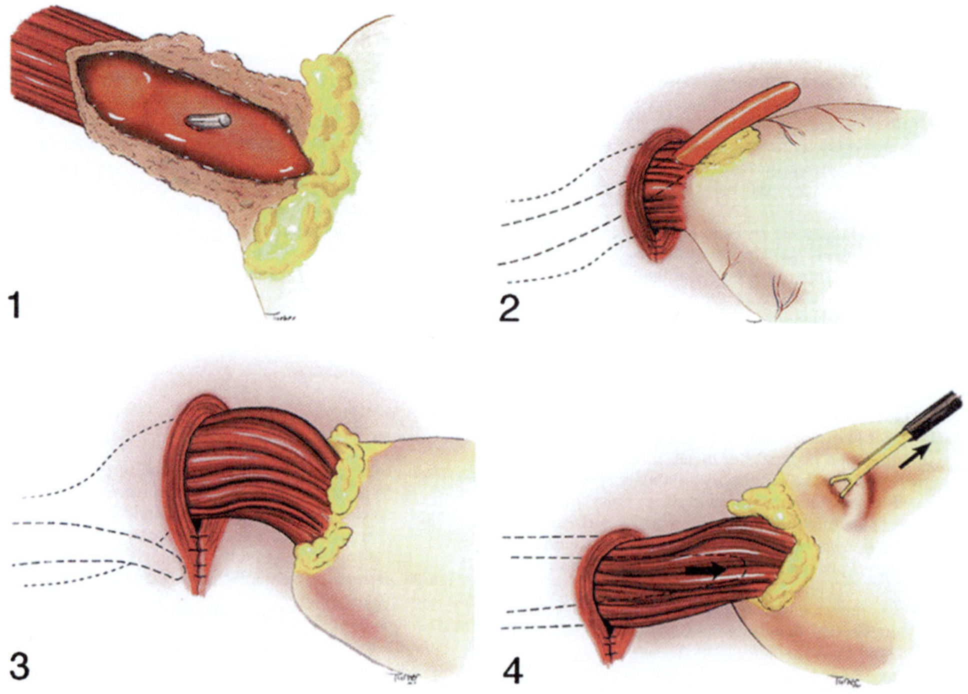

Fig. 17.2 Passage of a bougie or nasogastric tube must be done carefully after hiatal closure. Angulation of the distal esophagus must be controlled by axial traction or perforation can occur. (**1**) Nasogastric perforation of distal esophagus during laparoscopic Heller myotomy (**2**) Bougie perforation at the anterior GE junction due to closure of the hiatus and improper retraction (**3**) Bougie perforation of the posterior distal esophagus due to closure of the hiatus and improper retraction (**4**) Proper caudad and anterior laparoscopic retraction of the stomach during insertion of bougie (from Lowham et al. mechanisms and Avoidance of Esophageal Perforation by Personnel During Laparoscopic Foregut Surgery, Surg Endosc 1996, printed with permission) [12]

the wrap and the esophagus. If no obvious source of spillage is detected the fundoplication and the crural repair should still be taken down to fully assess the gastric and esophageal integrity as, on occasion, a small, contained leak may be the problem. In case of an esophageal leak which is not amenable to a sound primary suture repair, or a staple line leak after a Collis gastroplasty, the use of a covered self-expanding metal stent (SEMS) is recommended. Endoscopic stenting can be the sole form of treatment in the absence of large abscess or peritoneal contamination. Additional image-guided percutaneous drainage or re-operation should be performed to control significant mediastinal or abdominal contamination.

Prevention of these potentially serious complications requires a full understanding of the detailed anatomy of the gastroesophageal region, awareness of the recognized mechanisms of perforation and a meticulous surgical technique [13]. Subtle and possibly serious vital sign changes, combined with post-operative pain, increased narcotic medication use and antibiotics can obscure intra-abdominal processes, creating a diagnostic dilemma for even the most experienced surgeon. Surgeons should bear in mind that consequences accompanying esophageal perforation make this complication a prime litigation target. The requirement of surgical repair and a delay in diagnosis are two of the most common factors present in litigated cases resulting in a payment. All patients should therefore have a frank discussion about the possibility of complications such as esophageal perforation, during their informed consent for surgery.

Bleeding

Significant bleeding during surgery is uncommon and usually is easily controlled laparoscopically. It mainly occurs during short gastric division, when mobilizing the fundus of the stomach. Splenic injuries may occur during this dissection, but the need for incidental splenectomy is rare and dropped from 10 % during open surgery to less than 1 % for laparoscopic surgery [14]. This fortunate decrease is probably related to the improved exposure and vision provided by laparoscopy together with the dramatic change in energy instrumentation that allows a more straightforward technique to complete this step of the operation.

Acute Dysphagia

Dysphagia is a common side effect of fundoplication. Usually self-limiting, post-operative dysphagia is reported by 10–90 % of patients to varying degrees [15, 16]. Post-operative tightening of the gastroesophageal junction due to edema: with consequent slower emptying is normal due to

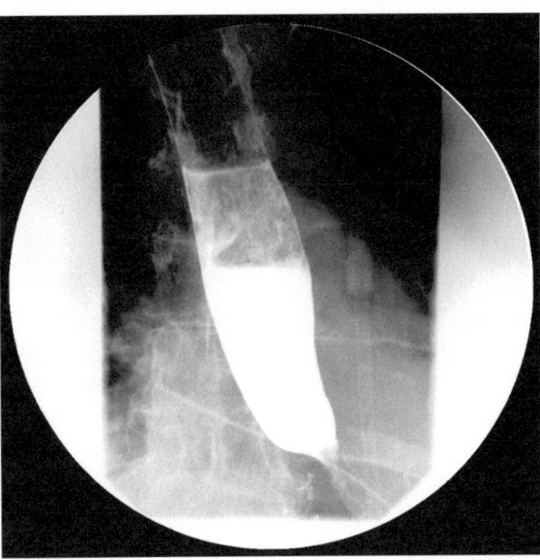

Fig. 17.3 Early dysphagia is normal post-fundoplication and an upper GI X-ray will often show slow emptying of the esophagus due to edema. This usually responds to conservative treatment with liquid diet and sometimes steroids

local edema and esophageal trauma. In fact, dysphagia should probably be considered a normal consequence of the fundoplication, and can typically last up to 6 weeks. It is usually well managed by dietary advice with a soft food diet being mandated by most surgeons for the first month or so. Severe dysphagia with important weight loss or dysphagia during this period should be investigated.

We believe that a water soluble upper X-ray study should be performed in every patient on post-operative day one to confirm the position of the fundoplication and assess the passage of the contrast into the stomach. If the exam shows contrast passing into the stomach, albeit slowly, and a correct sub-diaphragmatic position of the antireflux valve and stomach, a conservative approach can be followed even if the patient has significant dysphagia, and swallowing will usually improve over the ensuing few days (Fig. 17.3). Steroids are often effective for early dysphagia due to edema and can often relieve the obstruction and accelerate recovery. However, if absolutely no contrast passes into the stomach, early endoscopy and/or laparoscopic exploration is recommended to rule out technical flaws; such as too tight a crural repair, too tight or twisted a fundoplication, or too long a valve. In addition, other possible causes of dysphagia such as a malposition or a displacement of the valve (slippage) can only be ruled out by re-exploration.

The choice of early endoscopic dilatation in this setting is controversial. Severe acute dysphagia is not tremendously likely to respond to conservative treatments like dilatation, but it is a well tolerated, a benign intervention, helpful in the identification of the underlying problem, and occasionally works.

Pneumothorax

Pneumothorax, or more precisely capnothorax, is not to be considered a complication but rather a side effect of a complex mediastinal dissection. During such dissections, it is not unusual to tear one or both pleura when mobilizing the intrathoracic esophagus especially in patients with severe periesophagitis, large hiatal hernia, and previous operations. The consequences are negligible because the CO_2 is easily controlled with positive pressure ventilation and is quickly resorbed. In most patients pneumothorax is asymptomatic and does not compromise patients' hemodynamic and ventilatory status. Certain patients with poor pulmonary function or hemodynamic problems may represent more problematic management problems. Disciplined cooperation between anesthesiologists and surgeons is needed to ensure proper intra-operative management. PEEP modification can be used to manage the vast majority of cases of pneumothorax [16, 17]. Passage of CO_2 into the pleura after injury is facilitated due to the existence of a pressure gradient; intra-abdominal pressure > intrapleural end-expiratory pressure. Application of PEEP decreases or reverses the gradient which prevents further CO_2 build up. Being highly diffusible, the existing CO_2 in the pleura is rapidly removed by the circulating blood. Also, re-expansion of the lung with PEEP mechanically seals the surgically induced tear in the parietal pleura. An index of suspicion, close clinical observation of airway pressure and end-tidal CO_2, periodic auscultations of chest, and communication with the surgeon are needed to detect the rare occurrence of a tension pneumothorax which is potentially life threatening and needs prompt management with decompression by chest tube insertion or widening the pleural defect laparoscopically. Any attempt to seal a pleural tear should be avoided in order to prevent an iatrogenic tension pneumothorax.

Acute Migration

Intrathoracic gastric herniation after LF is an uncommon but potentially life-threatening event that can present in the early post-operative period. Acute intrathoracic migration can occur due to events that raise intra-abdominal pressure capable of forcing or disrupting the crural closure. This sudden raise of pressure usually happens during extubation or in the immediate post-operative period particularly in the recovery room. It is related to the not uncommon occurrence of "Bucking" against an endotracheal tube if the patient was not extubated immediately or from post-operative retching and vomiting. Intratracheal administration of lidocaine (10 %) has shown significant benefit for the suppression of bucking during the recovery of general anesthesia [18]. Post-operative nausea and vomiting efforts can also be avoided or minimized after LF with routine prophylactic administration of antiemetics in or before the recovery room.

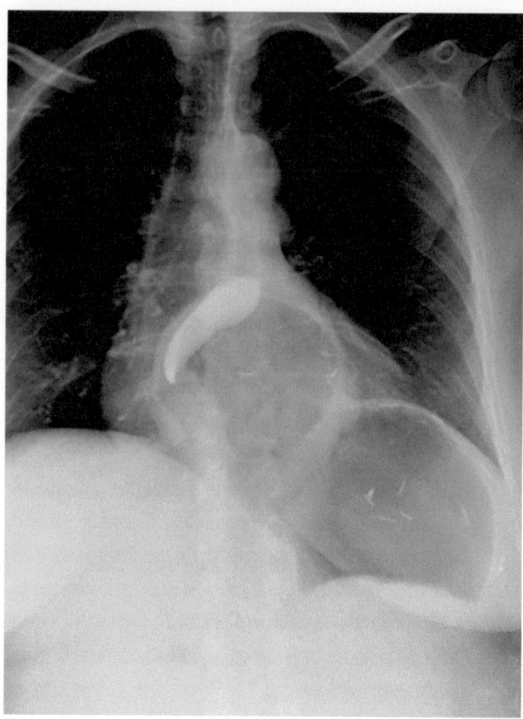

Fig. 17.4 Acute wrap herniation due to post-anesthesia retching can be a dangerous occurrence and needs immediate re-operation

Satisfactory outcomes in the management of wrap migration depend on early recognition and prompt surgical intervention. Many patients will report minor or no symptoms, and may complain just of a vague epigastric discomfort. Others will present with obvious signs of organ strangulation and ischemia. Awareness of this potential complication is necessary to detect and treat the condition early and so allow its correction by a laparoscopic approach. In most cases the crural repair is usually intact in spite of the migration of the fundoplication into the thorax. The wrap should be reduced back into the abdomen after undoing the crural closure (to prevent any injury to the herniated stomach). A new cruroplasty should then be carried out. Early diagnosis and timely surgical reduction of the hernia results in prompt recovery and an unchanged post-operative course. A routine post-operative gastrografin swallow should be performed in all patients to detect asymptomatic early migration (Fig. 17.4). Delay in recognition can result in strangulation, necrosis, and perforation of the stomach in the posterior mediastinum with resulting dreadful consequences [19].

Vagal Injury

The actual incidence of this complication is almost impossible to establish due to the vagaries of symptoms related to post-operative vagal function. Identification and preservation of the vagal nerves should be systematically attempted during esophageal dissection. Consequences of vagal injury may include early satiety, dumping/diarrhea, and post-prandial fullness due to iatrogenic gastroparesis. A problem is that these symptoms are also common after a fundoplication due to the impaired fundic accommodation. In short, an operative complication is only one possible etiology for delayed gastric emptying. This means that, evaluation and management should be comprehensive and well documented as this is a common medical-legal problem in Western counties. It is important to distinguish whether symptoms are, in fact, related to any surgical procedure [8, 20]. Patients presenting with suspected gastroparesis should be further characterized by whether symptoms were pre-existing or subsequent to the fundoplication. Vagal damage can occur during the initial dissection at the hiatus or later during the intramediastinal dissection. If the surgeon is careful, well educated, and experienced this should be an extremely rare "complication." The analysis of the literature would imply that fundoplication, complicated by vagal injury or vagotomy, accounts for 52 % of iatrogenic gastroparesis [8]. Of course this data does not take into account the possibility of pre-existing gastroparesis as a cause of the reflux.

Conclusions

Laparoscopic antireflux surgery is complex, in so far as it not only demands good surgical skills but also skillful patient selection. Poor patient selection, mediocre surgical technique, and the natural learning curve have created the impression that laparoscopic fundoplication is dangerous and complication "ridden." Standardization of the preoperative work-up as well as surgical technique is absolutely necessary. The lessons learned over 20 years of laparoscopic experience call for a systematization of the key operative steps, no matter what kind of valve is performed and no matter the surgeon's experience. Antireflux surgery is never an emergency operation and leaves no room for approximation. Its success requires a frank discussion about all the potential perioperative and post-operative problems, aggressive intervention when indicated, and a realistic understanding between the patient and the surgeon.

References

1. Dallemagne B. Clinical results of laparoscopic fundoplication at ten years after surgery. Surg Endosc. 2006;20:159–65.

2. Engstrom C, Cai W, Irvine T, et al. Twenty years of experience with laparoscopic antireflux surgery. Br J Surg. 2012;99:1415–21.

3. Wang YR, Dempsey DT, Richter JE. Trends and perioperative outcomes of inpatient antireflux surgery in the United States, 1993–2006. Dis Esophagus. 2011;24:215–23.

4. Rantanen TK, Salo JA, Sipponen JT. Fatal and life-threatening complications in antireflux surgery: analysis of 5,502 operations. Br J Surg. 1999;86:1573–7.

5. Brown CN, Smith LT, Watson DI, Devitt PG, Thompson SK, Jamieson GG. Outcomes for trainees vs experienced surgeons undertaking laparoscopic antireflux surgery – is equipoise achieved? J Gastrointest Surg. 2013;17:1173–80.

6. Dallemagne B, Perretta S. Twenty years of laparoscopic fundoplication for GERD. World J Surg. 2011;35:1428–35.

7. Rantanen T. Complications in antireflux surgery: national-based analysis of laparoscopic and open fundoplications. Arch Surg. 2008;143:359–65.

8. Je R. Gastroesophageal reflux disease treatment: side effects and complications of fundoplication. Clin Gastroenterol Hepatol. 2013;11:465–71.

9. Dominitz JA, Dire CA, Billingsley KG, Todd-Stenberg JA. Complications and antireflux medication use after antireflux surgery. Clin Gastroenterol Hepatol. 2006;4:299–305.

10. Schauer PR, Meyers WC, Eubanks S, Norem RF, Franklin M, Pappas TN. Mechanisms of gastric and esophageal perforations during laparoscopic Nissen fundoplication. Ann Surg. 1996;223:43–52.

11. Dr F. The nationwide frequency of major adverse outcomes in antireflux surgery and the role of surgeon experience, 1992–1997. J Am Coll Surg. 2002;195:611–8.

12. Lowham AS1, Filipi CJ, Hinder RA, Swanstrom LL, Stalter K, dePaula A, Hunter JG, Buglewicz TG, Haake K. Mechanisms and avoidance of esophageal perforation by anesthesia personnel during laparoscopic foregut surgery. Surg Endosc. 1996;10(10):979–82.

13. Svider PF, et al. Esophageal perforation and rupture: a comprehensive medicolegal examination of 59 jury verdicts and settlements. J Gastrointest Surg. 2013;17:1732–8.

14. Rogers DM, Herrington Jr JL, Morton C. Incidental splenectomy associated with Nissen fundoplication. Ann Surg. 1980;191:153–6.

15. Lundell L. Complications after anti-reflux surgery. Best Pract Res Clin Gastroenterol. 2004;18:935–45.

16. Dallemagne B, Arenas Sanchez M, Francart D, et al. Long-term results after laparoscopic reoperation for failed antireflux procedures. Br J Surg. 2011;98:1581–7.

17. Joris JL, Chiche JD, Lamy ML. Pneumothorax during laparoscopic fundoplication: diagnosis and treatment with positive end-expiratory pressure. Anesth Analg. 1995;81:993–1000.

18. Altintas F. Lidocaine 10 % in the endotracheal tube cuff: blood concentrations, haemodynamic and clinical effects. Eur J Anaesthesiol. 2000;17:436–42.

19. Balakrishnan SA. Acute transhiatal migration and herniation of fundic wrap following laparoscopic Nissen fundoplication. J Laparoendosc Adv Surg Tech. 2007;17:209–12.

20. McCallum RW, Berkowitz DM, Lerner E. Gastric emptying in patients with gastroesophageal reflux. Gastroenterology. 1981;80:285–91.

The Use of Mesh in Hiatal Hernia Repair

Marcelo W. Hinojosa, Andrew S. Wright, and Brant K. Oelschlager

Introduction

At its most basic, hiatal hernia can either be defined by the presence of stomach within the mediastinum—where it obviously doesn't belong—or as the defect in the diaphragm that allows the stomach to migrate. For the surgeon, the later is the primary concern as it is the size of the defect and the quality of the tissues surrounding the defect that will determine the success of the anatomic repair. Hiatal hernias are classified as four types. The most common, a type I hernia or sliding hiatal hernia is formed by the migration of the gastroesophageal junction (GEJ) cephalad through the hiatus into the mediastinum. A type II hiatal hernia, which is the most rare variation, is when the fundus of the stomach migrates through the hiatus into the mediastinum while the GEJ remains in the normal anatomical position. A type III hiatal hernia is a combination of a type I and type II hernia, where both the gastric fundus and the GEJ migrate through the hiatus into the mediastinum. A type IV hiatal hernia is a type III hernia with the migration of other organs (small bowel, colon, spleen, etc.) into the mediastinum. Some have also described a Type V hernia which is defined as one that occurs post previous hiatal hernia repair. Types II–V hiatus hernias are also typically referred to as paraesophageal hernias. They often present with obstructive or other mechanical symptoms and are at risk for volvulus or other complications. This is one of the main differentiations between these and type I, or sliding hernias. Furthermore, while some surgeons reinforce type 1 HH repairs with mesh based on an axiom that "all hernias should be meshed," for the most part Type I hiatal hernias less commonly involve massive diaphragm defects or abnormal tissues and therefore are most commonly repaired primarily.

Hiatal hernias (HH) are probably a result of a combination of mechanical "stressors" and biogenetic factors. Mechanical factors include those that increase intra-abdominal pressure such as chronic cough, obesity, pregnancy, heavy physical labor, and chronic constipation. Also these factors contribute to the natural history of HH which tend to slowly increase in size, though this is not universally true. The surgeon must not only repair the hernia well but also mitigate these inciting factors after surgery to minimize recurrences.

Truly giant hiatal hernias, especially paraesophageal hernias, probably also involve a connective tissue or cellular disorder as they are often familial and/or associated with other hernias. Exactly what this genetic defect is, or what components of the diaphragm it affects is unknown. Direct measurements show quantitative and qualitative defects in both the elastin and collagen content of the crura [1, 2].

There is evidence, as for inguinal and ventral hernias, that metalloproteinase metabolism may play a role as well [3]. Finally, structural differences at the cellular level between hiatal hernias and non-hiatal hernia reflux patients have been noted [4]. The number and significance of these etiologic factors have led many to believe that primary hiatal hernia repair is doomed to a high recurrence rate unless the repair is reinforced by a supplemental material.

M.W. Hinojosa, MD
Department of Surgery, University of Washington,
1959 NE Pacific Street, Box 356410, Seattle, WA 98195, USA
e-mail: hinojosa@u.washington.edu

A.S. Wright, MD
Department of Surgery, Center for Videoendoscopic Surgery,
University of Washington, 1959 NE Pacific Street,
Box 356410, Seattle, WA 98195, USA
e-mail: awright2@uw.edu

B.K. Oelschlager, MD (⊠)
Division of General Surgery, Department of Surgery,
Center for Esophageal and Gastric Surgery, Byers Endowed
Professor of Esophageal Research, University of Washington,
1959 NE Pacific Street, Box 356410, Seattle, WA 98195, USA
e-mail: brant@u.washington.edu

Operative Approach: Historical Perspective

Postemski performed the first hiatal hernia repair in 1889, which was followed by Aukeland's description of the first paraesophageal hernia repair in 1926. These repairs were

L.L. Swanstrom and C.M. Dunst (eds.), *Antireflux Surgery*,
DOI 10.1007/978-1-4939-1749-5_18, © Springer New York 2015

performed via an open thoracic or transabdominal approach and were associated with significant morbidity and mortality. The advent of laparoscopic surgery and its use in the treatment of gastroesophageal reflux revolutionized hiatal hernia repair. Today, hiatal hernia repair is one of the most common surgical procedures performed in the United States with over 40,000 cases performed each year [5].

In 1991, Congreve performed the first laparoscopic hiatal hernia repair [6]. Although laparoscopic repair was associated with lower morbidity and mortality, initial reports of high recurrence rates impacted the acceptance of the laparoscopic approach as the preferred approach. Hashemi et al. [7] documented, by video esophagram 17 months after repair, a 42 % recurrence with laparoscopic repair of giant hiatal hernias compared to 15 % with the open repair in 54 patients. Similarly, Mattar et al. and Khaitan et al. both found high recurrence rates with laparoscopic paraesophageal hernia repair when studied with esophagram postoperatively: 33 and 40 %, respectively [8, 9]. Since these reports were published, laparoscopic hiatal hernia repair has evolved. Tenets such as total hernia sac excision, achieving adequate intra-abdominal esophagus length, intra-abdominal anchoring, and the minimization of tension during reapproximation of hiatus with or without mesh reinforcement have become the corner stone of efforts to minimize recurrences. As experience has increased and recurrence rates have dropped, so has the acceptance of the laparoscopic technique. In a recent survey of SAGES members, 94 % of surgeons who perform hiatal hernia repair reported performing the procedure laparoscopically [10].

Hiatal reinforcement has been an area of interest in the last decade. The low recurrence rates associated with prosthetic mesh in the repair of inguinal and ventral hernias have raised interest in the use of mesh for reinforcement of hiatal hernia repair. Interestingly, the use of prosthetic material in the repair of hiatal hernia is not new. Reports of the use of synthetic materials date back to 1957 when Cooley et al. used a polyvinyl sponge to reinforce hiatal closure in dogs [11]. In 1960 Fusco described the use of a tantalum mesh in a patient [12]. In a case series of ten patients, Merendino and Dillard used Teflon mesh for hiatal reinforcement, noting only one small recurrence [13]. Freidman and MacKenzie used Ivalon in 17 patients and noted no recurrence [14]. Although these studies originated from the era of open surgery, it was not until reports of high recurrence rates associated with the laparoscopic repair surfaced that hiatal reinforcement has been revisited. However, to date, there is no consensus regarding the need or wisdom of using mesh in the hiatus, let alone which type of mesh to use or which technique should be used to implant it.

Prosthetic Mesh

In an effort to reduce recurrence rates, a number of prosthetic meshes have been used to reinforce the hiatus during laparoscopic hiatal hernia repair. Kuster and Gilroy reported the first six cases of laparoscopic paraesophageal hernia repair with synthetic mesh reinforcement placed anteriorly on the hiatus [15]. In this short-term study, they reported no mesh-related complications and two small asymptomatic posterior recurrences. Since then, most reports have shown similar results. In a prospective randomized trial of 72 patients with large hiatal hernias Frantzides et al. randomized 36 patients to laparoscopic repair with simple crural closure and 36 patients to laparoscopic repair with crural closure and polytetrafluoroethylene (PTFE) mesh reinforcement. This study was limited to patient with hernias greater than 8 cm [16]. A keyhole mesh was used for closure in the mesh reinforcement group (Fig. 18.1). There were no complications and at a median follow-up of 2.5 years, 22 % of patients that underwent paraesophageal hernia repair with primary closure had a radiographic recurrence compared to none in the PTFE group. In a similar study, Granderath et al. used polypropylene mesh as a posterior hiatal reinforcement (Fig. 18.2). He showed an 8 % recurrence rate in patients who underwent hiatal reinforcement with polypropylene compared to 26 % recurrence rate in those who underwent primary closure [17]. Although synthetic mesh appears to reduce hernia recurrence, it has come with a price as many complications from nonabsorbable mesh have been reported. Multiple case reports have identified problems such as dysphagia, ulceration, stricture, and mesh erosion related to the use of synthetic mesh for hiatal hernia reinforcement.

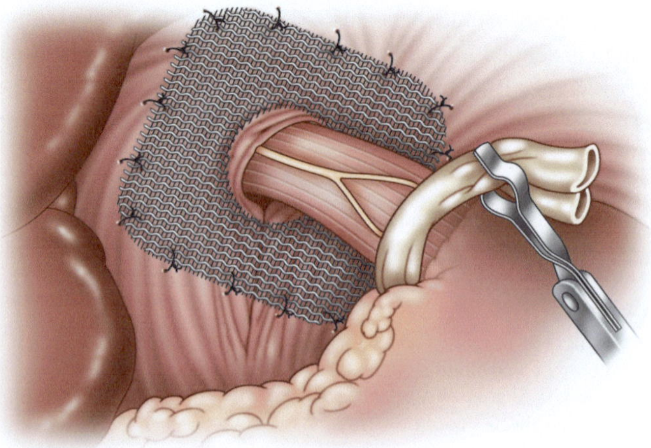

Fig. 18.1 Laparoscopic hiatal hernia repair with PTFE mesh reinforcement using keyhole configuration

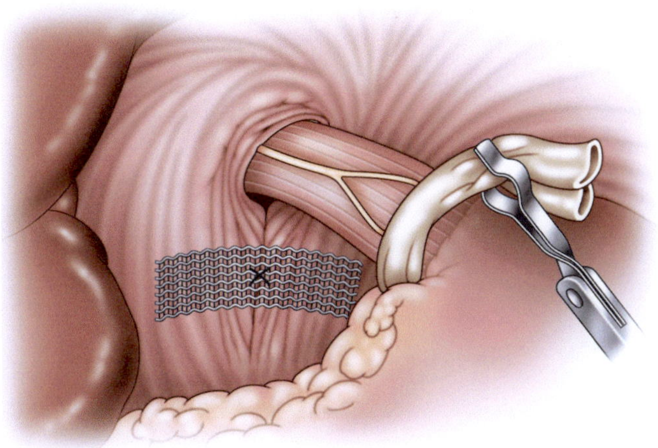

Fig. 18.2 Laparoscopic hiatal hernia repair with posterior polypropylene mesh

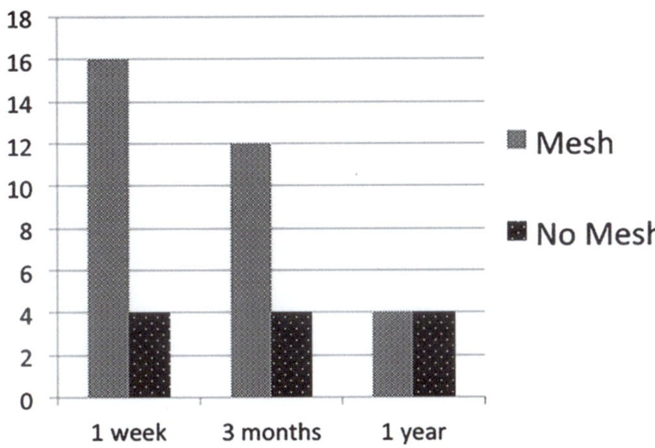

Post operative Dysphagia: Prosthetic Mesh vs No Mesh

Fig. 18.3 There can be a trade-off between recurrence rates and early postoperative dysphagia (data adapted from Granderath FA, et al. Arch Surg. 2005;140(1):40–8)

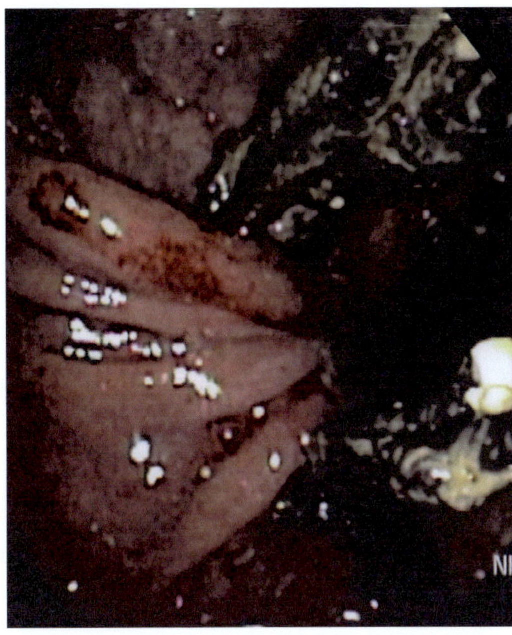

Fig. 18.4 Endoscopic view of laparoscopic hiatal hernia repair with polypropylene mesh erosion after paraesophageal hernia repair

Although Granderath's report showed a low recurrence with mesh reinforcement, the rate of postoperative dysphagia was three times greater after hiatal hernia repair with polypropylene when compared to the nonmesh group at 3 months postoperatively, even though the dysphagia was 4 % in both groups at 1 year (Fig. 18.3). Trus et al. [18] also noted a case of refractory dysphagia after mesh closure and formation of cicatrix of scar, which was treated with excision of mesh and myotomy of distal esophagus. Erosion of mesh into either esophagus or stomach has also been described (Fig. 18.4). Tatum et al. reported two complications that occurred after the placement of PTFE mesh for hiatal reinforcement during repair of large paraesophageal hernias. One patient had erosion of the PTFE mesh into the esophagogastric junction and

gastric cardia that required a gastrectomy. A second patient developed severe dysphagia from a stricture thought to be caused by PTFE mesh closure of the hiatus. In this patient, the mesh was removed and the Nissen fundoplication was taken down and converted to a partial fundoplication [19]. Coluccio et al. [20] also reported a case of PTFE mesh eroding into the gastric cardia which was treated with a distal esophagectomy. In a multi-institutional study Stadlhuder et al. [21] noted 28 patients who had complications after hiatal reinforcement with prosthetic mesh. In this series 17 patients presented with mesh erosion, 11 were found to have stenosis or dense adhesions, and nine patients underwent reoperation for resection and excision of mesh.

Biologic Mesh

In an attempt to avoid the complications that can occur with prosthetic mesh, while still providing the benefits of reinforcement of the hiatal closure in reducing recurrence, biologic mesh has been used with increasing frequency over the last decade. Biologic mesh is designed to serve as a temporary extracellular matrix scaffold for native tissue ingrowth which theoretically results in stronger tissue through normal healing [22, 23]. A number of biologic hernia mesh implants have been developed: porcine small intestine submucosa, bovine pericardium, human cadaveric dermis, cross-linked porcine dermal collagen, and non cross-linked porcine epithelium, etc. Each of these commercial products has various "benefits" ascribed to them: longevity, workability, native growth factors to stimulate healing, etc, but the true clinical benefits of these elements have not been scientifically proven to date. Of all biologic implants, those derived from human cadaveric dermis and porcine small intestine submucosa have been the most widely studied. Although other implants have been used for reinforcement of hiatal closure, most have been reported only as single case reports.

Acellular dermal matrix has been subject of multiple studies that have shown a low rate of hiatal hernia recurrence [24, 25]. Ringley et al. prospectively studied 44 patients with hiatal hernias >5 cm, 22 who underwent hiatal hernia repair with primary closure, and 22 who underwent hiatal hernia repair with reinforcement of primary closure with onlay human acellular dermis. The authors found no difference in postoperative dysphagia in each group. They noted 9 % recurrence of hiatal hernia at 6-month follow-up in the primary closure group and none in the human acellular dermis group [26]. In a more recent retrospective study of a cohort of 52 consecutive patients who had primary closure reinforcement with onlay human acellular dermal matrix, the same group found a hernia recurrence rate of 3.8 %. In follow-up of 16 months, one patient underwent reoperation due to recurrent symptoms [25]. Similarly Diaz et al. [27] examined 46 patients with large hiatal hernias (>5 cm) who had laparoscopic hiatal hernia repair with reinforcement of crural closure and found a recurrence rate of 4.3 % at a mean follow-up of 3.6 months.

In 2003, we reported on nine patients who underwent laparoscopic repair of large paraesophageal hernias with porcine small intestinal submucosa (SIS) [28]. Eight patients had follow-up at a median of 8 months with barium esophagram and endoscopy. Only one patient had evidence of anatomical recurrence and one patient reported mild dysphagia that resolved after one endoscopic dilation. This led to a multicenter, prospective randomized trial which has recently reported long-term results [29]. In all, 108 patients with hiatal hernia >5 cm were enrolled and randomized to primary repair versus SIS-reinforcement of primary repair (57 patients with and 51 patients without biomesh reinforcement). At 6 months, 95 patients had an upper gastrointestinal study. There was a significant decrease in hernia recurrence in the biomesh group (9 %) and the primary closure group (24 %). Although initial results were promising with regards to hiatal hernia recurrence using biologic mesh reinforcement, long-term data showed that the benefit diminished over time [30] (Fig. 18.5). Seventy-two patients from the initial 108 were followed-up at a median follow-up of 58 months. Sixty patients underwent repeat upper gastrointestinal series (34 patients in the primary repair group and 26 patients in the biomesh group). There was a 59 % recurrence in the primary repair group compared to 54 % recurrence in the biomesh group and there were no reported cases of erosions, strictures, dysphagia, or other complications related to

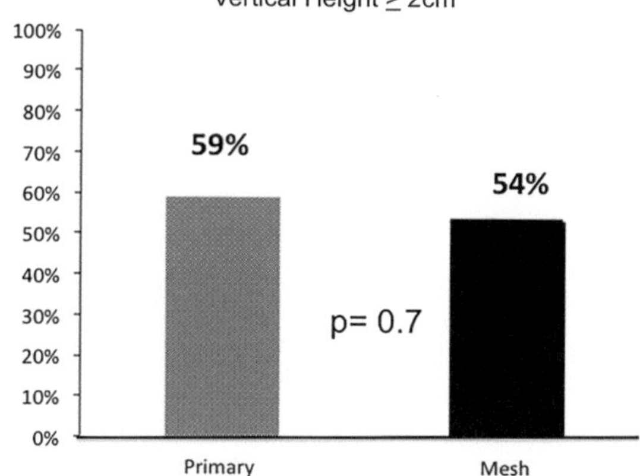

Fig. 18.5 RCT data showing 5-year results of biomesh vs no mesh during paraesophageal hernia repair [30]

the biologic mesh. There was also not a significant difference in relevant symptom severity or quality of life scores between groups. Interestingly there were two reoperations for hiatal hernia recurrence in the primary repair group and none in the biomesh group. To date this is the only long-term randomized prospective clinical trial using a biologic mesh.

Absorbable Mesh

More recently, absorbable mesh has been studied in hiatal hernia repair. They presumably work by providing shortterm structural reinforcement and by causing an inflammatory response during their resorption that results in a thicker scar. Parsak et al. [31] conducted a prospective randomized study with 75 patients who underwent LARS with polypropylene hiatal reinforcement and 75 who underwent polyglactin (Vicryl) mesh reinforcement. They showed that at a median follow-up of 38 months recurrence was similar between the polypropylene group and the absorbable mesh group: 5 and 4 %, respectively. These initial results are promising, however a major limitation of this study was that not all patients had objective studies to determine radiographic recurrence. Another problem is that, unlike recurrence with prosthetic mesh which occurs in less than 1 year, recurrence can occur much later with biologic and presumably absorbable meshes.

Operative Technique; Mesh Overlay

The best position and method of fixation of mesh remain poorly understood and there is no evidence to date to support one approach over another. The majority of practitioners

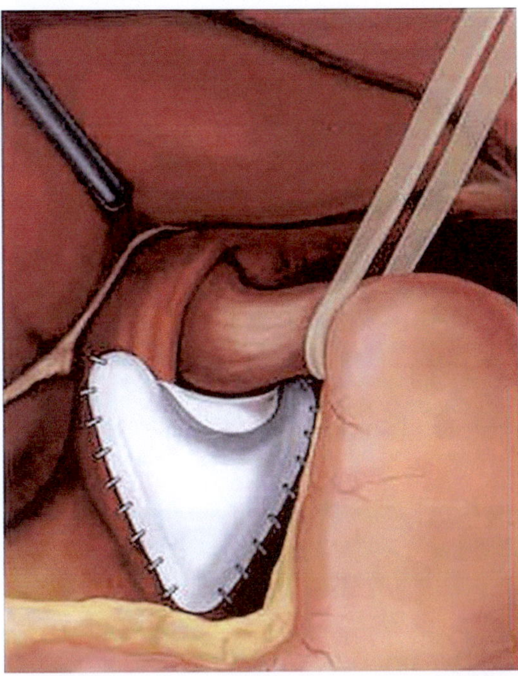

Fig. 18.6 Bridging plastic mesh is commercially available but is widely considered to be a bad idea

perform primary closure and then reinforcement with an onlay mesh. This is obviously the only method possible with absorbable and biologic meshes. There are reports describing "bridging" techniques with synthetic mesh and there are even commercial meshes designed specifically to bridge (Fig. 18.6). In general, experts question (admittedly without evidence) the wisdom of placing mesh directly in contact with the esophagus. We describe below one mesh overlay technique using biologic mesh.

A standard laparoscopic set up is used. The patient is placed in a modified lithotomy or split-leg position with a beanbag allowing for steep reverse Trendelenburg position. We begin with the left upper quadrant port, placed just lateral to the mid-clavicular line at the costal margin. Pneumoperitoneum is obtained using Veress needle followed by placement of a 10 mm optical trocar. A 5 mm camera port is positioned at 10–12 cm from the costal margin in a line that is 2 3 cm to the left of the umbilicus. Two additional 5 mm ports are then placed, one in the right upper quadrant and the other at the left anterior axillary line at the level of the camera port. Finally, a Nathanson liver retractor is placed through a stab wound just to the left of midline high in the epigastrium and used to retract the left liver lobe. This can be substituted with a paddle retractor if the left lobe of the liver is large. The short gastric and retro gastric vessels are divided to the level of the left crus. Circumferential dissection of the hernia sac from the hiatus and mediastinal structures is then performed. The mediastinal dissection is carried proximal until there is at least 3 cm of intra-abdominal esophagus.

The sac is then everted over the GEJ and partially excised (to the left of the anterior vagus to avoid its transection). The hiatus is closed posteriorly with interrupted permanent sutures. The suture pattern can be interrupted, figure-of-8 or horizontal mattress sutures.

For reinforcement of these large defects—by nature repaired under tension—a U-configured biologic mesh is placed at the hiatus with the U base overlying the posterior hiatal closure. It is then sutured to the diaphragm with interrupted sutures or secured with fibrin glue to provide good contact between the SIS and diaphragm (Fig. 18.7a–d). A Nissen fundoplication of between 2.5 and 3 cm in length is created over a lighted 50–54 Fr Bougie. As the fundoplication is completed, it is positioned onto the esophagus and the top of the fundoplication is secured to the lateral aspects of the esophagus and to the left and the right crus. Additional sutures are placed to the undersurface of the diaphragm to secure the position of the fundoplication and prevent it from sliding. After the fundoplication, upper endoscopy is performed to examine the esophagus, discover accidental injuries, and thoroughly evaluate the fundoplication in terms of its shape, position, and tightness.

Operative Technique—Incorporated Mesh Implantation

Swanstrom and colleagues described an alternative technique called the incorporated technique [32]. Using this method, the mesh implantation is performed simultaneously with the diaphragmatic closure using horizontal pledgeted sutures. The first suture, with pledget loaded, passes through the lower left side of the mesh then the left crus. The needle is passed through the hiatus and the right crus and finally through the back right side of the mesh. The needle is brought back out through the trocar and exchanged for the second needle of a double-armed heavy braided permanent suture. This needle is then run through the same sequence again. Once both needles are outside the trocar, they are passed though a second pledget and the mattress suture is secured. These steps are repeated for each suture until the closure is complete (usually 3 mattress sutures total) (Fig. 18.8a–f).

Operative Technique—Difficult Closures

On occasion, the diaphragmatic crura are under too much tension to close primarily. This can be seen with extremely large diameter hernias or when fibrosis has occurred, usually due to reoperations. Some have attempted to place permanent mesh to "bridge the gap," but long-term results are plagued with failures and erosions. An alternative is to create one or more relaxing incisions in the diaphragm to allow

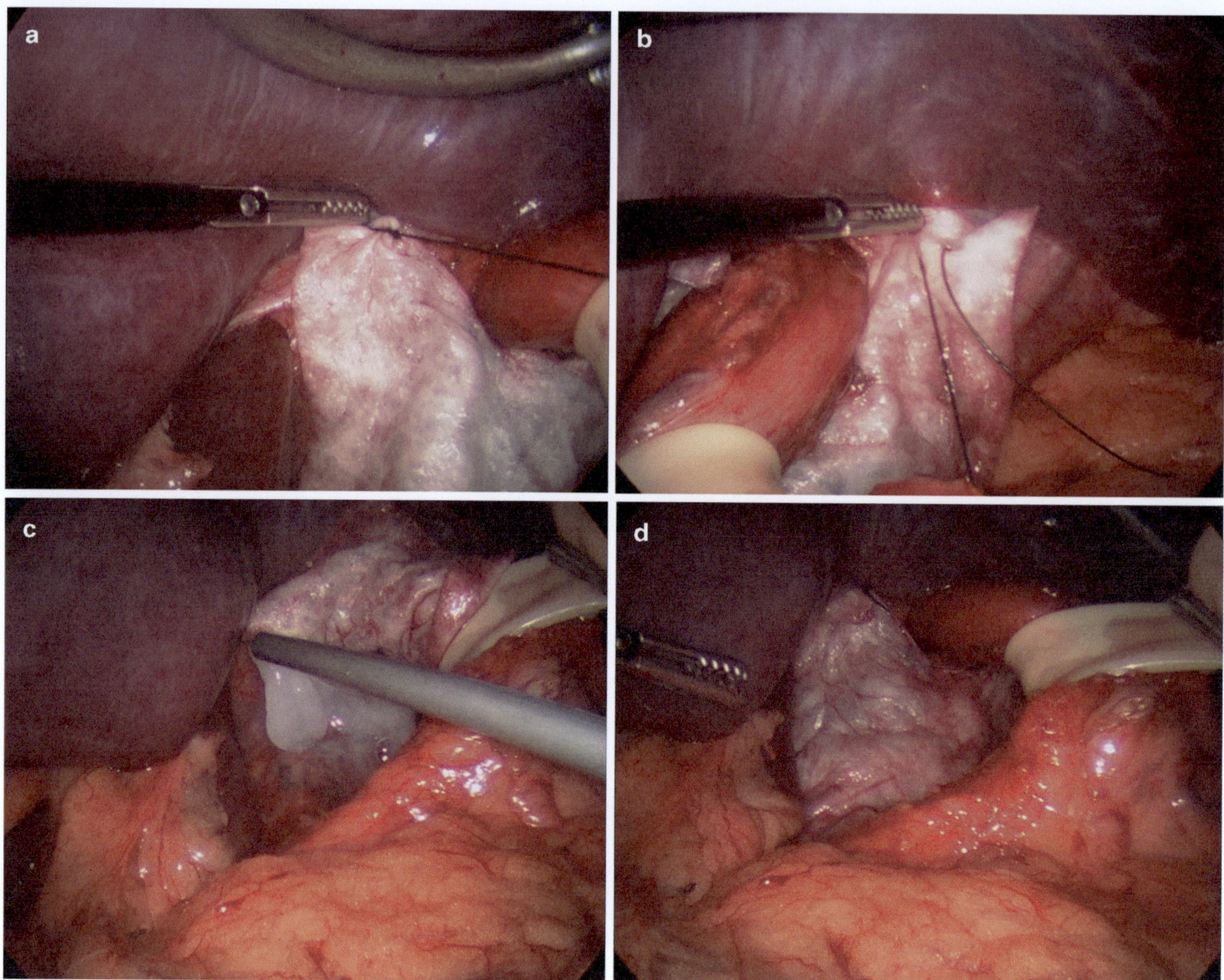

Fig. 18.7 Laparoscopic posterior crural closure with mesh overlay technique. The mesh is sutured in place at the top of the right crus (**a**) and to the left (**b**). Fibrin glue is placed between the mesh and the posterior closure (**c**). The complete repair (**d**)

primary closure of native tissue, with the resulting defects covered with mesh. The most commonly described technique, first described by Huntington, splits the right crus between the hiatus and the inferior vena cava [33].

The full thickness incision typically starts in the mid portion of the right crus. It is important to carry the incision high enough (anterior) to allow the entire closure to be free from tension though one must take care of the left hepatic vein near the upper limit. A permanent mesh is then used to close the diaphragmatic defect. Some argue that the risk of herniation through a right-sided relaxing incision is minimal due to the overlying presence of the liver and a mesh is not needed. We prefer to overlay a biologic mesh to reinforce the posterior closure as well as the right relaxing incision defect. A similar relaxing technique can be employed on the left side, behind the spleen, if there is insufficient space between the crura and the inferior vena cava for a right-sided proce-

dure. However, patching the defect with permanent mesh is mandatory on the left side to prevent diaphragmatic hernia formation. Recently, Greene et al. [34] have reported results of 15 patients undergoing various relaxing incisions (Fig. 18.9).

Small reports have described leaving the hiatus open, if it can't be closed, and using the mobilized left lateral hepatic segment placed behind the esophagus, as a "biologic" blockade to the partly closed hiatus. Obviously this is rather an extraordinary circumstance and its long-term success unknown.

Postoperative Care

Particularly with synthetic mesh, at least a single dose of postoperative antibiotics is reasonable. Patients generally start liquids the night of their procedure and are advanced to

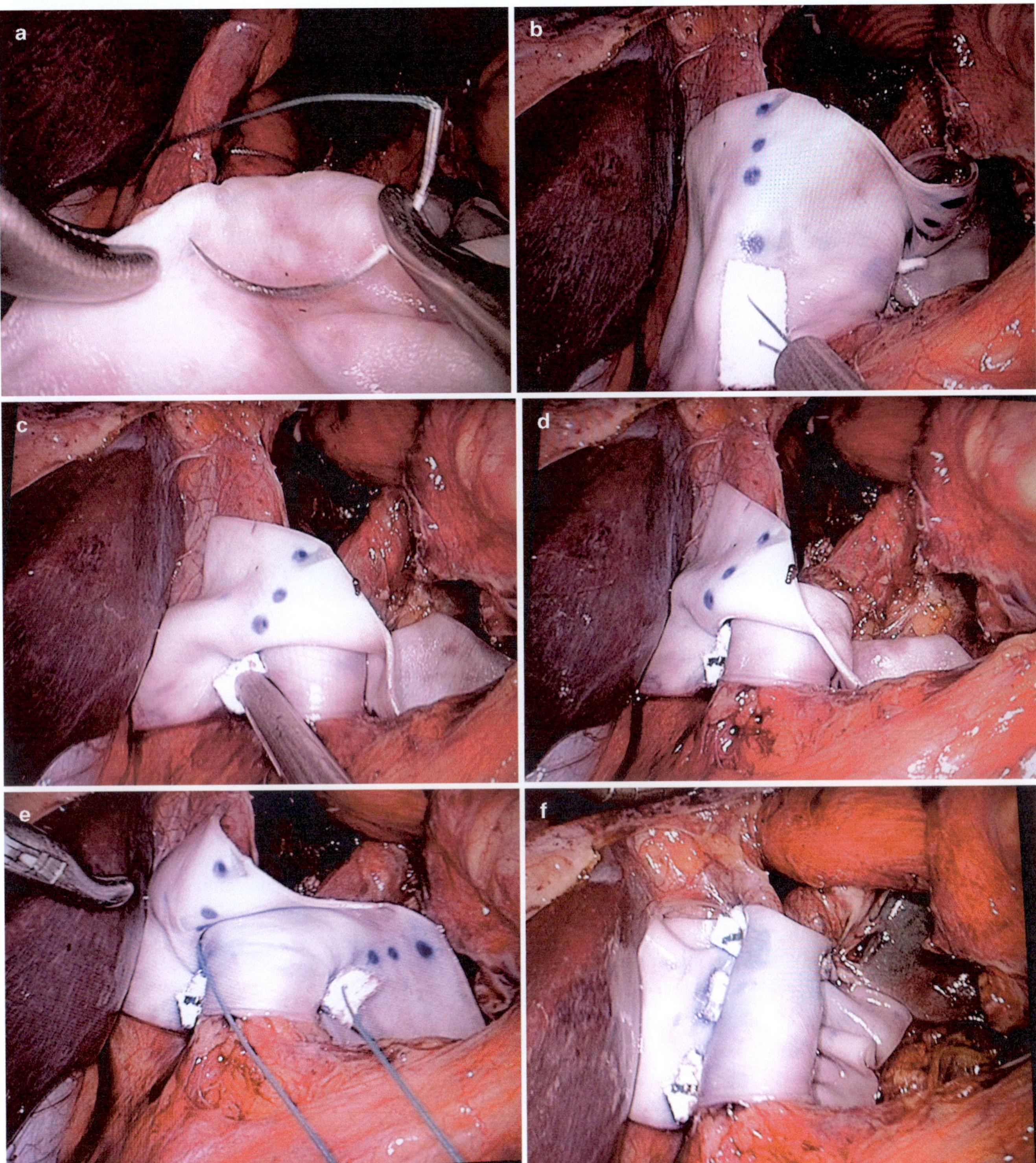

Fig. 18.8 Technique of incorporated mesh crural repair using 3 pledgeted horizontal mattress heavy braided polyester sutures. After passing through the left side of the mesh, the left crus, and the right crus, the needle is passed from back to front of the right side of the mesh (**a**). After loading second pledget, the suture is secured with a titanium crimp (Ti-knot, Redmond California) (**b**, **c**). Completed first pledgeted horizontal mattress suture (**d**). Second stitch in progress (**e**). Completed closure (**f**)

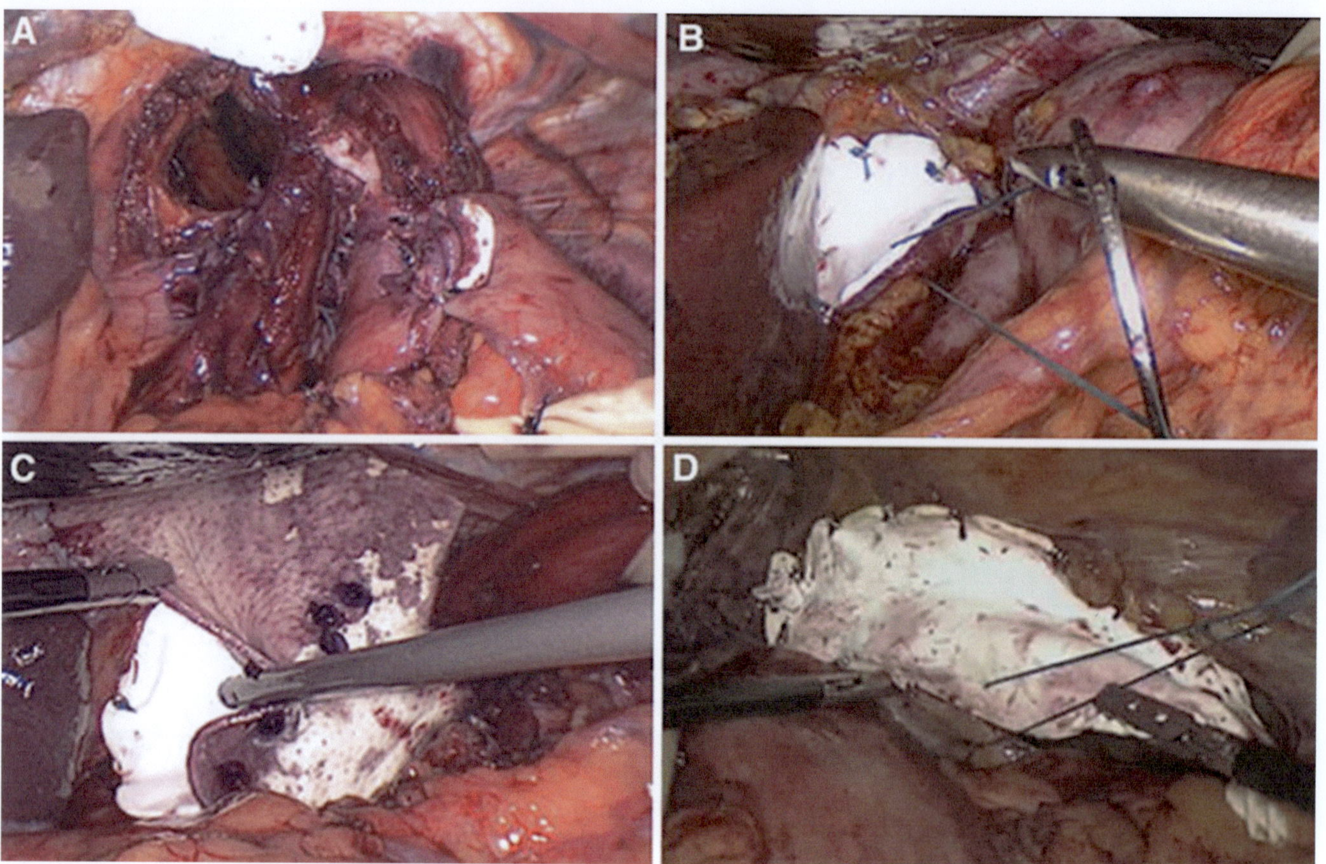

Fig. 18.9 Relaxing incisions for paraesophageal hiatal closure. (**A**) After a right relaxing incision, the hiatus is closed nicely with minimal tension. (**B**) The defect is closed with 1-mm polytetrafluoroethylene (PTFE) mesh. (**C**) The primary crural closure is reinforced with an absorbable (Allomax) mesh that also covers the PTFE patch. (**D**) A left relaxing incision is closed with 1-mm PTFE mesh (from Greene et al. 2013, published with permission from Surg Endosc)

a soft diet on postoperative day one. Median hospital stay is 1 day, and resumption of normal diet and activities occurs within 3–4 weeks. Considering the relatively high risk of recurrence and unknown natural history of even asymptomatic recurrences, objective follow-up by upper gastrointestinal series, and if needed, esophageal manometry and 24-h pH studies, can be considered mandatory.

Recommendations and Conclusion

Paraesophageal hernias are a complex surgical problem that can be plagued with high radiographic recurrence rates. In an effort to minimize recurrence, hiatal closure reinforcement has been advocated using synthetic, absorbable or biologic materials. Hiatal reinforcement using synthetic mesh has shown dramatically improved recurrence rates when compared to primary closure alone. However, devastating complications have been documented and for this reason many do not advocate its routine use. Biologic mesh reinforcement on the other hand seems to improve early rate of radiographic recurrence when compared to primary hiatal closure but is expensive. This improvement diminishes at long-term follow-up, which begs the question of whether it should be used routinely or at all?

Our current practice is to use biologic mesh reinforcement for large paraesophageal hernias (>5 cm) or in reoperative hernias in which the crura is thin or damaged. We believe that although the long-term recurrence with biologic mesh is similar to that of primary closure, it is possible that the biologic mesh helps minimize the size of recurrence and the reoperative rate, while minimizing the risk of complications seen with synthetic mesh. It may be that with newer biomesh materials and evolving techniques, the long-term recurrence rates may be improved. Nonetheless, it is our belief that if surgeons follow the tenets that have been described in the literature for repair of hiatal hernias including total hernia sac excision, achieving adequate intra-abdominal esophagus length, intra-abdominal anchoring with fundoplication, tension minimized reapproximation of hiatus with relaxing incisions when necessary, and selective use of biologic or absorbable mesh, recurrence rates will improve and postoperative complications remain rare.

References

1. Curci JA, Melman LM, Thompson RW, Soper NJ, Matthews BD. Elastic fiber depletion in the supporting ligaments of the gastro-esophageal junction: a structural basis for the development of hiatal hernia. J Am Coll Surg. 2008;207:191–6.

2. Asling B, Jirholt J, Hammond P, Knutsson M, Walentinsson A, Davidson G, Agreus L, Lehmann A, Lagerström-Fermer M. Collagen type III alpha I is a gastro-oesophageal reflux disease susceptibility gene and a male risk factor for hiatus hernia. Gut. 2009;58(8):1063–9.

3. Melman L, Chisholm PR, Curci JA, Arif B, Pierce R, Jenkins ED, Brunt LM, Eagon C, Frisella M, Miller K, Matthews BD. Differential regulation of MMP-2 in the gastrohepatic ligament of the gastro-esophageal junction. Surg Endosc. 2010;24(7):1562–5.

4. Fei L, del Genio G, Rossetti G, Sampaolo S, Moccia F, Trapani V, Cimmino M, del Genio A. Hiatal hernia recurrence: surgical complication or disease? Electron microscope findings of the diaphragmatic pillars. J Gastrointest Surg. 2009;13(3):459–64.

5. Colavita PD, Belyansky I, Walters AL, Tsirline VB, Zemlyak AY, Lincourt AE, Heniford BT. Nationwide inpatient sample: have anti-reflux procedures undergone regionalization? J Gastrointest Surg. 2013;17(1):6–13. discussion p. 13.

6. Congreve DP. Laparoscopic paraesophageal hernia repair. J Laparoendosc Surg. 1992;2:45–8.

7. Hashemi M, Peters JH, DeMeestr TR, et al. Laparoscopic repair of large type III hiatal hernia: objective followup reveals high recurrence rate. J Am Coll Surg. 2000;190:554–61.

8. Mattar SG, Bowers SP, Galloway KD, Hunter JG, Smith CD. Long-term outcome of laparoscopic repair of paraesophageal hernia. Surg Endosc. 2002;16(5):745–9.

9. Khaitan L, Houston H, Sharp K, Holzman M, Richards W. Laparoscopic paraesophageal hernia repair has an acceptable recurrence rate. Am Surg. 2002;68(6):546–51.

10. Pfluke JM, Parker M, Bowers SP, et al. Use of mesh for hiatal hernia repair: a survey of SAGES members. Surg Endosc. 2010;24(5):1017–24.

11. Cooley JC, Grindlay JH, Clagett OT. Esophageal hiatal hernia: anatomic and surgical concepts, with special reference to the experimental use of an ivalon prosthesis in the repair. Surgery. 1957;41(5):714–22.

12. Fusco EM. The repair of hiatus hernia with tantalum mesh. Mil Med. 1960;125:189–90.

13. Merendino KA, Dillar DH. Permanent fixation by teflosn mesh of the size of the esophageal diaphragmatic aperture in hiatus hernioplasty: a concept in a repair. Am J Surg. 1965;110:416–20.

14. Friedman MH, Mackenzie WC. The clinical use of polyvinyl sponge (ivalon) in the repair of oesophageal hiatus hernia. Can J Surg. 1961;4:176–82.

15. Frantzides CT, Madan AK, Carlson MA, Stavropoulos GP. A prospective, randomized trial of laparoscopic polytetrafluoroethylene (PTFE) patch repair vs simple cruroplasty for large hiatal hernia. Arch Surg. 2002;137(6):649–52.

16. Granderath FA, Schweiger UM, Kamolz T, Asche KU, Pointner R. Laparoscopic Nissen fundoplication with prosthetic hiatal closure reduces postoperative intrathoracic wrap herniation: preliminary results of a prospective randomized functional and clinical study. Arch Surg. 2005;140(1):40–8.

17. Trus TL, Bax T, Richardson WS, Branum GD, Mauren SJ, Swanstrom LL, Hunter JG. Complications of laparoscopic paraesophageal hernia repair. J Gastrointest Surg. 1997;1(3):221–7.

18. Tatum RP, Shalhub S, Oelschlager BK, Pellegrini CA. Complications of PTFE mesh at the diaphragmatic hiatus. J Gastrointest Surg. 2008;12(5):953–7. Epub 2007 Sep 18.

19. Coluccio G, Ponzio S, Ambu V, Tramontano R, Cuomo G. Dislocation into the cardial lumen of a PTFE prosthesis used in the treatment of voluminous hiatal sliding hernia, a case report. Minerva Chir. 2000;55(5):341–5.

20. Stadlhuber RJ, Sherif AE, Mittal SK, Fitzgibbons Jr RJ, Michael Brunt L, Hunter JG, Demeester TR, Swanstrom LL, Daniel Smith C, Filipi CJ. Mesh complications after prosthetic reinforcement of hiatal closure: a 28-case series. Surg Endosc. 2009;23(6):1219–26.

21. Gloeckner DC, Sacks MS, Billiar KL, Bachrach N. Mechanical evaluation and design of a multilayered collagenous repair biomaterial. J Biomed Mater Res. 2000;52(2):365–73.

22. Badylak S, Kokini K, Tullius B, Whitson B. Strength over time of a resorbable bioscaffold for body wall repair in a dog model. J Surg Res. 2001;99(2):282–7.

23. Lee YK, James E, Bochkarev V, Vitamvas M, Oleynikov D. Long-term outcome of cruroplasty reinforcement with human acellular dermal matrix in large paraesophageal hiatal hernia. J Gastrointest Surg. 2008;12(5):811–5.

24. Lee E, Frisella MM, Matthews BD, Brunt LM. Evaluation of acellular human dermis reinforcement of the crural closure in patients with difficult hiatal hernias. Surg Endosc. 2007;21(4):641–5.

25. Ringley CD, Bochkarev V, Ahmed SI, Vitamvas ML, Oleynikov D. Laparoscopic hiatal hernia repair with human acellular dermal matrix patch: our initial experience. Am J Surg. 2006;192(6):767–72.

26. Diaz DF, Roth JS. Laparoscopic paraesophageal hernia repair with acellular dermal matrix cruroplasty. JSLS. 2011;15(3):355–60.

27. Oelschlager BK, Barreca M, Chang L, Pellegrini CA. The use of small intestine submucosa in the repair of paraesophageal hernias: initial observations of a new technique. Am J Surg. 2003;186(1):4–8.

28. Oelschlager BK, Pellegrini CA, Hunter J, Soper N, Brunt M, Sheppard B, Jobe B, Polissar N, Mitsumori L, Nelson J, Swanstrom L. Biologic prosthesis reduces recurrence after laparoscopic paraesophageal hernia repair: a multicenter, prospective, randomized trial. Ann Surg. 2006;244(4):481–90.

29. Oelschlager BK, Pellegrini CA, Hunter JG, Brunt ML, Soper NJ, Sheppard BC, Polissar NL, Neradilek MB, Mitsumori LM, Rohrmann CA, Swanstrom LL. Biologic prosthesis to prevent recurrence after laparoscopic paraesophageal hernia repair: long-term follow-up from a multicenter, prospective, randomized trial. J Am Coll Surg. 2011;213(6):461–8. Epub 2011 Jun 29. Erratum in: J Am Coll Surg. 2011 Dec;213(6):815.

30. Parsak CK, Erel S, Seydaoglu G, Akcam T, Sakman G. Laparoscopic antireflux surgery with polyglactin (vicryl) mesh. Surg Laparosc Endosc Percutan Tech. 2011;21(6):443–9.

31. Diwan TS, Ujiki MB, Dunst CM, Swanström LL. Biomesh placement in laparoscopic repair of paraesophageal hernias. Surg Innov. 2008;15(3):184–7.

32. Huntington TR. Laparoscopic mesh repair of the esophageal hiatus. J Am Coll Surg. 1997;184(4):399–400.

33. Greene CL1, DeMeester SR, Zehetner J, Worrell SG, Oh DS, Hagen JA. Diaphragmatic relaxing incisions during laparoscopic paraesophageal hernia repair. Surg Endosc. 2013;27(12):4532–8.

34. Quilici PJ, McVay C, Tovar A. Laparoscopic antireflux procedures with hepatic shoulder technique for the surgical management of large paraesophageal hernias and gastroesophageal reflux disease. Surg Endosc. 2009;23(11):2620–3.

The Short Esophagus

Ezra N. Teitelbaum and Nathaniel J. Soper

Abbreviations

GEJ	Gastroesophageal junction
GER	Gastroesophageal reflux
GERD	Gastroesophageal reflux disease
SE	Short esophagus
LARS	Laparoscopic antireflux surgery
PPI	Proton-pump inhibitor
PEH	Paraesophageal hernia
ELI	Esophageal length index
LES	Lower esophageal sphincter
HRM	High-resolution manometry

Introduction

The goal of any antireflux surgery is to create a fundoplication that provides a permanent functional and non-obstructive barrier to gastric contents moving cephalad past the gastroesophageal junction (GEJ) and into the intrathoracic esophagus. No matter what fundoplication technique or surgical approach is employed, all operations must adhere to the sample basic principles:

(1) *The fundus must be used for the wrap, rather than the body of the stomach.* Only the fundus exhibits vagally mediated receptive relaxation and will relax during a swallowing episode.

(2) *The fundoplication must be formed around esophagus, rather than stomach.* A "low fundoplication" placed incorrectly around gastric body or a "slipped fundoplication" that migrates caudally postoperatively will both result in dysphagia and over time, dilation of the segment of stomach proximal to the wrap. This will subsequently cause pooling of gastric contents in this proximal portion and their reflux back into the esophagus, worsening the problem that the operation was intended to fix.

(3) *The fundoplication should be situated below the diaphragmatic hiatus.* An intraabdominal fundoplication works physiologically to increase GEJ pressure when intraabdominal pressure is elevated, the condition under which pathologic gastroesophageal reflux (GER) occurs. If the wrap migrates into the thoracic cavity, not only is this physiologic mechanism lost, but a hiatal hernia has been created that puts the patient at higher risk for obstructive symptoms or recurrent GER and even possible incarceration and strangulation.

(4) *The portion of intraabdominal esophagus around which the fundoplication is formed cannot be under axial tension.* As with any hernia repair or fascial closure, tension is the enemy. If there is axial tension from a short esophagus, it will predispose a newly formed fundoplication to migration of the wrap into the chest, thus violating the previously mentioned tenant and again creating a hiatal hernia, or cause wrap disruption.

In order to comply with these key principles, the initial steps of any antireflux operation must involve creation of an intraabdominal length of esophagus that is long enough for a tension-free fundoplication to be formed around it. If one is not able to mobilize this length by various maneuvers, the result is by definition a "short esophagus" which must be addressed before the operation can progress to the creation of an antireflux barrier. Keep in mind, the distance used to define what constitutes a short esophagus (SE) is not a measure of the entire length of the esophagus, but only its intraabdominal component. Additionally, this "diagnosis" by definition cannot be made preoperatively, but only after a mediastinal dissection has been performed in an attempt to mobilize an adequate intraabdominal esophageal segment. Although authors have used various cutoffs for this length, the most accepted value is 2.5–3 cm. This is a utilitarian number, derived from the fact that a standard fundoplication is approximately 2 cm long, and therefore a slightly longer

---

E.N. Teitelbaum, MD (✉) • N.J. Soper, MD
Department of Surgery, Northwestern University,
251 E. Huron St., Galter 3-150, Chicago, IL 60611, USA
e-mail: e-teitelbaum@northwestern.edu; nsoper@nmh.org

L.L. Swanstrom and C.M. Dunst (eds.), *Antireflux Surgery*,
DOI 10.1007/978-1-4939-1749-5_19, © Springer New York 2015

Table 19.1 Minimally invasive SE series

Authors	Indication	Total number	Requiring a lengthening procedure (%)	Type of lengthening procedure
Madan et. al [3]	GERD	628	0	None
Bochkarev et al. [2]	GERD	106	0	None
Swanstrom et al. [24]	GERD+PEH	238	3	Laparoscopic-thoracoscopic gastroplasty
Oelschlager et al. [27]	Redo LARS+PEH	166	7	Vagotomy
Terry et al. [26]	GERD+PEH	143	10	Laparoscopic wedge-gastroplasty
Mattioli et al. [4]	GERD	180	14	Laparoscopic or laparoscopic-thoracoscopic gastroplasty

intraabdominal esophageal length allows the wrap to be comfortably formed around it.

While most surgeons are in agreement regarding the previously outlined principles that guide antireflux operations, when it comes to the prevalence of SE there exists considerable debate. In historic open series, use of an esophageal lengthening procedure for SE was reported in some centers in up to 60 % [1] of cases. Other authors have claimed that SE does not even exist, that is to say, that with adequate esophageal mobilization, an intraabdominal length of >2.5 cm can be obtained in all cases [2, 3]. Most contemporary authors describe rates of SE during laparoscopic antireflux surgery (LARS) occurring between 3 and 15 % [4] (Table 19.1) with some outliers reporting higher or lower rates. These differences are likely due in part to disparities in patient populations, disease severity, operative technique, and the comfort level of the surgeons with complex laparoscopic surgery of the mediastinum.

Additionally, there remains considerable debate over the optimal surgical method to deal with SE after esophageal mobilization has been exhausted, as several approaches have been described. Regardless of these unanswered questions, it is essential for any surgeon who is currently performing LARS to have a firm grasp of the preoperative predictors of SE and have a technical plan in place in the event that one is encountered intraoperatively.

Pathophysiology

Early in the twentieth century, it was believed that SE was a congenital, rather than acquired, disease entity [5]. Moersch first postulated that SE developed as a result of chronic scarring of the esophagus [6]. However, at that time GERD was believed to be a consequence, rather than the cause, of SE [7]. Subsequent laboratory work was able to demonstrate that long-standing GERD is primarily responsible for the inflammatory pathway that ultimately leads to SE.

Uncontrolled gastric acid, as well as biliary and pancreatic secretions, refluxing from the stomach into the distal esophagus causes a burn injury that can penetrate the full thickness of the esophageal wall [8–11]. This injury initiates an acute inflammatory response with release of cytokines and recruitment of neutrophils. As with any burn injury, this inflammatory cascade leads to healing by way of fibroblast infiltration, collagen production, and ultimately fibrosis. When this fibrotic scar is formed in the inner circular muscle layer of the esophagus, it causes a radial contraction. The result is a peptic stricture that narrows the esophageal lumen and is identifiable on endoscopic examination. When the fibrosis occurs in the outer longitudinal muscle layer, the contracture occurs in a cephalad–caudad orientation, producing a shortening of overall esophageal length and predisposing to SE. While peptic stricture and SE often appear in concert, each can be present independent of one another. The pathophysiologic mechanism by which some patients suffering from long-standing GERD go on to develop one but not the other has yet to be elucidated.

With the widespread introduction of proton-pump inhibitors (PPIs), complications of long-standing and severe GERD have dramatically decreased in frequency. These include both peptic stricture and SE. This change accounts in a large part for the decreased prevalence of SE in the LARS literature of the past 20 years, as compared with descriptions of open, and largely transthoracic, earlier series. While a significant percentage of patients with GERD may eventually fail medical therapy and go on to require surgery, the pathologic effect of their reflux on the distal esophagus will have likely been partially attenuated by PPIs, making SE less likely.

SE can also be associated with a paraesophageal hernia (PEH) by way of a different mechanism. Rather than repeated acute inflammatory insults leading to longitudinal fibrosis, a PEH results in an anatomic distortion of the normal anatomic relationships of the distal esophagus, GEJ, and stomach. In a type III hiatal hernia, the GEJ and stomach body both migrate through the diaphragmatic hiatus and into the chest. This leads to a kinking, or so-called "accordioning," of the distal esophagus (Fig. 19.1). Over time, dense adhesions can form within the hernia sac, tethering the bent esophagus to itself and the surrounding structures. This may lead to an irreversible compression and shortening of esophageal length, although some authors argue that these adhesions can always be lysed and the esophagus can be uniformly unfolded and restored to its original length in almost all cases [2, 3].

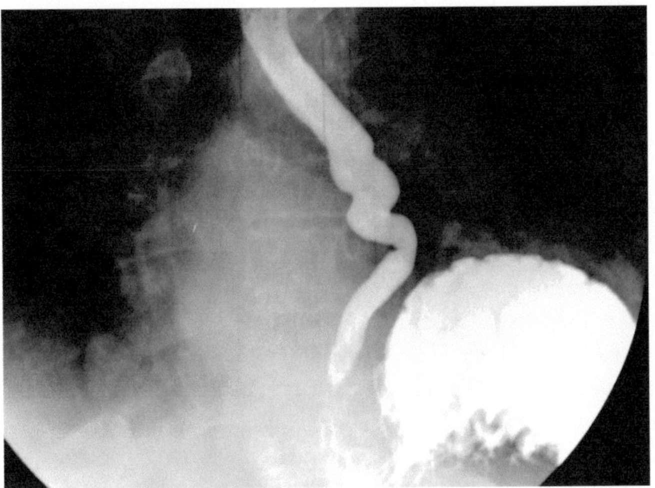

Fig. 19.1 Radiograph of paraesophageal hernia with "accordion" esophagus

Table 19.2 Preoperative predictors of SE

History
– Long-standing GERD
– Prior esophageal or antireflux surgery
Contrast radiograph
– Hiatal hernia >5 cm
– Non-reducing hiatal hernia
– Type III PEH
Endoscopy
– Peptic stricture
– Barrett's esophagus
– ELI < 19.5
Manometry
– Aperistalsis
– GEJ to crura distance >5 cm

Historical Treatment

Surgeons in the early to mid twentieth century dealt with the problem of SE using a variety of methods, almost entirely through an open transthoracic approach. Harrington divided the phrenic nerve and pexied the diaphragm in order to reduce the GEJ into the abdomen—essentially moving the hiatus to fit the esophagus [12]. Other surgeons performed a partial gastrectomy as a primary acid-reducing operation in order to eliminate the need for an effective antireflux barrier [13]. After use of a fundoplication to stop reflux became popular in the mid-twentieth century, Krupp and Rossetti simply performed an intrathoracic fundoplication in cases where the GEJ could not be mobilized due to SE, and this technique is still used in some centers [14, 15]. These solutions, however, were associated with significant morbidity, as well as suboptimal postoperative physiology.

Collis was an english thoracic surgeon who in 1957 described the first operation to "lengthen" the esophagus by performing a vertical gastroplasty to create a tubular length of neo-esophagus from gastric fundus [16]. After fully mobilizing the esophagus via a left thoracoabdominal incision, a bougie-type tube was passed into the stomach. The proximal fundus was then divided between two clamps placed in parallel to the bougie and the divided fundal edges were sutured closed. Collis did not perform a fundoplication or any other antireflux operation, believing that a hiatal repair and reduction of the newly created GEJ below the diaphragm would be sufficient to protect against GER.

Modifications of the Collis operation remain the primary means to lengthen the esophagus and the preferred method for treating SE. Since its original description, the Collis gastroplasty has been modified by using a linear cutting stapler to divide the stomach and almost always includes the addition of an antireflux fundoplication, typically a 360-degree Nissen (the Collis–Nissen). The operation has also been adapted so that it can be performed via a minimally invasive laparoscopic approach.

Preoperative Evaluation

Although one is less likely to encounter a SE in the current era of LARS and PPIs, it is still extremely important to risk-stratify patients preoperatively so that adequate preparations can be made if SE is suspected. Although no single preoperative finding is pathognomonic for SE, patients at higher risk can be identified by way of careful history taking and via suggestive findings on upper endoscopy, contrast radiograph, and manometry (Table 19.2). Patients with a long-standing history of heartburn are at greater risk, especially if they have not been treated with PPIs. Patients who additionally complain of dysphagia, nausea, chest pain, or regurgitation are more likely to have complicated GERD caused by a PEH, peptic stricture, or Barrett's esophagus, all of which are associated with an increased incidence of SE. Patients with a history of prior esophageal surgery, especially a failed antireflux operation, are at a significantly increased risk of SE due to adhesions and scaring. In evaluating such patients, it should be kept in mind that an inadequately addressed SE may have been the cause of their operative failure in the first place.

Endoscopy

An upper endoscopy should be performed on all patients prior to antireflux surgery. The primary goal is to evaluate for malignancy, Barrett esophagus, peptic stricture, ulcers, esophagitis, and/or gastritis, but the findings of this study can also be used to help determine the risk for SE. While contrast radiographs can evaluate the distance between the GEJ and diaphragmatic crura, this measure is much less clear during endoscopy. For this reason, the presence of a hiatal hernia observed endoscopically should not be given as much weight as the findings on fluoroscopic evaluation. It should be kept in mind that radiographs provide the best anatomic description, whereas endoscopy should be used primarily as an examination of intraluminal pathology.

Yano and colleagues conducted an analysis of preoperative endoscopic findings in patients who went on to require an esophageal lengthening procedure for SE and compared these with patients who underwent antireflux surgery without SE [17]. They found that the presence of a peptic stricture on endoscopy was a significant risk factor for SE, with an odds ratio of 7.5 compared with non-SE patients. Interestingly, there was no difference in the rates of esophagitis on endoscopy between the two groups, a result corroborated by a second study [18]. These findings support the concept that SE is not caused by acute mucosal injury to the esophagus, but rather results from the chronic healing and stricture process that comes with repeated insults over a sustained period of time.

Esophageal length was measured endoscopically by Yano et al. and was defined as the scope distance from the incisors to the GEJ [17]. There was an association of increased length with increased patient height, so in order to account for this baseline anatomic variation, esophageal length (in cm) was divided by height (in meters) to produce an "esophageal length index" (ELI). Based on these values, a cutoff of ELI < 19.5 was determined to produce a specificity of 95 % in predicting SE preoperatively. This resulted in a positive predictive value of 81 % and a negative predictive value of 83 %, although a sensitivity of only 56 %.

Contrast Radiograph

A contrast radiograph (i.e., barium esophagram or "upper GI series") should also be included in the routine evaluation of any patient with a sizable hiatal hernia prior to LARS. This study provides the best anatomic evaluation of the esophagus, GEJ, diaphragmatic hiatus, stomach, and their relationships to one another. The first thing that should be noted is the presence of a hiatal hernia, demonstrated by a GEJ that is situated superior to the diaphragmatic hiatus. The precise distance between these two points should be measured. This requires the X-ray images to be calibrated to a ruler, which although intuitive, is not the case in all fluoroscopy protocols and systems. The width of the hiatal defect should also be measured, and the presence of the stomach and/or other abdominal viscera above the hiatus noted, defining the presence of a PEH. If a hiatal hernia or PEH is present, it is important to obtain a series of x-ray images over time and throughout the course of several swallows, in order to elucidate whether the GEJ is mobile in relationship to the hiatus

(i.e., "sliding") or fixed in a supradiaphragmatic position. A type III PEH (where both the GEJ and stomach body protrude through the hiatus) increases the risk for SE. Additionally, patients with a fixed GEJ are more likely to have a chronically incarcerated hiatal hernia, which will be less amenable to operative mobilization, and may further increase the likelihood of encountering a SE.

Gastal and colleagues retrospectively analyzed preoperative studies performed on patients prior to antireflux surgery, of whom 16 % required an esophageal lengthening procedure for SE [19]. They found that the presence of a hiatal hernia >5 cm (defined as the vertical distance between the GEJ and the diaphragmatic hiatus) was predictive of intraoperative SE, although with a positive predictive value of only 58 %. It should also be noted that patients in this series suspected of having SE preoperatively were approached via thoracotomy, whereas all other operations were performed laparoscopically, which introduces a potentially confounding variable into these data. In another study of patients who were all operated on laparoscopically, the same cutoff of a hiatal hernia >5 cm had a sensitivity of 66 % and a positive predictive value of 37 % for predicting SE [20].

Manometry

Manometry provides the best functional examination of the esophagus and lower esophageal sphincter (LES), allowing for both qualitative and quantitative evaluation of esophageal peristalsis and LES basal and relaxation pressures. Some authors argue that manometry need not be included in the routine evaluation of patients prior to antireflux surgery. However, we prefer to obtain one if possible on all patients for several reasons. Although rare, patients presenting with what symptomatically appears to be GERD can have an underlying motility disorder such as achalasia, which will become apparent only on manometry. Additionally, many GERD patients will have subtle changes in both esophageal body and LES function. Non-specific spastic contractions can lead to postoperative symptoms that may cause dissatisfaction. A motility study allows preoperative counseling regarding this possibility [21]. As many patients will have some degree of dysphagia after their operation, it is also important to have a preoperative manometry to serve as a functional baseline, allowing the surgeon to more accurately evaluate the cause of any postoperative complaints.

In addition to these important functional descriptions, manometry provides anatomic delineations that can add to an analysis of the potential for SE. The most basic manometric determination is that of esophageal length, measured from upper to lower esophageal sphincter. Mittal and colleagues performed manometry on 32 patients with suspected SE preoperatively, based on the criteria of an irreducible hiatal hernia or peptic stricture. In this patient subgroup, a higher percentage of patients who required an esophageal lengthening procedure had a short esophageal length on preoperative manometry (defined as two standard deviations below the mean of healthy subjects), but this criterion had both a low sensitivity (43 %) and positive predictive value (25 %).

It should be noted that in this study, the manometric measurements were performed using the then-standard pull-through method. The recent technological advance of high-resolution manometry (HRM) has allowed these studies to provide a more detailed picture of both esophageal and LES function, as well as anatomic delineations. The HRM catheter has pressures sensors spaced at 1 cm intervals along its entire length, allowing for simultaneous measurements to be performed from UES to LES without need for catheter repositioning. This provides a more accurate anatomic picture, as length can be measured at a single point in time, as opposed to the pull-through technique of standard manometry which introduces the variables of both time and probe movement.

These differences become even more crucial in the setting of a hiatal hernia. HRM is able to detect fluctuations in esophageal length as the GEJ moves vertically in the case of a mobile hernia, in addition to measuring the distance between LES and the diaphragmatic crural contraction point [22]. The end result is a more complex anatomic picture that can help to corroborate radiographic and endoscopic findings to quantitatively assess the size and reducibility of a hiatal hernia, giving yet another indicator of the probability of encountering a SE intraoperatively. Other authors have suggested that decreased GEJ pressures and hypo or aperistalsis are also predictive of SE, and certainly the functional component of the esophagus as measured by HRM must be taken into account prior to any LARS [4, 23].

Operative Technique

Preoperative Planning and Operative Setup

If a SE is suspected based on preoperative studies, it is important to make adequate preparations in order to be prepared to address it. Although we inform all patients undergoing LARS and PEH repair that an esophageal lengthening procedure may be necessary, this point is emphasized in patients with a higher suspicion for SE. The added perioperative risk of staple-line leak should be discussed, as well as the long-term outcomes of this modification to the procedure. It is equally important to inform the anesthesia and nursing teams so that all necessary equipment, such as endoscopic staplers and bariatric length laparoscopic instruments, is available and everyone is prepared for a potentially longer operation.

Although some authors argue that patients undergoing antireflux surgery who have a high likelihood of SE should be approached transthoracically [19], most surgeons today proceed laparoscopically in almost all cases. Some alterations are made to our routine LARS protocol, including the placement of a Foley catheter and administration of preoperative antibiotic prophylaxis, due to the increased potential for a longer operative time and inadvertent esophageal or gastric perforation. Operating room setup, patient positioning, and port placement in any LARS should be designed to facilitate easy access to, and visualization of, the esophageal hiatus and mediastinum. This is especially true when undertaking an operation that may include an esophageal lengthening procedure. Patients are positioned supine on a vacuum bean-bag in order to provide evenly distributed support and facilitate a steep reverse Trendelenburg tilt. The patient's legs are abducted on padded straight leg boards and the surgeon stands between the patient's legs, with the assistant to the patient's right and the camera operator seated on a stool on the patient's left side. An orogastric tube is placed to decompress the stomach.

Laparoscopic ports should be positioned to create a "triangulation" or "diamond" orientation with the camera viewing the operative field straight on and the surgeon's two operating instruments coming in from either side at 30–60° angles. To achieve this configuration, we first place the camera port approximately 12 cm caudad to the xiphoid process and just to the left of midline using a Veress needle technique. The surgeon's right-hand port is placed 10 cm from the xiphoid and a few centimeters below the left costal margin, and the left-hand port is placed just below and to the right of the xiphoid. A self-retaining liver retractor is used to elevate the left lateral segment to fully expose the hiatus, and it is placed through a port 15 cm from the xiphoid and just below the right costal margin. We typically have the assistant stand to the patient's right and place their operating port in the right mid-rectus region, between the liver retractor and camera ports. A 30° or 45° angled laparoscope should be used in order to provide a dynamic view of the mediastinum. Bariatric length laparoscopic instruments may be needed for higher mediastinal dissection, especially in larger patients.

Mediastinal Dissection and Esophageal Mobilization

The importance of a circumferential hiatal dissection and esophageal mobilization during LARS cannot be overemphasized, especially in the context of SE. With extensive mobilization, an adequate intraabdominal esophageal length can be obtained in the vast majority of cases, obviating the need for a lengthening procedure. The most accurate measurement of esophageal length during LARS was performed by Mattioli and colleagues using intraoperative endoscopy during a series of 180 operations [4]. They found that only 17 % of patients had an intraabdominal length of esophagus >2.5 cm prior to mediastinal dissection, but that this proportion was increased to 68 % after full esophageal mobilization. This should be considered the goal in this initial phase of the operation.

After port placement and liver retraction, the patient is placed in steep reverse Trendenelburg position to facilitate exposure of the hiatus. The pars flaccida of the hepatogastric ligament is opened using an ultrasonic energy device and the base of the right crus is approached. After the thin peritoneal layer overlying the crus is opened, blunt dissection is used to develop a mediastinal plane between the right crus (lateral) and esophageal wall (medial). If a type III PEH is present, this dissection is modified slightly, as the GEJ and stomach will be situated in the chest and surrounded by hernia sac. In these cases, the correct initial plane is created between the right crus and the right-lateral border of the hernia sac, so that mediastinal dissection proceeds outside of the sac. This allows for reduction of the sac, and the stomach will thus be reduced simultaneously.

Once entered on the right side, the mediastinum is opened anteriorly by dividing the phrenoesophageal membrane completely, across to the left crus. Dissection then proceeds cephalad to open the hiatus and develop the space between the esophagus and the surrounding structures. We use a blunt two-handed technique, employing a "breast-stroke" motion to separate the esophagus from the bilateral parietal pleura, the pericardium, and aorta. The ultrasonic dissector (or other energy device or electrocautery) is used sparingly to divide small mediastinal blood vessels, and only after the vagus nerves have been identified and protected. It is important to keep the active blade away from the esophageal body, and to be aware that it will remain hot for a period of time after inactivation. During this dissection, the assistant places caudad traction on the esophagus by grasping the anterior gastric fat pad or gastric fundus. It is extremely important that neither the assistant nor surgeon directly grasp the esophageal body at any point during the operation to avoid traction injury and perforation.

After initial anterior mediastinal dissection, we shift our attention away from the hiatus to divide the short gastric vessels. We prefer to completely divide the short gastric arteries at this point in the operation, as it allows for creation of a tension-free fundoplication later on and increases fundal mobility, which facilitates both further anterior and posterior esophageal mobilization. With the short gastrics divided, the assistant then rolls the fundus anteriorly to the patient's right. This allows the surgeon access to the base of the left crus in order to create a posterior "window" behind the esophagus, essentially connecting with the area at the base of the right crus where the hiatal dissection was initiated. At this point, a

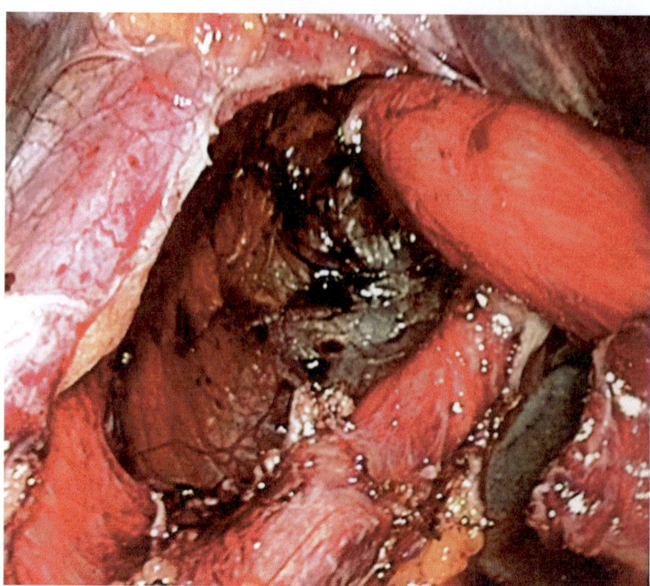

Fig. 19.2 Intraoperative photo of intraabdominal esophageal length after hiatal hernia reduction

Penrose drain can be placed around the GEJ in order to facilitate caudad retraction, but generally we find that this is not required and that grasping the gastric fat pad or fundus is both sufficient and safe.

After access is obtained to the posterior mediastinum, a similar blunt dissection technique is used to elevate the esophagus off of the posterior structures. Once a circumferential esophageal mobilization has been performed, intraabdominal esophageal length should be assessed. During this measurement, it is important that any caudad retraction be completely released so that the intraabdominal distance is not falsely elongated. If the GEJ cannot be accurately identified, the anterior gastric fat pad can be excised in order to more clearly visualize this anatomy or an intraoperative endoscopy can be performed and the GEJ transilluminated. If a large PEH was present, as much of the hernia sac should be resected as possible, as this will help to more accurately identify the true location of the GEJ, as well as make the later fundoplication easier. We use the gap between the open jaws of a Hunter grasper, which is 2.5 cm, as a ruler to measure the intraabdominal esophageal length (Fig. 19.2). However, it is important to note that this distance will be shortened if the instrument shaft and longitudinal esophageal axis are not at a right angle with one another. If any question exists, a sterile tape-measure should be used to precisely measure this distance, especially if the surgeon is in the beginning of his or her learning curve and is not experienced with visualizing the hiatus laparoscopically.

If at this point, if the length is less than 2.5 cm, additional mediastinal dissection should be performed. Starting anteriorly, the esophagus is mobilized circumferentially further cephalad again using a primarily blunt spreading technique.

As this dissection proceeds further superiorly, the laparoscope can be passed through the hiatus to provide an adequate working view. It may be necessary to switch to instruments with extended bariatric-length shafts to avoid creating excessive torque at the level of the abdominal wall. This dissection should proceed to the level of the pulmonary veins, or even the carina, as needed.

Swanstrom and colleagues have described a system for classifying the extent of dissection needed for this mobilization [24, 25]: a type I dissection extends less than 5 cm past the level of the hiatus, whereas a type II progresses beyond 5 cm cephalad. A type III dissection is defined as a case in which the GEJ cannot be mobilized to >2 cm below the hiatus despite complete esophageal mobilization laparoscopically. While this classification system is useful for research purposes and should be recorded in any prospective esophageal surgery database, we do not uniformly dissect to a predetermined level during either uncomplicated LARS cases or in the instance of SE. Even in straightforward LARS operations we routinely perform a type II dissection. In cases of SE, we employ a tailored approach in which mediastinal dissection is incrementally extended and the intraabdominal esophageal length re-measured periodically, so that an overly aggressive mobilization is not performed unnecessarily. If after complete, maximal type II mobilization, the intraabdominal length of esophagus is still less than 2.5 cm, an esophageal lengthening procedure should be performed.

Stapled-Wedge Gastroplasty

We prefer a modified stapled-wedge gastroplasty (or "wedge fundectomy") as originally described by Terry et al. [26]. This technique allows for the procedure to be performed entirely through transabdominal trocars, which eliminates the need for a chest port, single-lung ventilation, and postoperative tube thoracostomy. Additionally, surgeons already experienced with laparoscopic bariatric procedures and the use of endoscopic articulating staplers should have little difficulty translating those skills towards this usage.

The epiphrenic fat pad and any residual hernia sac are first removed from the GEJ. After removal of the orogastric tube, a bougie is placed under laparoscopic visualization and passed into the distal stomach. We prefer a size 50 French, but other authors have described the use of other size tubes, from 48 to 58 French. With the bougie snug against the lesser curvature of the stomach, a point on the fundus is marked with a suture placed at the left edge of the bougie, usually ~3 cm distal to the GEJ. This point will serve as a guide, marking the distal extent of the eventual neo-esophagus. Its distance from the GEJ should be determined to ensure that at least 3 cm of esophagus and/or neo-esophagus lies comfortably below the hiatus.

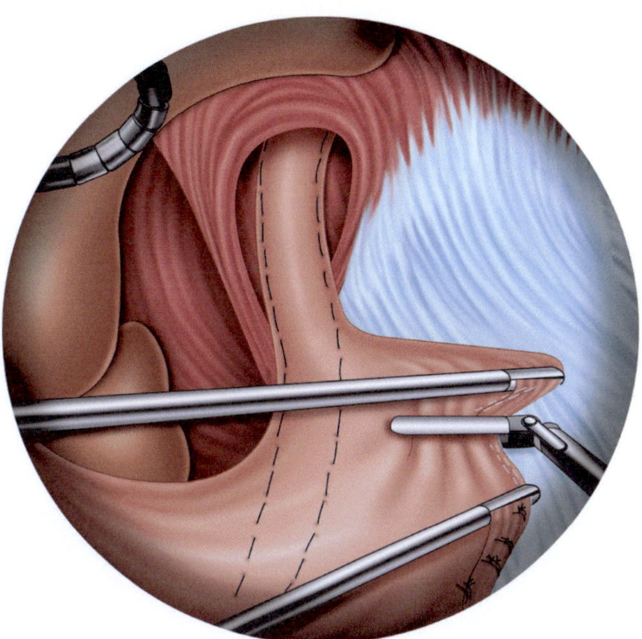

Fig. 19.3 Laparoscopic stapled-wedge gastroplasty: initial staple-line aimed towards the "guide" suture

The surgeon's right-hand port is then upsized to a 12 mm trocar in order to accommodate an endoscopic stapler. The surgeon's left-hand grasper retracts the proximal fundus and the assistant grasps lower on the greater curvature, which should have already been completed mobilized. These points of retraction are used in concert to stretch the fundus laterally to the patient's left, in effect fanning the stomach out in a flat, horizontal plane. An endoscopic articulating stapler is then introduced through the surgeon's right-hand port and articulated completely to the left (counterclockwise). A 45 mm length stapler with 2.5 mm height staples is passed across the fundus between the two grasping instruments at approximately 90° to the greater curvature. If this orientation cannot be achieved through the surgeon's right-hand port, an additional trocar can be placed more laterally below the left costal margin in order to create a less severe angle of stapler introduction.

The stapler is aimed towards the previously marked point and several fires are typically required to reach the bougie (Fig. 19.3). The last application of the stapler should directly abut the bougie and adequate left-lateral retraction on the stomach is required to ensure that excess tissue is not left undivided close to the lesser curvature. Before firing this stapler load, the anesthesiologist should gently slide the bougie in and out to ensure that the tube has not been caught in the stapler jaws.

Once the last lateral-to-medial stapler load is fired, the stapler is dearticulated in a clockwise direction and a second staple line is begun, following the left edge of the bougie proximally to the angle of His (Fig. 19.4). Again, lateral retraction is important to ensure that the neo-esophagus tube

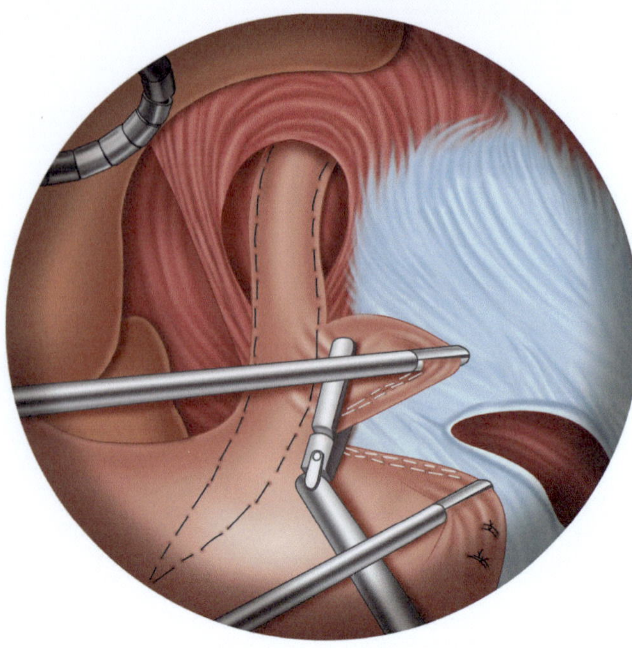

Fig. 19.4 Laparoscopic stapled-wedge gastroplasty: second staple-line formed parallel to the bougie

is created flush against the exterior of the bougie. After locking the stapler in position, but before firing, the posterior aspect of the stomach should be examined for redundant tissue. The fat of the hepatogastric ligament overlaps with the lesser curve at this point, potentially creating the illusion that little stomach is left to the anatomic right of the stapler. However, as long as the bougie is in position and the stapler is tight against it, the neo-esophagus will be of adequate diameter. The goal should be to make the neo-esophagus as narrow as the native esophagus to prevent increased intraluminal pressure that can lead to eventual dilatation of this segment. Once this staple line has reached the angle of His, the small, resected portion of the proximal fundus is removed through the 12 mm trocar.

Combined Laparoscopic–Thoracoscopic Collis Gastroplasty

Another technique for creating a Collis gastroplasty was developed by Swanstrom and subsequently modified by Filipi and involves a combined laparoscopic and thoracoscopic approach [24, 25]. This operation best approximates the original Collis technique through minimally invasive access, as it does not involve resection of a wedge of fundus, and thus creates a potentially shorter stapler line that may be less prone to leak. However, this procedure has gained less widespread acceptance than the one previously described because it requires thoracic surgery privileges and familiarity with thoracoscopic techniques, as well as potentially

resulting in increased pain from a chest incision and a higher risk of postoperative pneumothorax.

The diaphragmatic hiatus is opened and the mediastinum dissected in an identical fashion to that which has been previously described. Once the esophagus has been fully mobilized and it is determined that there is less than 2.5 cm of intraabdominal esophagus, a roll is placed under the patient's left shoulder and the left chest is prepped and redraped. If there was a high preoperative suspicion of a SE, the prep can be done at the beginning of the case. An incision is made at the third or fourth intercostal space at the lateral edge of the pectoralis major and a 12 mm trocar is introduced into the chest. This is done under dual-lung ventilation and the lung is collapsed by initiating low pressure CO_2 insufflation (10 mm/Hg). A laparoscope is then introduced into the chest to evaluate for adhesions and judge the path towards the mediastinal parietal pleura just above the hiatus. The laparoscope is withdrawn and an endoscopic stapler with a 3 cm load is introduced through the thoracic port. The authors pass this stapler blindly along the anterior thoracic wall, identifying the location of its tip laparoscopically when it causes an indentation in the mediastinal pleura. This is an advanced technique, requiring substantial experience with video assisted thoracic surgery (VATS), and during any surgeon's initial experience with this procedure, a second trocar and laparoscope should be introduced into the left chest to allow for passage of the stapler to be visualized directly.

Once the stapler is in place, the overlying pleura is incised laparoscopically and the stapler is advanced into the abdomen anterior to the esophagus. A 48 French bougie is placed into the stomach and the fundus is then grasped and rotated anteriorly to allow for the stapler to slide adjacent to the bougie (Fig. 19.5). Following identical principles to the previously described wedge-gastroplasty, having adequate fundal retraction is essential prior to locking the stapler to avoid being left with a dilated neo-esophagus. Using this technique, a single stapler fire creates a 3 cm segment of neo-esophagus. The pleural defect is left open and the thoracic trocar left in place to prevent deinsufflation of pneumoperitoneum. Generally a chest tube is not required.

Vagotomy

Typically during LARS, a meticulous mediastinal dissection is carried out in order to identify and preserve both the anterior and posterior vagus nerves. This is based on the physiologic repercussions of dividing one or both of the vagi, including delayed gastric emptying and dumping syndrome. However, Oelschlager and colleagues have proposed intentional truncal vagotomy as a technique for lengthening the esophagus and their outcome data seem to suggest that these traditional fears of vagotomy complications are over

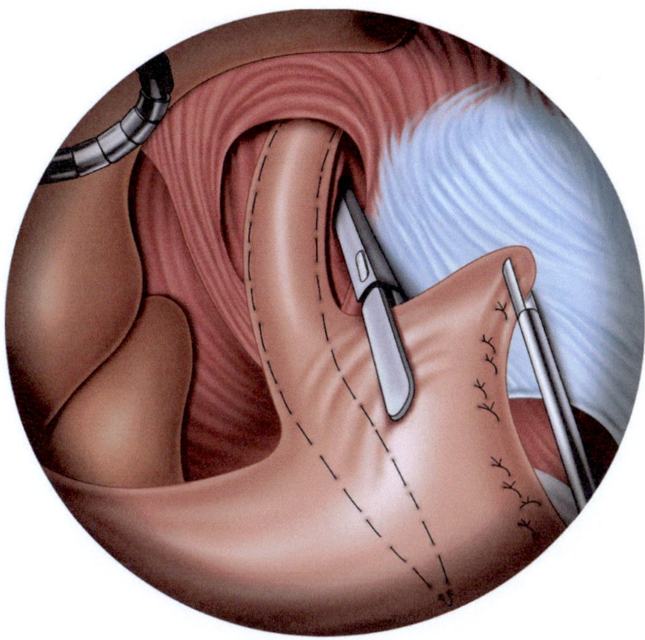

Fig. 19.5 Combined laparoscopic–thoracoscopic Collis gastroplasty: stapler introduced through the left chest

emphasized [27]. Using their technique, the esophagus is fully mobilized as previously described. If an adequate infra-diaphragmatic length of esophagus cannot be obtained, a posterior vagotomy is performed to further release cephalad tension. If this maneuver is not successful in achieving enough added length, an anterior vagotomy is performed. Only after failure of bilateral vagotomy, would they proceed to a wedge-gastroplasty as a last resort. However, in an experience of 166 patients undergoing redo LARS or PEH repairs, an additional SE lengthening procedure was never required using this technique.

During their follow-up, they found no difference in heartburn, bloating, nausea, or diarrhea symptoms between patients who had a vagotomy and those who did not. However, all of the patients who underwent *bilateral* vagotomy developed some degree of dumping syndrome postoperatively. Therefore we would recommend that if this technique is employed, only a single vagus should be divided, and that if this maneuver fails to adequately lengthen the esophagus, a Collis procedure, rather than a bilateral vagotomy, would be preferred.

Crural Closure and Fundoplication

After the SE has been lengthened the diaphragmatic crura must be closed in order to recreate a natural antiflux barrier and prevent herniation of the new GEJ and eventual fundoplication into the chest. Interrupted size 0 or 2–0 braided,

non-absorbable sutures are placed starting at the base of the hiatus at 1 cm intervals. Generally three or four sutures are required posterior to the esophagus, and anterior sutures are not placed unless a completely posterior closure would create an abnormal esophageal angulation ventrally. Reducing the pressure of the pneumoperitoneum may facilitate closure of the crura without tension. If closure is accompanied by significant tension, it may be necessary to perform a relaxing incision by dividing the diaphragm just lateral to the right crus using an ultrasonic shears, covering the resulting defect with a biological or resorbable prosthetic mesh.

After the crura are closed, we proceed with creation of an antireflux barrier. In the case of an esophageal lengthening procedure, the fundoplication performed should adhere to the same principles as in a routine operation for GERD. The wrap should be formed around the neo-esophagus, rather than stomach body, and it should lie entirely below the level of the hiatus without tension when completed.

With the surgeon's left hand, an instrument is passed posterior to the esophagus from the anatomic right side, and the most proximal portion of the remaining fundus is grasped and pulled back through the posterior window. The right-hand instrument grasps slightly anterior to the greater curvature on the fundus that remains to the left of the neo-esophagus, and the surgeon's two instruments are brought together to approximately a 360-degree fundoplication. A back-and-forth "shoe shine" maneuver is used to check for abnormal torque or tension on the fundoplication. When released, the anatomic right side of the fundoplication should remain in position, rather than be pulled back through the posterior esophageal window. If such tension exists, further mobilization of the greater curvature distally may be necessary.

The fundoplication is secured with three interrupted 2–0 braided non-absorbable sutures that incorporate seromuscular fundal bites on either side. The middle suture is placed first and then the cephalad–caudad position of the wrap can be adjusted. Under ordinary circumstances, the two staplelines should be buried beneath the enveloping fundus, decreasing the likelihood of leak (Fig. 19.6). The most proximal suture should incorporate a bite of native esophageal wall to improve propulsion through the neo-esophagus. We do not place sutures between the fundoplication and crura, as this tethering may adversely affect normal distal esophageal axial motility during swallowing.

After the fundoplication is complete, the bougie is removed and the staple lines are checked for leak. This can be done by injecting air and/or blue dye through a nasogastric tube or by endoscopic visual and insufflation inspection. After the staple lines are deemed satisfactory, the liver retractor is removed under direct visualization, the 12 mm port closed with fascial sutures, and the skin incisions closed with subcuticular sutures.

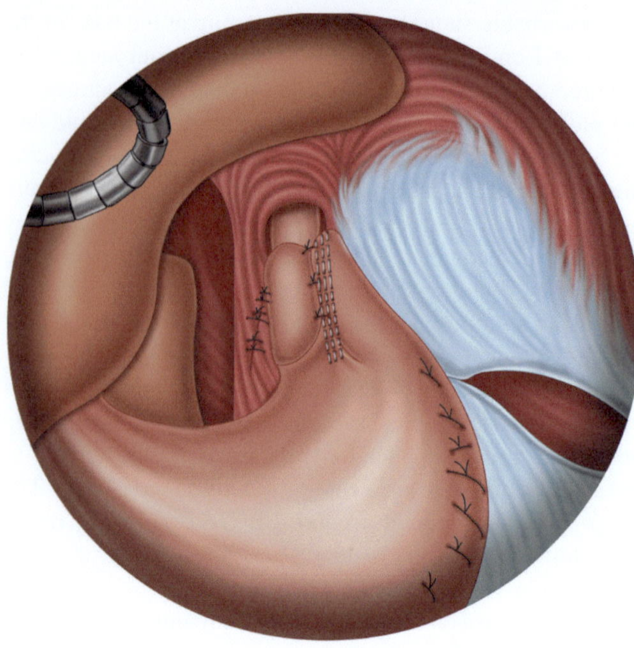

Fig. 19.6 Completed Collis procedure with fundoplication around the neo-esophagus and covering the staple-line

Postoperative Care

Patients are extubated following surgery and we do not routinely leave a nasogastric tube. Scheduled intravenous ketorolac and ondansetron are administered, as well as intravenous opioids for breakthrough pain. Patients are kept NPO immediately after surgery and undergo a contrast swallow study on the morning after surgery to check for staple-line leak. If that study is negative and contrast moves freely past the GEJ and wrap, a liquid diet is started and advanced to a soft diet for lunch if tolerated. Patients are typically discharged on the afternoon of the first postoperative day if progressing as expected. A soft diet is maintained until follow-up in the clinic in two weeks.

Long-Term Follow-Up and Outcomes

Several physiologic differences between the anatomy created by an esophageal lengthening procedure and that after normal LARS must be noted and applied to the long-term postoperative care of these patients. The first is that the neo-esophagus is amotile, which may predispose to dysphagia postoperatively. On follow-up manometry, Jobe and colleagues found that 43 % of patients undergoing combined laparoscopic-thoracoscopic Collis gastroplasty and fundoplication had an aperistaltic segment of distal esophagus (likely neo-esophagus) [28]. However, there was no difference between preoperative and postoperative frequencies of dysphagia in that same patient cohort.

Secondly, the segment of neo-esophagus is composed of native gastric tissue and may contain acid-producing parietal cells. The previously mentioned study found that endoscopic biopsy proximal to the new high-pressure zone (i.e., location of the fundoplication) revealed positive Congo red staining for parietal cells in 100 % of patients, and 50 % had abnormal esophageal acid exposure on 24-h pH monitoring studies [28]. Based on this variant physiology, we modify our routine LARS follow-up protocol for patients who have had a lengthening procedure, performing a full battery of testing at one-year postoperatively that includes a contrast radiograph, endoscopy, HRM, and 24-h pH monitoring study. Any patient with evidence of abnormal GER (esophagitis on endoscopy, or an abnormal 24-h pH study) is placed on lifelong PPI therapy.

Despite these potential physiologic disruptions that arise from the abnormal anatomy of the Collis gastroplasty, results in most series in the laparoscopic era have been encouraging. Complication rates remain on par with those after PEH repair or redo LARS without a lengthening procedure. Similarly, excellent long-term symptom resolution with respect to heartburn, regurgitation, dysphagia, and chest pain has been reported in both open and laparoscopic series [28–31]. It should be noted that patients who require a lengthening procedure for SE are more likely to have had severe symptoms preoperatively due to long-standing and often complicated GERD. Therefore it is our opinion that anticipation of a SE preoperatively should not serve as a deterrent to proceeding with an antireflux operation, and in almost all cases, a laparoscopic approach is still feasible.

Conclusions

Although rarely encountered, SE constitutes an important aspect of LARS. Preoperative risk-stratification for SE based on a careful history and all available anatomic and physiologic studies is essential, and even if a SE is suspected preoperatively, a laparoscopic approach should be employed. Completing a full mediastinal esophageal mobilization is key to minimizing SE intraoperatively; however, when mobilization fails to deliver a 2.5 cm length of esophagus below the hiatus, a lengthening procedure is required. While several options exist, we feel that a laparoscopic stapled-wedge modification of the "Collis" gastroplasty is the most technically feasible procedure for surgeons already comfortable with laparoscopic foregut surgery. Postoperative management should be altered accordingly after a lengthening procedure and a strict schedule of follow-up studies must be adhered to, but overall, patients can expect excellence long-term symptomatic results.

References

1. Pearson FG, Cooper JD, Patterson GA, Ramirez J, Todd TR. Gastroplasty and fundoplication for complex reflux problems. Long-term results. Ann Surg. 1987;206:473–81.
2. Bochkarev V, Lee YK, Vitamvas M, Oleynikov D. Short esophagus: how much length can we get? Surg Endosc. 2008;22:2123–7.
3. Madan AK, Frantzides CT, Patsavas KL. The myth of the short esophagus. Surg Endosc. 2004;18:31–4.
4. Mattioli S, Lugaresi ML, Costantini M, et al. The short esophagus: intraoperative assessment of esophageal length. J Thorac Cardiovasc Surg. 2008;136:834–41.
5. Findlay L, Kelly AB. Congenital shortening of the oesophagus and the thoracic stomach resulting therefrom. Proc R Soc Med. 1931;24:1561–78.
6. Moersch HJ. Hiatal hernia. In: Ann Otol Rhinol Laryngol; 1938:754–67.
7. Herbella FA, Patti MG, Del Grande JC. When did the esophagus start shrinking? The history of the short esophagus. ISDE. 2009; 22:550–8.
8. Lillemoe KD, Johnson LF, Harmon JW. Role of the components of the gastroduodenal contents in experimental acid esophagitis. Surgery. 1982;92:276–84.
9. Lillemoe KD, Johnson LF, Harmon JW. Taurodeoxycholate modulates the effects of pepsin and trypsin in experimental esophagitis. Surgery. 1985;97:662–7.
10. Gozzetti G, Pilotti V, Spangaro M, et al. Pathophysiology and natural history of acquired short esophagus. Surgery. 1987;102: 507–14.
11. Hoang CD, Koh PS, Maddaus MA. Short esophagus and esophageal stricture. Surg Clin North Am. 2005;85:433–51.
12. Harrington SW. The diagnosis and treatment of diaphragmatic hernia. J Thoracic Surg 1931;24–40.
13. Wangensteen OH, Leven NL. Gastric resection for esophagitis and stricture of acid-peptic origin. Surg Gynecol Obstet. 1949;88: 560–70.
14. Krupp S, Rossetti M. Surgical treatment of hiatal hernias by fundoplication and gastropexy (Nissen repair). Ann Surg. 1966; 164:927–34.
15. Volonte F, Collard JM, Goncette L, Gutschow C, Strignano P. Intrathoracic periesophageal fundoplication for short esophagus: a 20-year experience. Ann Thorac Surg. 2007;83:265–71.
16. Collis JL. An operation for hiatus hernia with short oesophagus. Thorax. 1957;12:181–8.
17. Yano F, Stadlhuber RJ, Tsuboi K, Garg N, Filipi CJ, Mittal SK. Preoperative predictability of the short esophagus: endoscopic criteria. Surg Endosc. 2009;23:1308–12.
18. Yau P, Watson DI, Jamieson GG, Myers J, Ascott N. The influence of esophageal length on outcomes after laparoscopic fundoplication. J Am Coll Surg. 2000;191:360–5.
19. Gastal OL, Hagen JA, Peters JH, et al. Short esophagus: analysis of predictors and clinical implications. Arch Surg. 1999;134:633–6. discussion 7–8.
20. Mittal SK, Awad ZT, Tasset M, et al. The preoperative predictability of the short esophagus in patients with stricture or paraesophageal hernia. Surg Endosc. 2000;14:464–8.
21. Winslow ER, Clouse RE, Desai KM, et al. Influence of spastic motor disorders of the esophageal body on outcomes from laparoscopic antireflux surgery. Surg Endosc. 2003;17:738–45.
22. Kahrilas PJ, Kim HC, Pandolfino JE. Approaches to the diagnosis and grading of hiatal hernia. Best Pract Res Clin Gastroenterol. 2008;22:601–16.
23. Horvath KD, Swanstrom LL, Jobe BA. The short esophagus: pathophysiology, incidence, presentation, and treatment in the era of laparoscopic antireflux surgery. Ann Surg. 2000;232:630–40.
24. Swanstrom LL, Marcus DR, Galloway GQ. Laparoscopic Collis gastroplasty is the treatment of choice for the shortened esophagus. Am J Surg. 1996;171:477–81.
25. O'Rourke RW, Khajanchee YS, Urbach DR, et al. Extended transmediastinal dissection: an alternative to gastroplasty for short esophagus. Arch Surg. 2003;138:735–40.
26. Terry ML, Vernon A, Hunter JG. Stapled-wedge Collis gastroplasty for the shortened esophagus. Am J Surg. 2004;188:195–9.
27. Oelschlager BK, Yamamoto K, Woltman T, Pellegrini C. Vagotomy during hiatal hernia repair: a benign esophageal lengthening procedure. J Gastrointest Surg. 2008;12:1155–62.
28. Jobe BA, Horvath KD, Swanstrom LL. Postoperative function following laparoscopic Collis gastroplasty for shortened esophagus. Arch Surg. 1998;133:867–74.
29. Nason KS, Luketich JD, Awais O, et al. Quality of life after Collis gastroplasty for short esophagus in patients with paraesophageal hernia. Ann Thorac Surg. 2011;92:1854–60. discussion 60–1.
30. Durand L, De Anton R, Caracoche M, et al. Short esophagus: selection of patients for surgery and long-term results. Surg Endosc. 2012;26:704–13.
31. Cooper JD, Gill SS, Nelems JM, Pearson FG. Intraoperative and postoperative esophageal manometric findings with Collis gastroplasty and Belsey hiatal hernia repair for gastroesophageal reflux. J Thorac Cardiovasc Surg. 1977;74:744–51.

Poor Esophageal Motility: A Tailored Approach?

Stefan Niebisch and Jeffrey H. Peters

Introduction

Creating an effective gastroesophageal barrier with long-term subjective and objective reflux control without side effects such as dysphagia is the challenge of antireflux surgery. The relation between esophageal motility and antireflux surgery has been of interest for decades. Patient variables such as the size of hiatal hernia and presence of esophageal stricture as well as the surgical technique including type and degree of hiatal closure, the length and shape of the fundic wrap, and the use of a Bougie or not have long been recognized to influence outcomes. Poor esophageal motility likely influences both symptomatic relief and the propensity for side effects, particularly postoperative dysphagia. Reflux in the setting of poor motility and delayed esophageal clearance predisposes to continued symptoms and increased mucosal injury. On the other hand, it is established that outflow resistance at the gastroesophageal junction is proportional to the degree of a gastric wrap around the distal esophagus. These opposing concerns frame the concepts of "tailored" antireflux surgery. While controversial, and still debated, the rationale for altering the degree of fundoplication based upon adequacy of esophageal motility, so called "tailoring", is substantial and includes:

(1) Ex-vivo studies of the outflow resistance afforded by complete versus partial fundoplication
(2) Recurrent dysphagia and esophageal dilation in patients with achalasia treated with Nissen fundoplication
(3) Physiologic studies of peristaltic wave and contraction amplitudes necessary for liquid bolus transport
(4) The propensity for new onset dysphagia in any patient post Nissen fundoplication
(5) Physiologic studies of the esophagogastric junction in patients with post Nissen dysphagia.

Experiments with ex-vivo human esophagogastric specimens (no esophageal motility) in which either a complete or partial fundoplication is created around the lower esophagus reveal free flow through a partial fundoplication while a complete Nissen results in a 20–30 cm of water outflow resistance. Wills and Hunt [1] compared the long-term outcomes of patients undergoing Heller myotomy and either partial or complete fundoplication. Nissen fundoplication resulted in progressively higher prevalence of recurrent dysphagia and slow esophageal dilation when compared to those with partial fundoplication.

Many terms for poor esophageal motility are used in the literature: "esophageal dysmotility," "ineffective esophageal motility (IEM)," "weak peristalsis," and "impaired peristalsis." In the context of circular muscle strength, they all describe an esophageal body contraction pattern that is below the 5th percentile threshold observed in healthy volunteers without a history of foregut symptoms or surgery. Controversy of the benefits of "tailoring" the fundoplication in the presence of poor esophageal motility is partially driven by the isolated focus on esophageal circular muscle function. In fact, the risk of postoperative dysphagia is dependent upon many factors including:

- The presence of dysphagia preoperatively
- Poor bolus transit assessed via esophagram or impedance
- Esophageal body contractility
- Surgical technique

The presence of preoperative dysphagia has been shown to be among the most significant predictors for persistent dysphagia postoperatively [2–4]. Montenovo et al. reported a significant difference in the prevalence of postoperative dysphagia in patients with (77 %) and without (23 %) dysphagia prior to surgery ($p<0.01$). Similar findings have been described by Herron and colleagues; 47 % of patients with post-op dysphagia had pre-op dysphagia compared to 11 %

S. Niebisch, MD (✉)
University of Mainz Medical Center, Gerneral-, Viszeral- and Transplant-Surgery, Langenbeckstr. 1, Mainz 55131, Germany
e-mail: stefanniebisch@googlemail.com

J.H. Peters, MD
Department of Surgery, University of Rochester Medical Center, 601 Elmwood Avenue, Box SURG, Rochester, NY 14642, USA
e-mail: jeffrey_peters@urmc.rochester.edu

L.L. Swanstrom and C.M. Dunst (eds.), *Antireflux Surgery*,
DOI 10.1007/978-1-4939-1749-5_20, © Springer New York 2015

in patients without preoperative dysphagia ($p=0.029$). In a multivariate analysis of 219 patients, Tsuboi et al. found that preoperative dysphagia was an independent predictor for postoperative dysphagia (OR 4.4, 95 % CI 1.2–15.5; $p=0.023$). They further identified delayed esophageal emptying on video esophagram (OR 8.2, 95 % CI 1.6–42.2; $p=0.012$) as a risk factor for postoperative dysphagia. Combined high-resolution impedance manometry studies in patients with non-obstructive/unexplained dysphagia reveal that peristaltic breaks are more frequently observed in patients with dysphagia and that patients with peristaltic defects had a higher incidence of incomplete bolus transit [5]. Whether these findings have an impact on predicting postoperative dysphagia is unknown and is certainly a topic of future study.

Defining Poor Esophageal Motility

Conventional Manometry

Classification of IEM using conventional manometry was reported by Spechler and Castel in 2001. Hypocontractility was defined as at least 30 % of wet swallows with contraction amplitudes below 30 mmHg, with or without peristaltic wave propagation, or 30 % peristaltic waves that are not propagated to the distal esophagus or absence of peristalsis [6]. The threshold of 30 mmHg is based on classic studies of combined manometry and video barium bolus transport reported by Kahrilas et al. [7]. Contraction amplitudes less than 30 mmHg were frequently associated with incomplete bolus clearance and bolus escape. Others have suggested that the 30 mmHg threshold might be too high. For example Tutuian and Castell using combined multichannel intraluminal impedance manometry have shown that 48 % of swallows with contraction amplitudes less than 30 mmHg still achieved complete bolus transit. An important limitation of conventional manometry catheters relates to the assessment of contraction amplitudes at one or two levels along the distal esophagus, which may miss segments of weak peristalsis [8]. This technical limitation is eliminated with closely distributed pressure channels characteristic of current high-resolution manometry (HRM) catheters.

High-Resolution Manometry

The recently published Chicago classification representing a consensus of international esophageal motility experts redefined esophageal peristalsis using HRM. Ineffective motility or hypocontractility is defined as frequent failed peristalsis (>30 % but < 100 % of wet swallows) and/or weak peristalsis with small (2–5 cm) breaks in more than 20 % of swallows, or large breaks (>5 cm) in more than 30 % given an isobaric contour of 20 mmHg. Failed peristalsis is defined as less than 3 cm integrity of the 20 mmHg isobaric contour distal to the transition zone (Fig. 20.1) [9]. Using HRM, the Northwestern group has shown that large breaks are virtually always, and small breaks frequently, associated with bolus escape, and that both occur significantly more often in patients with dysphagia. Incomplete bolus transit never occurred in the absence of peristaltic breaks (Fig. 20.2) [5].

Although not part of the current classification of ineffective or weak esophageal motility, the distal contractile integral (DCI) provides further assessment of global distal esophageal circular muscle strength. The DCI is calculated as the product of mean amplitude of the contraction (excluding pressure below 20 mmHg) from the transition of the striated to smooth esophageal muscles (proximal pressure trough) to the proximal border of the LES by duration and by length and gives an overall value of the circular muscle strength of the distal esophagus. To date, the DCI has largely been used to define hypercontractility, focusing on the upper limits of normal, differentiating hypercontractility from normal contractions, rather than the lower limits of esophageal motility. Figure 20.3 shows a normal esophageal body contraction in esophageal pressure topography and its corresponding line tracing in a patient with distal contraction amplitude and DCI within normal limits. A limitation of the automated DCI calculation provided by the analysis software is that repetitive pressure signals separated from the esophageal contractile complex such as vascular artifacts are included in this calculation. This may lead to artifactual overestimation of the circular contraction strength in patients with a hypocontractile esophagus [10]. The lower limit of the DCI, expressed by the 5th percentile of asymptomatic controls is 500 mmHg • cm • s.

The Tailored Approach in the Current Literature

The benefits of tailoring the degree of fundoplication, either by performing an alternative wrap or by altering the Nissen wrap in some way, based upon the patients esophageal motility remain unknown mostly due to insufficient and poor quality data to date. Nearly all published studies (Tables 20.1 and 20.2) suffer from one or more of the following problems.

(1) Small sample size and not enough patients to answer the question, i.e., a type II error
(2) Differences in defining preoperative poor esophageal motility
(3) Variability and difficulty in measuring the primary outcome, i.e., dysphagia
(4) Variability in the technique of both partial and complete fundoplication.

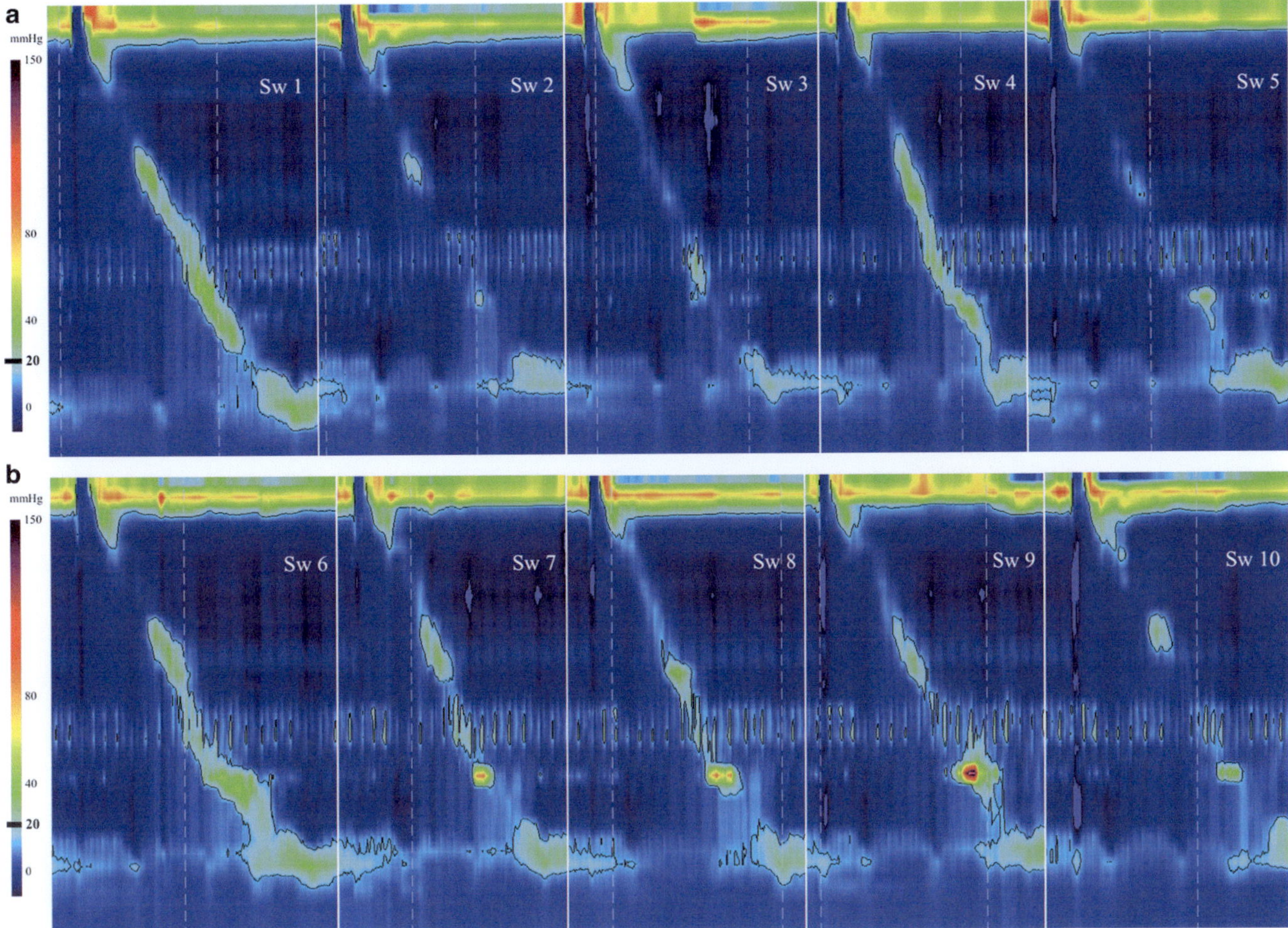

Fig. 20.1 Example of ineffective esophageal motility, Swallow (Sw) 1–10: *Hypotensive contraction* (Swallow 1, 4, 6, 7, 8, 9); *Failed peristalsis* (Swallow 2, 3, 5, 10); *Weak peristalsis* with small (2–5 cm) and large (>5 cm) breaks in the isobaric contour of 20 mmHg (Swallow 7–9)

Outcome of Partial Fundoplication

Fundamental to the concept of a tailored approach is an acceptable record of reflux control and symptomatic relief following partial fundoplication. Recent long-term data would suggest that the outcomes of partial fundoplication when applied to the broad population of patients undergoing antireflux surgery are good [11].

Granderath and colleagues analyzed 155 patients with either contraction amplitudes less than 30 mmHg, or more than 40 % simultaneous contractions who underwent Toupet fundoplication [12]. At 1-year follow-up, 2.6 % had moderate dysphagia and all had control of heartburn and regurgitation. They concluded that partial fundoplication in patients with impaired motility is well tolerated and effectively relieves GERD symptoms. The same group compared 32 patients with poor motility that underwent partial fundoplication and 17 patients with normal esophageal motility after

Nissen fundoplication [13]. Postoperative dysphagia occurred in one patient in each group (3.1 vs. 5.9 %). Two patients (7.4 %) in the partial group had positive pH studies post-op, compared to none after a Nissen. The conclusions are confounded however by a relatively "mild" definition of poor motility. Contraction amplitudes of less than 30 mmHg at one distal level in more than 10 % of swallows were considered as poor motility.

Partial vs Complete Fundoplication in the Presence of IEM

Kauer et al. suggested a tailored approach in antireflux surgery in 1995 [14]. Symptomatic patients underwent preoperative endoscopy, manometry, esophagram, and pH monitoring. Based on esophageal length and body contractility patients were allocated to an abdominal or thoracic Nissen fundoplication

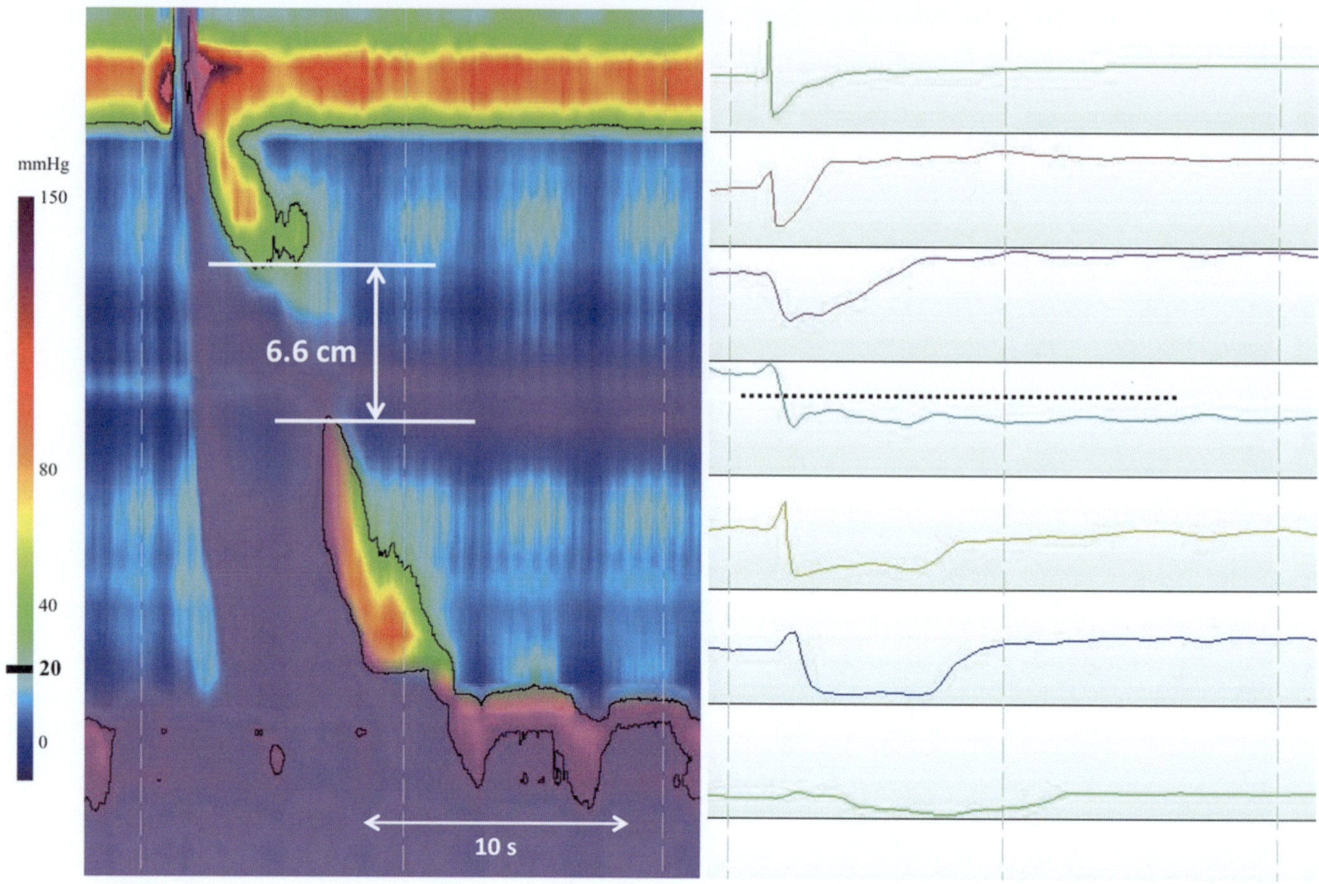

Fig. 20.2 Incomplete bolus transit due to a large break in the 20 mmHg isobaric contour in high-resolution impedance manometry. The *pink* shaded area indicates bolus presence in the esophageal pressure topog- raphy. The corresponding line tracing shows inadequate recovery (<50 %), which indicates incomplete clearance (*dashed line*)

when both appeared normal or to a thoracic approach with a Belsey partial fundoplication in cases of poor esophageal motility. Interestingly, patients with a Belsey fundoplication had less symptomatic improvement than those with Nissen fundoplication. Abdominal and thoracic Nissen had a cure rate of 90 and 95 % respectively, compared to partial fundo- plication following which 67 % of patients had symptomatic improvement. It must be remembered however that patients with poor esophageal motility likely have more severe reflux disease on average than those in which a Nissen fundoplica- tion may have been performed.

Booth and colleagues reported 1-year symptomatic out- comes of 52 patients with IEM who were randomized to either Nissen or Toupet fundoplication [15]. The overall prevalence of postoperative dysphagia was higher in the Nissen group, although there was no difference in new onset or worsened dysphagia. Surprisingly, de novo or worsened postoperative dysphagia occurred less often in the poor motility group compared to those with normal motility (15 vs. 23 %). Chrysos et al. randomly assigned 33 patients with poor motility (contraction amplitude <35 mmHg) to Nissen

($n = 14$) or Toupet ($n = 19$) fundoplication. Early dysphagia after 3 months was significantly higher after a total fundopli- cation (57 vs. 16 %). However, at 1-year follow-up the preva- lence of dysphagia (grade 1–3) was similar in both groups (14 vs. 16 %) [16].

Assessing the possibility of pursing a Nissen fundoplica- tion in all patients, Patti et al. reported outcomes of a tailored approach compared to a second group in which all patients underwent laparoscopic Nissen fundoplication regardless the quality of esophageal peristalsis. All fundoplications were cre- ated over a 56 French Bougie, and poor motility was defined as mean contraction amplitudes less than 40 mmHg. There was no difference in new onset postoperative dysphagia in patients with IEM regardless of the surgical approach. However, significantly more patients with poor motility had postoperative heartburn following a Toupet than a Nissen fun- doplication [17]. Strate et al. and Shaw et al. used similar defi- nitions for ineffective motility including contraction amplitudes of less than 40 mmHg and/or failed peristalsis in more than 40 % of swallows. Patients with and without poor motility were allocated to either total or partial fundoplication.

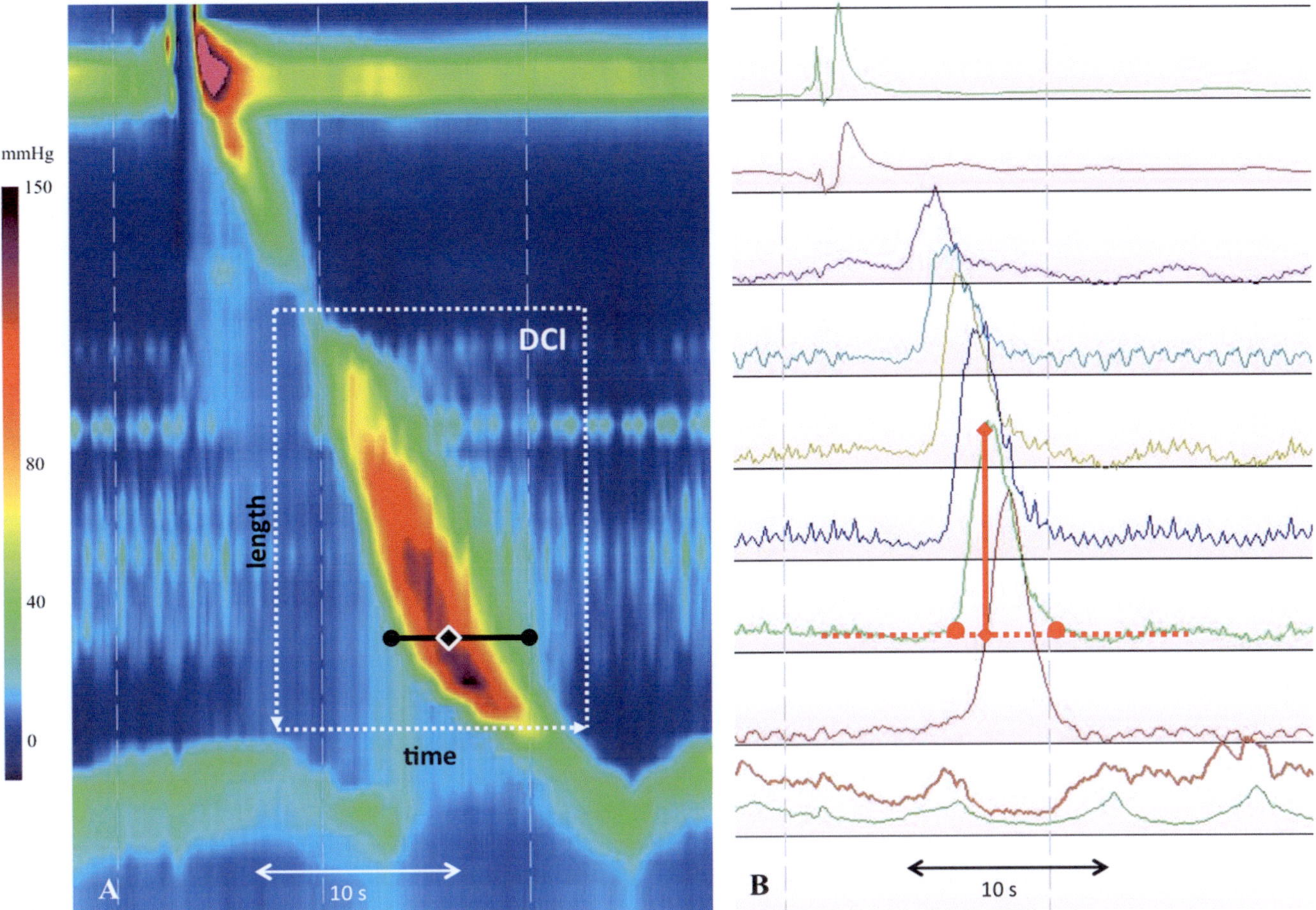

Fig. 20.3 Normal contraction amplitude and distal contractile integral (DCI): Color plot (**A**) and corresponding line tracing (**B**). *Black* and *red dots* indicate begin and end of contraction. Peak of contraction (contraction amplitude) displayed by *white square* in **A** and as *vertical red line* in **B**. DCI is calculated by average pressure (in an isobaric contour of 20 mmHg) × time × length (*doted white box*). Contraction amplitude: 120 mmHg; DCI 1,800 mmHg • s • cm

Table 20.1 Dysphagia after Nissen fundoplication in patients with ineffective esophageal motility (IEM) vs. normal motility (N); CA: Contraction Amplitude

	Definition of poor motility	IEM	N	OP	Use of Bougie	Hiatal closure	f/u	Postoperative dysphagia
Biertho [20]	Mean CA < 30 mmHg	38	533	Nissen	No	n/r	Up to 5 years	No difference in dysphagia score
Ravi [21]	CA < 30 mmHg or failed in ≥30 %	38	60	Nissen	No	Yes	Six months	Moderate/severe: 13 % (IEM) vs. 8 % (N)
Munitiz [22]	CA < 30 mmHg in ≥50 %	41	52	Open Nissen	48–50 Fr	Yes	Median 5–6.5 years	New onset: 7.3 % (IEM) vs. 3.9 % (N)

Postoperatively, new onset dysphagia in patients with IEM was noted in 2/14 who underwent a Nissen versus 0/11 in the Toupet group ($p=0.6$) [18]. In the 2-year follow-up data of Strate et al., 13.5 % (27/200) of patients complained of moderate to severe dysphagia 26 % (13/50) after Nissen and 10 % (5/50) after Toupet fundoplication. Of note the authors utilized a 36 French nasogastric tube instead of a Bougie [19].

IEM Versus Normal Motility

Biertho and colleagues reported 38 patients with poor motility versus 533 patients with normal motility undergoing laparoscopic Nissen fundoplication [20]. IEM was defined as mean contraction amplitudes less than 30 mmHg; however, the authors did not describe the frequency of failed peristalsis

Table 20.2 Postoperative dysphagia after total (Nissen) and partial (Toupet) fundoplication in a cohort of ineffective esophageal motility (IEM) and normal motility (N); CA: Contraction Amplitude

	Definition of poor motility	IEM	N	OP	Use of Bougie	Hiatal closure	f/u	Postoperative dysphagia
Strate [19]	CA < 40 mmHg and/or failed peristalsis > 40 %	50	50	Nissen	36 Fr	Yes	2 years	IEM: 26 % (Nissen) vs. 10 % (Toupet) N: 12 % (Nissen) vs. 6 % (Toupet)
		50	50	Toupet				
Booth [15]	CA < 30 mmHg and/or non-propagating ≥ 30 %	26	38	Nissen	56 Fr	Yes	1 year	No difference in prevalence of new onset of worsened dysphagia
		26	37	Toupet				
Shaw [18]	CA < 40 mmHg and/or failed peristalsis > 40 %	14	36	Nissen	52 Fr	Yes	~5 years	IEM: 14 % (Nissen) vs. 0 % (Toupet)
		11	39	Toupet				
Patti [17]	mean CA ≤ 40 mmHg	55	67	Nissen	56 Fr	Yes	Mean 70 months	IEM: 9 % (Nissen) vs. 8 % (Toupet)
		141	–	Toupet				
Chrysos [16]	CA < 35 mmHg	14	–	Nissen	No	Yes	1 year	IEM: 14 % (Nissen) vs. 16 % (Toupet)
		19	–	Toupet				
Wetscher [13]	CA < 30 mmHg or simultaneous or interrupted > 10 %	–	17	Nissen	58–60 Fr	Yes	Median 15 months	5.9 % (Nissen) vs. 3.1 % (Toupet)
		32	–	Toupet				

or abnormal wave propagation. They further described that they performed a "looser" fundoplication in patients with esophageal dysmotility but did not use a Bougie intraoperatively, suggesting technical alterations in those with poor motility, a form of a tailored approach. No differences in postoperative dysphagia score were noted in a 5-year follow-up. They concluded that a Nissen fundoplication is not contraindicated in patients with poor motility. However, only 26 % of patients were available for 5-year follow-up evaluation.

Investigators from Ireland reported no difference in postoperative dysphagia 6 months after Nissen fundoplication. Defining IEM as amplitudes below 30 mmHg or failed peristalsis in ≥ 30 % of swallows, 68 % with IEM versus 72 % with normal motility had no dysphagia and 18 % (IEM) vs. 20 % (Normal) had grade 1 dysphagia. Three patients (9 %) in the dysmotility group had severe dysphagia compared to 0 % in the normal motility group. Both groups showed similar overall symptom improvement (88 vs. 89 %) [21].

Contraction amplitudes of less than 30 mmHg were required in at least 50 % of swallows to be considered IEM in the report of Munitiz et al. Forty-one patients with IEM and 52 with normal motility underwent an open Nissen fundoplication with excellent or good clinical results in 90 and 94 % respectively. Preoperative dysphagia resolved in 90 % of patients with IEM after surgery. New onset dysphagia tended to be higher in the poor motility group (7.3 vs. 3.9 %), however did not reach statistical significance. They concluded that Nissen fundoplication is appropriate in the setting of IEM [22].

Conclusions

While most of the studies suggest that a Nissen fundoplication is reasonably well tolerated in the setting of poor esophageal peristalsis, nearly all published data to date have significant limitations. The appropriate definition of poor motility is lacking, although it seems clear that patients with contraction amplitudes < 30 mmHg and/or up to 50 % failed peristalsis on average will not have an unacceptable prevalence of new onset dysphagia following Nissen fundoplication. As such most experts currently suggest consideration of a partial fundoplication in the setting of nearly or completely absent motility of the distal esophagus. Furthermore it is important to remember that esophageal motility assessment is only one piece of the puzzle. Combining other key elements almost certainly play a role including the presence of dysphagia prior to surgery and an assessment of bolus transport via contrast esophagram or multichannel impedance studies.

The published data to date suggest that in the presence of reduced esophageal circular muscle strength secondary to advanced GERD (DeMeester Score > 50, Barrett's esophagus, stricture, esophagitis LA grade III–IV), a partial fundoplication is associated with an increased failure rate. [12, 23, 24]. Given the limitations of defining esophageal body motility with conventional manometry, studies using HRM thresholds are lacking and needed. The higher distribution of pressure channels and easy identification of segments of weak peristalsis as well as utilizing combined

HRM-Impedance catheters might help to identify patients with end-stage GERD and poor motility that are likely to suffer from postoperative dysphagia. Taken together, the data suggest that any combination of reduced circular muscle strength and preoperative symptoms of dysphagia and/or poor bolus transit should be approached with caution, and a partial fundoplication seriously considered.

References

1. Wills VL, Hunt DR. Functional outcome after Heller myotomy and fundoplication for achalasia. J Gastrointest Surg. 2001;5:408–13.
2. Tsuboi K, Lee TH, Legner A, Yano F, Dworak T, Mittal SK. Identification of risk factors for postoperative dysphagia after primary anti-reflux surgery. Surg Endosc. 2011;25:923–9.
3. Herron DM, Swanstrom LL, Ramzi N, Hansen PD. Factors predictive of dysphagia after laparoscopic Nissen fundoplication. Surg Endosc. 1999;13:1180–3.
4. Montenovo M, Tatum RP, Figueredo E, Martin AV, Vu H, Quiroga E, Pellegrini CA, Oelschlager BK. Does combined multichannel intraluminal esophageal impedance and manometry predict postoperative dysphagia after laparoscopic Nissen fundoplication? Dis Esophagus. 2009;22:656–63.
5. Roman S, Lin Z, Kwiatek MA, Pandolfino JE, Kahrilas PJ. Weak peristalsis in esophageal pressure topography: classification and association with Dysphagia. Am J Gastroenterol. 2011;106:349–56.
6. Spechler SJ, Castell DO. Classification of oesophageal motility abnormalities. Gut. 2001;49:145–51.
7. Kahrilas PJ, Dodds WJ, Hogan WJ. Effect of peristaltic dysfunction on esophageal volume clearance. Gastroenterology. 1988;94:73–80.
8. Fox M, Hebbard G, Janiak P, Brasseur JG, Ghosh S, Thumshirn M, Fried M, Schwizer W. High-resolution manometry predicts the success of oesophageal bolus transport and identifies clinically important abnormalities not detected by conventional manometry. Neurogastroenterol Motil. 2004;16:533–42.
9. Bredenoord AJ, Fox M, Kahrilas PJ, Pandolfino JE, Schwizer W, Smout AJ, International High Resolution Manometry Working Group. Chicago classification criteria of esophageal motility disorders defined in high resolution esophageal pressure topography. Neurogastroenterol Motil. 2012;24:57–65.
10. Lin Z, Roman S, Pandolfino JE, Kahrilas PJ. Automated calculation of the distal contractile integral in esophageal pressure topography with a region-growing algorithm. Neurogastroenterol Motil. 2012;24:e4–10.
11. Mardani J, Lundell L, Engstrom C. Total or posterior partial fundoplication in the treatment of GERD: results of a randomized trial after 2 decades of follow-up. Ann Surg. 2011;253:875–8.
12. Granderath FA, Kamolz T, Schweiger UM, Pasiut M, Wykypiel Jr H, Pointner R. Quality of life and symptomatic outcome three to five years after laparoscopic Toupet fundoplication in gastroesophageal reflux disease patients with impaired esophageal motility. Am J Surg. 2002;183:110–6.
13. Wetscher GJ, Glaser K, Wieschemeyer T, Gadenstaetter M, Prommegger R, Profanter C. Tailored antireflux surgery for gastroesophageal reflux disease: effectiveness and risk of postoperative dysphagia. World J Surg. 1997;21:605–10.
14. Kauer WK, Peters JH, DeMeester TR, Heimbucher J, Ireland AP, Bremner CG. A tailored approach to antireflux surgery. J Thorac Cardiovasc Surg. 1995;110:141–6. discussion 146–7.
15. Booth MI, Stratford J, Jones L, Dehn TC. Randomized clinical trial of laparoscopic total (Nissen) versus posterior partial (Toupet) fundoplication for gastro-oesophageal reflux disease based on preoperative oesophageal manometry. Br J Surg. 2008;95:57–63.
16. Chrysos E, Tsiaoussis J, Zoras OJ, Athanasakis E, Mantides A, Katsamouris A, Xynos E. Laparoscopic surgery for gastroesophageal reflux disease patients with impaired esophageal peristalsis: total or partial fundoplication? J Am Coll Surg. 2003;197:8–15.
17. Patti MG, Robinson T, Galvani C, Gorodner MV, Fisichella PM, Way LW. Total fundoplication is superior to partial fundoplication even when esophageal peristalsis is weak. J Am Coll Surg. 2004;198:863–9. discussion 869–70.
18. Shaw JM, Bornman PC, Callanan MD, Beckingham IJ, Metz DC. Long-term outcome of laparoscopic Nissen and laparoscopic Toupet fundoplication for gastroesophageal reflux disease: a prospective, randomized trial. Surg Endosc. 2010;24:924–32.
19. Strate U, Emmermann A, Fibbe C, Layer P, Zornig C. Laparoscopic fundoplication: Nissen versus Toupet two-year outcome of a prospective randomized study of 200 patients regarding preoperative esophageal motility. Surg Endosc. 2008;22:21–30.
20. Biertho L, Sebajang H, Anvari M. Effects of laparoscopic Nissen fundoplication on esophageal motility: long-term results. Surg Endosc. 2006;20:619–23.
21. Ravi N, Al-Sarraf N, Moran T, O'Riordan J, Rowley S, Byrne PJ, Reynolds JV. Acid normalization and improved esophageal motility after Nissen fundoplication: equivalent outcomes in patients with normal and ineffective esophageal motility. Am J Surg. 2005;190:445–50.
22. Munitiz V, Ortiz A, Martinez de Haro LF, Molina J, Parrilla P. Ineffective oesophageal motility does not affect the clinical outcome of open Nissen fundoplication. Br J Surg. 2004;91:1010–4.
23. Horvath KD, Jobe BA, Herron DM, Swanstrom LL. Laparoscopic Toupet fundoplication is an inadequate procedure for patients with severe reflux disease. J Gastrointest Surg. 1999;3:583–91.
24. Stein HJ, Bremner RM, Jamieson J, DeMeester TR. Effect of Nissen fundoplication on esophageal motor function. Arch Surg. 1992;127:788–91.

Delayed Gastric Emptying and Reflux Disease

Steven G. Leeds, Radu Pescarus, and Christy M. Dunst

Introduction

An important consideration for patients with so-called "refractory" or "medication unresponsive" GERD is the possibility of underlying gastroparesis. Gastroparesis affects an estimated 4–5 % of the general population [1]. Up to 40 % of patients presenting for antireflux surgery have associated symptoms suggestive of gastroparesis [2] with many patients confirmed via objective abnormal radio-nuclide gastric emptying studies [3]. Gastroparesis is a chronic digestive disorder best defined by it symptoms: severe nausea, vomiting, bloating, and abdominal pain in the setting of objective confirmation of delayed gastric emptying without mechanical gastric outlet obstruction. Although its pathogenesis is poorly understood, gastroparesis is thought to result from a disturbance in the gastric autonomic innervation [4]. The three most common etiologies of this disease are diabetic gastropathy (29 %), post-surgical (vagal compromise) (13 %) and increasingly, idiopathic (36 %) [5]. Opioid dependence also likely has a role in the etiology of gastroparesis for some patients as an estimated 25–40 % of gastroparesis patients use narcotics [6].

In addition to the more typical symptoms of nausea, bloating, and abdominal pain, gastroparetic patients often report upper abdominal symptoms such as epigastric pain, heartburn, and reflux. The relationship between gastroparesis and GERD is a complex one and the symptomatic overlap often makes it quite difficult to sort out clinically. Gastroparesis, at least in theory, can cause GERD through multiple mechanisms: gastric distension can cause transient lower esophageal sphincter relaxations, food residues in the stomach stimulate gastric acid production, and the increase in gastric volume parallels an increase in the gastric pressure that results in higher volume of esophageal refluxate [7, 8]. Some patients have a generalized gastrointestinal motility disorder and others a true isolated gastroparesis (idiopathic or disease related) that can actually be the sole etiology of their GERD. Still others have symptoms consistent with gastroparesis but in fact have normal emptying and are merely dyspeptic, often due to maladaptive habits like aerophagia related to their GERD. Many of these patients will be treated for one disease or the other without objective testing. When they are finally referred to surgery for refractory symptoms it is important to perform a thorough foregut evaluation. A detailed history is paramount to obtain an accurate understanding of their symptom profile to identify the symptoms that are most troublesome and therefore should be the primary target of treatment. While antireflux surgery is highly successful at treating GERD, gastroparesis is a chronic disorder for which there is no cure. It is imperative to differentiate between patients with symptoms attributable to isolated gastroparesis and patients who have concomitant gastroesophageal reflux disease (GERD) because the treatment strategies and the goals of treatment differ (Fig. 21.1).

There have been studies in the adult and pediatric populations that have indicated delayed gastroparesis may adversely affect the outcome of antireflux surgery [9, 10]. Despite initial excellent reflux control, gastroparetic patients may be dissatisfied with the results of the surgery for many reasons. Gastroparesis has been linked to the failure of the procedure with regard to wrap disruption, gas bloating, severe nausea and vomiting, and unhappy patients [9–13]. If nausea and vomiting persist after surgery secondary to gastroparesis, the integrity and durability of the antireflux procedure are at risk.

S.G. Leeds, MD
Minimally Invasive Surgery Department, Advanced Gastrointestinal Surgery, Surgical Specialists Dallas, Baylor University Medical Center, 3410 Worth Street, Suite 235, Dallas, TX 75246, USA
e-mail: Steven.Leeds@BaylorHealth.edu

R. Pescarus, MD
Department of Surgery, Hopital Sacre Coeur, 5400 Blvd. Gouin Ouest, Montreal, QC, Canada H4J 1C5
e-mail: radupes@yahoo.com

C.M. Dunst, MD, FACS (✉)
Division of GI and MIS Surgery, The Oregon Clinic, 4805 SE Glisan St #6N60, Portland, OR 97213, USA
e-mail: cdunst@orclinic.com

L.L. Swanstrom and C.M. Dunst (eds.), *Antireflux Surgery*,
DOI 10.1007/978-1-4939-1749-5_21, © Springer New York 2015

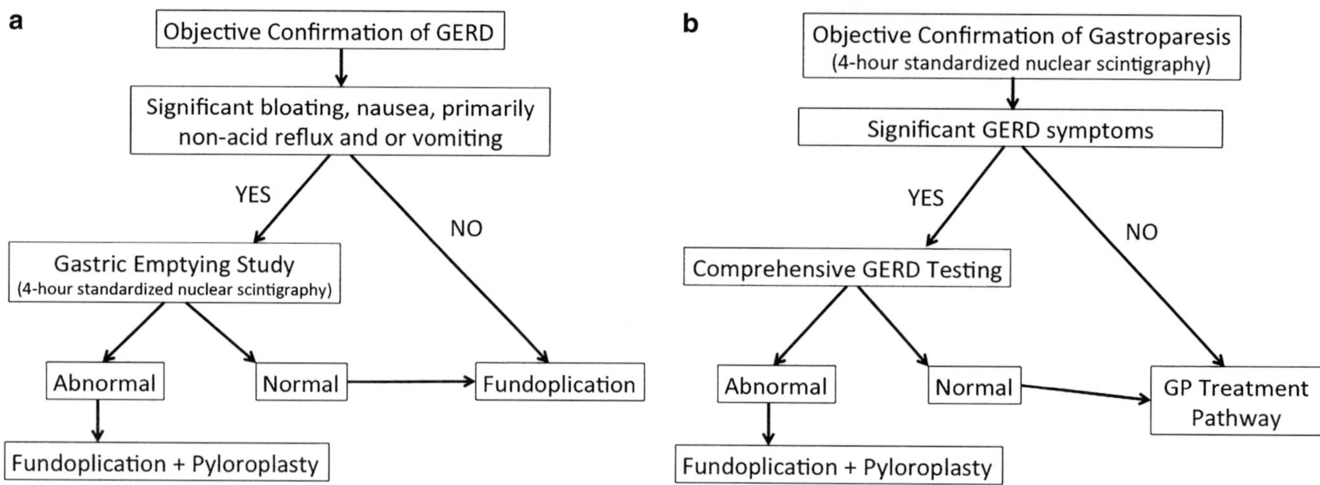

Fig. 21.1 Various evaluation and treatment algorithms for patients presenting with (**a**) primarily GERD or (**b**) primarily gastroparesis symptoms

In addition, recreating the reflux barrier with surgery may exacerbate gas bloating by preventing the release of trapped air in the stomach that would normally escape as belching. Patients recognize this as a failure of their antireflux surgery and return to clinic unhappy, despite resolution of reflux symptoms. Even worse, a fundoplication can even exacerbate gastroparesis symptoms. Overall, the presence of underlying gastroparesis complicates the care of the GERD patient and patients diagnosed with gastroparesis must be counseled carefully regarding expectations of surgery.

The goals of gastroparesis treatment are aimed at palliation of symptoms, not complete resolution that often relies on several modalities used in combination. Current first-line treatment strategies include prokinetic agents, antiemetic medications, glycemic control in diabetics, weaning of narcotics and dietary modifications. Endoscopic therapies directed at the pylorus such as dilation and intra-pyloric botulinum toxin A injection (Botox) have been shown to improve gastric emptying temporarily [14–16]. Options for surgical strategies range from decompressive gastrostomy tubes [17] and feeding jejunostomy to subtotal gastrectomy. Pyloroplasty is recognized as an effective and permanent gastric drainage procedure for primary gastroparesis with or without concurrent GERD [2, 18, 19]. Implantation of a neuro-gastric stimulator is another surgical option for refractory gastroparesis. As prokinetic options have been dramatically reduced over recent years due to safety concerns [20–22] surgical therapies are becoming more important.

Gastric Emptying Study

The most common scenario that the esophageal surgeon faces with respect to gastroparesis is the patient with severe, refractory GERD who is referred for antireflux surgery but

who has unrecognized gastroparesis. Alternatively, patients may be referred for surgical treatment of gastroparesis but have significant GERD, possible due to years of gastric distension and vomiting. Either way, a formal gastric emptying scintigraphy (GES) is mandatory for patients suspected to have gastroparesis as part of their standard comprehensive GERD evaluation, including upper endoscopy to rule out mechanical obstruction of the stomach. Adherence to published recommendations for standardized meals and a 4-h emptying measurement is important to maximize the accuracy of the test. The quality of radionucleide GES is known to differ amongst radiology centers due to a wide variability in testing protocols and normal values. Tougas et al. [3] and Ziessman et al. [23] have refined the test to create standardization of the test meal and imaging protocols at 0, 1, 2, and 4 h. Using this protocol, diagnosis of GP is based on retention of the tracer at each interval. Specifically, 90 % of persistent tracer remaining at one hour, 60 % at 2 h, or 10 % at 4 h are diagnostic of gastroparesis. This has shown to be more sensitive to detecting gastroparesis than the previously thought for only 2 h, and other interval protocols.

Treatment Options

Despite the various treatment options for isolated gastroparesis, we prefer to start with a pyloroplasty in patients with gastroparesis who are having antireflux surgery. Critics of this approach argue that fundoplication alone will improve gastric emptying [10–12, 24–28]. However, after following this advice for mild delays on scintigraphy, we have found that the addition of the pyloroplasty significantly improves outcomes and has an acceptable complication profile [2, 29]. Patients with objective evidence of gastroparesis, despite significant improvement in bloating, nausea, and abdominal pain/

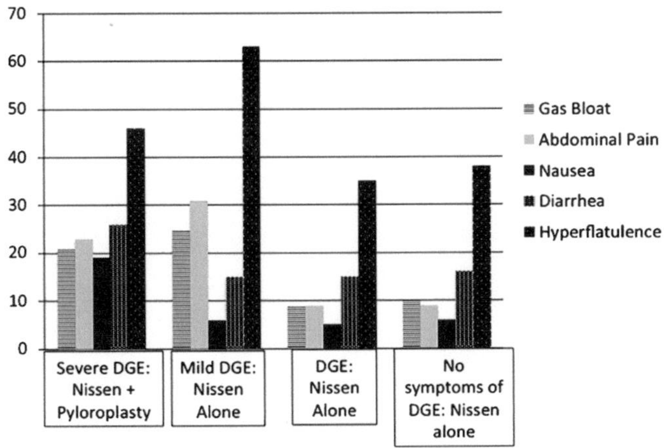

Fig. 21.2 Symptom profiles for GERD patients with concurrent delayed gastric emptying undergoing fundoplication with and without pyloroplasty

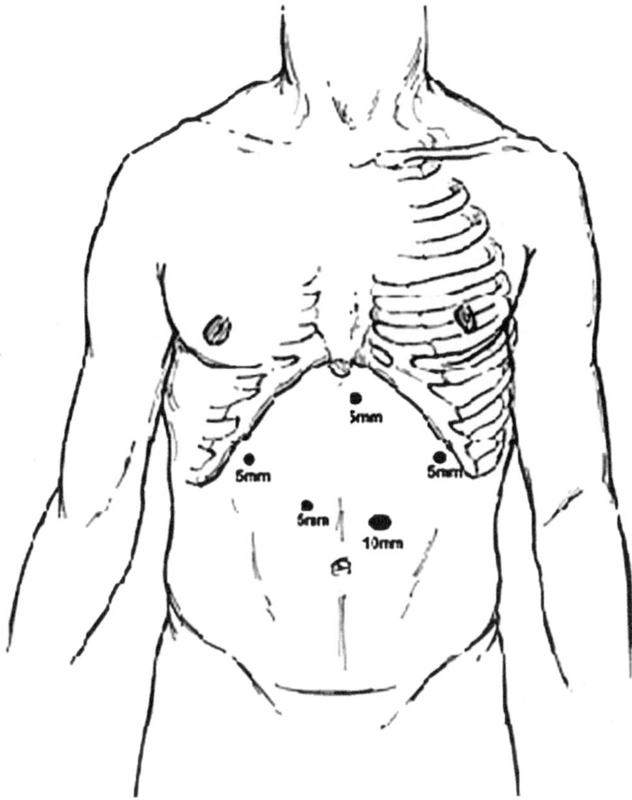

Fig. 21.3 Laparoscopic trocar arrangement for pyloroplasty. The surgeon's left hand is in the subxiphoid position while the right hand is in the left subcostal position. The assistant port is in the right upper abdomen and the camera is in the left and slightly cephalad to the umbilicus. The liver retractor is placed in the far right trocar

fullness, still had a significantly higher incidence of these symptoms post-operatively as compared to patients without gastroparesis [2]. While successful, symptomatic GERD outcomes are similar regardless of the presence or absence of objective gastroparesis (86 vs 91 %), but there is a 25 % failure rate for recurrent/persistent GERD symptoms among patients with objective gastroparesis who did not have a pyloroplasty compared to those who had a pyloroplasty. In fact this sub-group of patients, those with gastroparesis who had a fundoplication without a pyloroplasty, demonstrated worse control of reflux symptoms as compared to patients with gastroparesis who had fundoplication with pyloroplasty or to those without gastroparesis who underwent fundoplication alone (Fig. 21.2). Patients with concomitant fundoplication and pyloroplasty do have a higher incidence of transient post-operative diarrhea and should be counseled for this possibility. True dumping, on the other hand, is rare in the absence of a concomitant vagotomy.

Laparoscopic Pyloroplasty

Laparoscopic Heineke–Mikulicz pyloroplasty can be performed using the same trocar configuration as for the concurrent antireflux surgery (Fig. 21.3). The liver retractor is inserted through the far right trocar and used to expose the pylorus. With the surgeon standing at the patient's left side, a gentle Kocher maneuver is performed to mobilize the pylorus to decrease tension on the eventual suture line. The attachments on the cephalad and caudad sides of the pylorus are divided taking care to avoid the underlying portal structures and maintain adequate blood supply to the pylorus. Precise identification of the pylorus, usually aided by the location of the vein of Mayo, is mandatory and can be facilitated by intra-operative upper endoscopy. After mobilization, the

pylorus is grasped by the surgeon's left hand and the assistant using the subxiphoid trocar. Our preference is to use the ultrasonic shears in the surgeon's right hand, which enables tissue division, sealing, and dissection. Using the ultrasonic shears, a gastrotomy is created about 2–3 cm proximal to the pylorus. The gastrotomy is then extended across the pylorus for a 5 cm full thickness pyloromyotomy (Fig. 21.4). The assistant grasper is then repositioned with one jaw inside the lumen at the level of the pylorus on the cephalad edge to keep the suture line elevated and maximize the sewing angle for the surgeon. The complete myotomy is confirmed by viewing the muscular ridge in the center of the enterotomy. The defect is then closed transversely using a running 2-0 absorbable monofilament suture. This suture choice avoids chronic inflammation of the repair which can be seen with permanent alternatives. The first suture is placed to reapproximate the linear (proximal and distal) ends of the myotomy into the center of the future suture line and run cephalad, away from the surgeon, toward the assistant grasper (Fig. 21.5). Care should be taken to avoid "back-walling" the closure in the center but deeper bites can be taken as the end of the suture line is approached to decrease the dog-ear. When the end is reached,

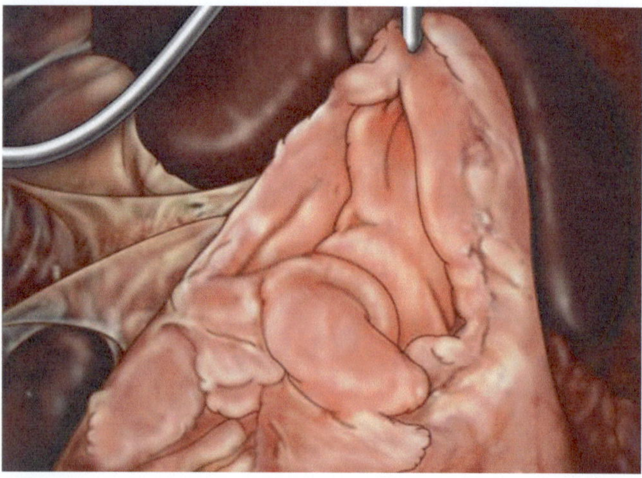

Fig. 21.4 Completed pyloromyotomy with assistant grasper retracting the center cephalad to facilitate transverse closure

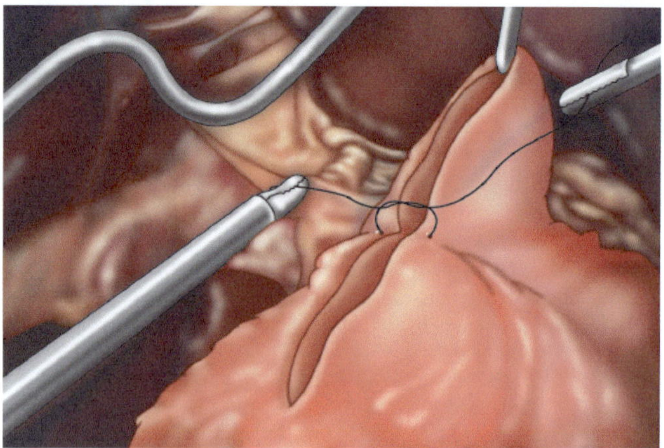

Fig. 21.5 First pyloroplasty suture re-approximating the linear (proximal and distal) ends of the pyloromyotomy incision

the assistant removes the grasper and the suture is tied to itself just past the end of the myotomy. The second suture is then placed, starting at the caudad end of the myotomy and running toward the start of the previous suture in the center of the suture line. The assistant retracts the original suture in the center using a needle driver. The suture is then secured to the tail of the first suture to complete the closure (Fig. 21.6). Intra-operative submersion air-leak and/or methylene blue tests are performed using the upper endoscope. No omental patch is placed. A 15f closed suction drain is then placed in the gastrohepatic ligament along the suture line. Contrast study is performed POD #1 to ensure patent pyloroplasty and confirm the absence of a suture line leak. Nausea is treated aggressively with IV antiemetics and the patients are kept on a PPI for 6 weeks. Routine 4 h GES is performed at 3 months and the patient's symptoms are reassessed.

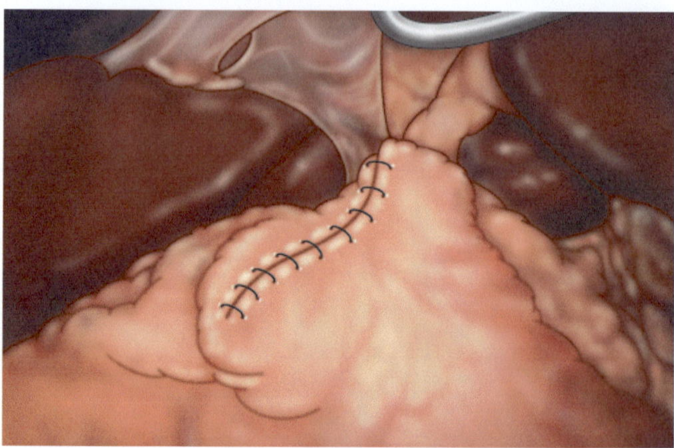

Fig. 21.6 Completed laparoscopic pyloroplasty

Feeding Tube and Gastrostomy Tube Placement

Feeding jejunostomy tubes and decompressive gastrostomy tubes can be helpful in the care of the gastroparetic patient. The paretic stomach is particularly sensitive to post-fundoplication gas-bloat. Decompressive gastrostomy tubes have been advocated for gastroparetics undergoing fundoplication [17, 30]. We also advocate this approach but reserve it for patients undergoing fundoplication and pyloroplasty who also report severe bloating and/or vomiting to assist with these symptoms during recovery. A majority of the tubes are successfully removed by 3 months when the swelling from the pylorus has resolved and the ability to belch, or naturally vent, recovers. Feeding jejunostomy tubes are also helpful in severe gastroparetics. In a selected group of gastroparetic patients presenting frequent admissions for dehydration and severe malnourishment, a laparoscopic jejunostomy tube can serve as an effective "life-line" [1, 31]. Usually, the fundoplication-pyloroplasty can be performed at the time of the feeding jejunostomy but occasionally, the feeding tube is placed alone if the patient is simply too debilitated to proceed with more surgery up front.

GERD in Obese Gastroparetic Patients

Special mention should be made regarding the obese patient with gastroparesis and GERD. The same considerations exist regarding recommendations for RY gastric bypass and are covered elsewhere in this book. The only difference is that we recommend removing the remnant stomach as it is diseased and if left behind it risks continuing to cause symptoms. This does increase the morbidity of the operation overall and should be discussed with the patient ahead of time.

Gastroparesis as a Complication of Antireflux Surgery

Iatrogenic gastroparesis is most often secondary to surgical procedures susceptible of causing a vagal nerve injury such as fundoplication, bariatric surgery, or procedures in which vagotomy is needed such as anti-ulcer operations [30]. As expected, the incidence of iatrogenic post-operative gastroparesis seems to increase with the number of re-operations in a given patient. It is important to be aware of gastroparetic symptoms in a post-fundoplication patient as the gastric dysfunction may eventually lead to a hiatal hernia recurrence or failed fundoplication.

Gastroparesis Refractory to Pyloroplasty

Perhaps the most challenging group of patients are those who are refractory to dietary modification, medical therapy, and pyloroplasty. Unfortunately, debilitating symptoms, particularly pain and nausea, may be persistent regardless of the impact of pyloroplasty on objective gastric emptying [32–34]. It is appropriate to consider gastrectomy for this group of patients [35–37]. Our group has recently presented our experience with 35 patients who underwent a laparoscopic subtotal or total gastrectomy for refractory gastroparesis. Of these, 46 % had previous pyloroplasties, 54 % had previous fundoplications, and 11 % had previous feeding or venting tubes that failed to result in clinical improvement [38]. At a median of 6 months follow-up, there was complete resolution in the pre-operative symptoms in 72 % of patients with nausea, 79 % of those with belching, 89 % of those with bloating, and in 50 % of those with chronic abdominal pain. While the results are promising, the operative morbidity of gastrectomy in gastroparesis is not trivial ranging from 20 to 40 % [35, 37, 38]. These patients often have severe gastritis, retained food in the stomach and in general are not healthy. Malnutrition or poor nutrition is not uncommon among patients with gastroparesis, making for tenuous anastomotic healing [39]. Because of these factors, the procedure should be reserved for refractory patients.

Another option for refractory gastroparesis is gastric nerve stimulation as the implant has been shown to reduce nausea and vomiting, and ameliorate chronic pain [40]. This is a particularly appealing option for high-risk patients with primary nausea. However, a recent study has demonstrated that gastrectomy may be superior to gastric stimulation in the primary treatment of gastroparesis [41]. The decision to proceed with gastrectomy or gastric stimulation after failed pyloroplasty is a challenge and one that needs to be individualized to the unique needs of the patient. There is little if any

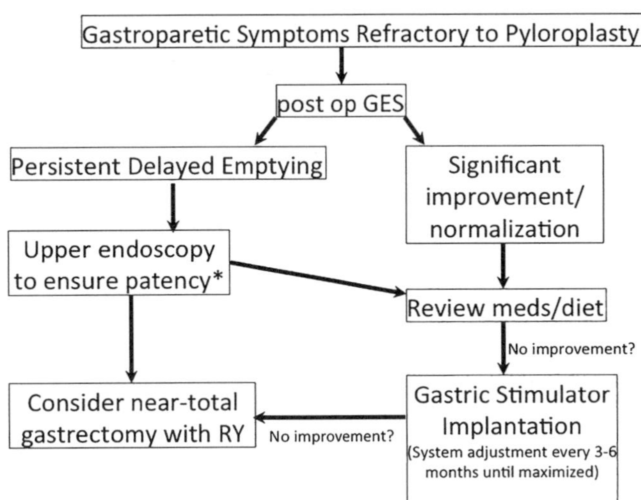

Fig. 21.7 Clinical algorithm for gastroparesis refractory to pyloroplasty. Only patients with persistent symptoms continue to move through the algorithm. *Patients who have gastric outlet obstruction or stenosis despite pyloroplasty should move on to gastrectomy but if the pyloroplasty is open some may consider GS prior to gastrectomy depending on the symptom profile and other patient factors

published literature to help guide the clinician. We have found that patients who suffer from predominantly bloating and retained food do well with a gastrectomy while primary nausea often responds to gastric stimulation. While more work needs to be done in this field, our current clinical algorithm for refractory gastroparesis is shown in Fig. 21.7.

Per-Oral Pyloroplasty

Investigators have been working on methods to perform an endoscopic technique for pyloroplasty for many years [42]. Our initial clinical experience used a trans-oral flexible circular stapler to perform a laparoscopic assisted pyloroplasty [18]. The technology was clumsy but promising. Unfortunately, the stapler was removed from the market shortly thereafter. Applying techniques from per-oral endoscopic myotomy (POEM) we were able to successfully perform endoscopic pyloroplasties on patients with gastroparesis. The feasibility and efficacy of this technique has recently been demonstrated in a porcine model [43] as well as in a single case report [44]. Endoscopic pyloromyotomy utilizing a different technique has also been previously evaluated for the treatment of congenital pyloric stenosis in the pediatric population [45]. Our early results suggest 86 % symptom improvement and statistically significant improvements in GES [46] Although preliminary, we are encouraged by the results that endoluminal pyloromyotomy, or Per-Oral Pyloroplasty (POP), technique could provide an incisionless, less invasive alternative to standard laparoscopic pyloroplasty.

POP Technique

The operative technique is similar in its basic principles to the endoscopic submucosal dissection and myotomy techniques that have been well described in the setting of POEM for the treatment of achalasia [47, 48]. Under general anesthesia, upper endoscopy is performed using a high definition gastroscope and carbon dioxide insufflation. A transparent dissection cap and a 50 cm gastric overtube are necessary. A mucosotomy site is selected approximately 5 cm proximal to the pylorus on the anterior wall of the stomach. Submucosal injection of a 5–10 cc lift solution creates a submucosal bleb. A 1–2 cm longitudinal mucosal incision is then performed using a triangle tip knife. A submucosal tunnel is created by dividing the loose submucosal fibrous tissue. Tunneling continues just past the pylorus into the duodenal bulb. After completion of the tunnel, the myotomy is initiated roughly 2 cm proximal to the pylorus leaving a 3 cm overlap of redundant tunnel. The myotomy is carried to the level of the serosa and extends across the pylorus. Considerable care must be taken when dividing the distal edge of the pylorus, as the duodenal mucosal drapes over perpendicularly. The scope is removed from the tunnel and the mucosotomy is closed using clips or an endoscopic suturing device (Fig. 21.8).

Following the procedure the patient is admitted for overnight observation. The next day, an upper GI contrast study confirms adequate pyloric opening and absence of a leak. A high dose proton pump inhibitor (PPI) is continued for a period of 6 weeks after the procedure.

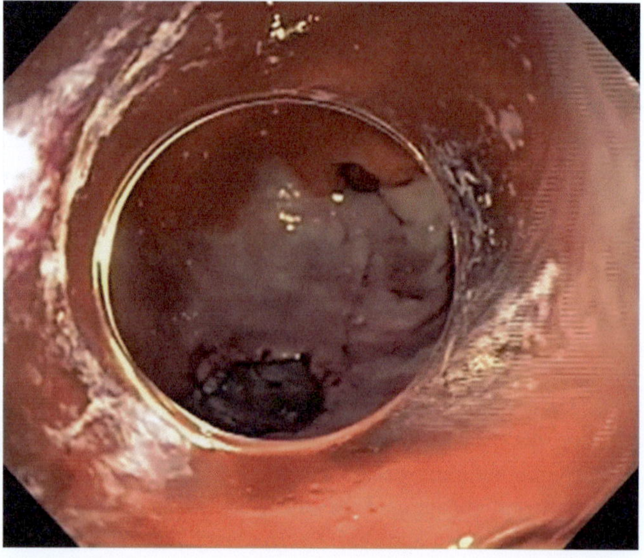

Fig. 21.8 Per-oral endoscopic pyloroplasty after completion of submucosal tunnel

Conclusions

Although our understanding of the complex mechanisms responsible for the recent epidemic of gastroparesis is incomplete, it is important for the foregut specialist to recognize this chronic debilitating disease and how it complicated antireflux surgery. Depending on their pre-operative work-up and symptomatology, the operative candidate may benefit from a gastroparesis treatment, GERD treatment, or a combined approach. A tailored approach is necessary in choosing the best operative approach in the individual patient suffering from gastroparesis and GERD.

References

1. Enweluzo C. Gastroparesis: a review of current and emerging treatment options. Clin Exp Gastroenterol. 2013;5(6):161–5.
2. Khajanchee YS, Dunst CM, Swanstrom LL. Outcomes of Nissen fundoplication in patients with gastroesophageal reflux disease and delayed gastric emptying. Arch Surg. 2009;144(9):823–8.
3. Tougas G, Eaker EY, Abell TL, et al. Assessment of gastric emptying using a low fat meal: establishment of international control values. Am J Gastroenterol. 2000;95:1456–62.
4. Oh JH¹, Pasricha PJ. Recent advances in the pathophysiology and treatment of gastroparesis. J Neurogastroenterol Motil. 2013;19(1): 18-24. doi: 10.5056/jnm.2013.19.1.18. Epub 2013 Jan 8.
5. Hyett B, Martinez FJ, Gill BM, Mehra S, Lembo A, Kelly CP, Leffler DA. Delayed radionucleotide gastric emptying studies predict morbidity in diabetics with symptoms of gastroparesis. Gastroenterology. 2009;137(2):445–52.
6. Bielefeldt K, Gastroparesis: concepts, controversies, and challenges. Scientifica Volume 2012, Article ID 424802.
7. Parkman HP. Pathophysiologic relationship between gastroparesis and GERD. Gastroenterol Hepatol. 2009;5(10):4–16.
8. McCallum RW, Berkowitz DM, Lerner E. Gastric emptying in patients with gastroesophageal reflux. Gastroenterology. 1981; 80(2):285–91.
9. Alexander F, Wyllie R, Jirousek K, Secic M, Porvasnik S. Delayed gastric emptying affects outcome of Nissen fundoplication in neurologically impaired children. Surgery. 1997;122(4):690–7. discussion 697–698.
10. Dunn JC, Lai EC, Webber MM, Ament ME, Fonkalsrud EW. Long-term quantitative results following fundoplication and antroplasty for gastroesophageal reflux and delayed gastric emptying in children. Am J Surg. 1998;175(1):27–9.
11. Brown RA, Wynchank S, Rode H, Millar AJ, Mann MD. Is a gastric drainage procedure necessary at the time of antireflux surgery? J Pediatr Gastroenterol Nutr. 1997;25(4):377–80.
12. Hinder RA, Stein HJ, Bremner CG, DeMeester TR. Relationship of a satisfactory outcome to normalization of delayed gastric emptying after Nissen fundoplication. Ann Surg. 1989;210(4):458–64. discussion 464-465.
13. Maddern GJ, Jamieson GG, Chatterton BE, Collins PJ. Is there an association between failed antireflux procedures and delayed gastric emptying? Ann Surg. 1985;202(2):162–5.
14. Bromer MQ, Friedenberg F, Miller LS, Fisher RS, Swartz K, Parkman HP. Endoscopic pyloric injection of botulinum toxin A for the treatment of refractory gastroparesis. Gastrointest Endosc. 2005;61:833–9.

15. Ezzeddine D, Jit R, Katz N, Gopalswamy N, Bhutani MS. Pyloric injection of botulinum toxin for treatment of diabetic gastroparesis. Gastrointest Endosc. 2002;55:920–3.

16. Miller LS, Szych GA, Kantor SB, et al. Treatment of idiopathic gastroparesis with injection of botulinum toxin into the pyloric sphincter muscle. Am J Gastroenterol. 2002;97:1653–60.

17. Van Sickle KR, McClusky DA, Swafford VA, Smith CD. Delayed gastric emptying in patients undergoing antireflux surgery: analysis of a treatment algorithm. J Laparoendosc Adv Surg Tech A. 2007;17(1):7–11.

18. Hibbard ML, Dunst CM, Swanström LL. Laparoscopic and endoscopic pyloroplasty for gastroparesis results in sustained symptom improvement. J Gastrointest Surg. 2011;15(9):1513–9.

19. Toro JP[1], Lytle NW[1], Patel AD[1], Davis SS Jr[1], Christie JA[1], Waring JP[1], Sweeney JF[1], Lin E[2]. Efficacy of laparoscopic pyloroplasty for the treatment of gastroparesis. J Am Coll Surg. 2014;218(4):652–60. doi: 10.1016/j.jamcollsurg.2013.12.024. Epub 2013 Dec 24.

20. Perkel M, Moore C, Hersh T, Davidson E. Metoclopramide therapy in patients with delayed gastric emptying: a randomized, double-blind study. Dig Dis Sci. 1979;24:662–6.

21. Tonini M, Cipollina L, Poluzzi E, Crema F, Corazza GR, De Ponti F. Review article: clinical implications of enteric and central D2 receptor blockade by antidopaminergic gastrointestinal prokinetics. Aliment Pharmacol Ther. 2004;19:379–90.

22. Shlomovitz E, Pescarus R, Cassera MA, Sharata AM, Reavis KM, Dunst CM, Swanström LL. http://www.ncbi.nlm.nih.gov/pubmed/25106716. Early human experience with per-oral endoscopic pyloromyotomy (POP). Surg Endosc. 2014. [Epub ahead of print] PMID: 25106716.

23. Ziessman HA, Bonta DV, Goetze S, Ravich WJ. Experience with a simplified, standardized 4-hour gastric-emptying protocol. J Nucl Med. 2007;48(4):568–72.

24. Bais JE, Samsom M, Boudesteijn EA, van Rijk PP, Akkermans LM, Gooszen HG. Impact of delayed gastric emptying on the outcome of antireflux surgery. Ann Surg. 2001;234(2):139–46.

25. Farrell TM, Richardson WS, Halkar R, et al. Nissen fundoplication improves gastric motility in patients with delayed gastric emptying. Surg Endosc. 2001;15(3):271–4.

26. Hui TT[1], Fass SM, Giurgiu DI, Iida A, Takagi S, Phillips EH. Gastroesophageal disease and nausea: does fundoplication help or hurt? Arch Surg. 2000;135(5):545–9.

27. Pacilli M[1], Pierro A, Lindley KJ, Curry JI, Eaton S. Gastric emptying is accelerated following laparoscopic Nissen fundoplication. Eur J Pediatr Surg. 2008;18(6):395–7. doi: 10.1055/s-2008-1038919. Epub 2008 Nov 27.

28. Schwizer W, Hinder RA, DeMeester TR. Does delayed gastric emptying contribute to gastroesophageal reflux disease? Am J Surg. 1989;157(1):74–81.

29. Masqusi S, Velanovich V. Pyloroplasty with fundoplication in the treatment of combined gastroesophageal reflux disease and bloating. World J Surg. 2007;31(2):332–6.

30. Camilleri M, et al. What are the important subsets of gastroparesis? Neurogastroenterol Motil. 2012;24:597–603.

31. Fontana RJ, et al. Jejunostomy tube placement in refractory diabetic gastroparesis: a retrospective review. Am J Gastroenterol. 1996;91(10):2174–8.

32. Camilleri M, et al. Clinical guideline: management of gastroparesis. Am J Gastroenterol. 2013;108(1):18–37.

33. Tack J, Bisschops R, Sarnelli G. Pathophysiology and treatment of functional dyspepsia. Gastroenterology. 2004;127(4):1239–55.

34. Sarnelli G, et al. Symptoms associated with impaired gastric emptying of solids and liquids in functional dyspepsia. Am J Gastroenterol. 2003;98(4):783–8.

35. Forstner-Barthell AW, Murr MM, Nitecki S, Camilleri M, Prather CM, Kelly KA, Sarr MG. Near-total completion gastrectomy for severe postvagotomy gastric stasis: analysis of early and long-term results in 62 patients. J Gastrointest Surg. 1999;3(1):15–21.

36. Watkins PJ, Buxton-Thomas MS, Howard ER. Long-term outcome after gastrectomy for intractable diabetic gastroparesis. Diabet Med. 2003;20(1):58–63. PubMed PMID: 12519321.

37. Speicher JE, Thirlby RC, Burggraaf J, Kelly C, Levasseur S. Results of completion gastrectomies in 44 patients with postsurgical gastric atony. J Gastrointest Surg. 2009;13(5):874–80. doi:10.1007/s11605-009-0821-y. Epub 2009 Feb 18. PubMed PMID: 19224297.

38. Bhayani N, Sharata A, Dunst CM, Kurian AA, Reavis KM, Swanstrom LL. End of the road for a dysfunctional end-organ: laparoscopic gastrectomy for *Refractory Gastroparesis* Presented at DDW May 5th; 2014 Chicago.

39. Parkman HP, Yates KP, Hasler WL, Nguyan L, Pasricha PJ, Snape WJ, Farrugia G, Calles J, Koch KL, Abell TL, McCallum RW, Petito D, Parrish CR, Duffy F, Lee L, Unalp-Arida A, Tonascia J, Hamilton F, NIDDK Gastroparesis Clinical Research Consortium. Dietary intake and nutritional deficiencies in patients with diabetic or idiopathic gastroparesis. Gastroenterology 2011;141(2):486–98, 498. e1-7. doi: 10.1053/j.gastro.2011.04.045. Epub 2011 Apr 28. PubMed PMID: 21684286; PubMed Central PMCID: PMC3499101.

40. McCallum RW, Lin Z, Forster J, Roeser K, Hou Q, Sarosiek I. Gastric electrical stimulation improves outcomes of patients with gastroparesis for up to 10 years. Clin Gastroenterol Hepatol. 2011;9(4):314–9.e1. doi: 10.1016/j.cgh.2010.12.013. Epub 2010 Dec 23. PubMed PMID: 21185396.

41. Zehetner J[1], Ravari F, Ayazi S, Skibba A, Darehzereshki A, Pelipad D, Mason RJ, Katkhouda N, Lipham JC, Minimally invasive surgical approach for the treatment of gastroparesis. Surg Endosc. 2013;27(1):61–6. doi: 10.1007/s00464-012-2407-0. Epub 2012 Jun 30.

42. Park P, Bergström M, Ikeda K, Fritscher-Ravens A, Mosse S, Kochman M, et al. Endoscopic pyloroplasty with full-thickness transgastric and transduodenal myotomy with sutured closure. Gastrointest Endosc. 2007;66(1):116–20.

43. Kawai M, et al. Endoscopic pyloromyotomy: a new concept of minimally invasive surgery for pyloric stenosis. Endoscopy. 2012;44(2):169–73.

44. Khashab MA, et al. Gastric peroral endoscopic myotomy for refractory gastroparesis: first human endoscopic pyloromyotomy (with video). Gastrointest Endosc. 2013;78(5):764–8.

45. Ibarguen-Secchia E. Endoscopic pyloromyotomy for congenital pyloric stenosis. Gastrointest Endosc. 2005;61(4):598–600.

46. Shlomovitz E, Pescarus R, Maria A. Cassera, Sharata A, Reavis KM, Dunst CM, Swanstrom LL. Early human experience with Per-Oral Endoscopic Pyloromyotomy (POP). Presented at SAGES; 2014.

47. Swanström LL, Rieder E, Dunst CM. A stepwise approach and early clinical experience in peroral endoscopic myotomy for the treatment of achalasia and esophageal motility disorders. J Am Coll Surg. 2011;213(6):751–6.

48. Swanstrom LL, Kurian A, Dunst CM, Sharata A, Bhayani N, Rieder E. Long-term outcomes of an endoscopic myotomy for achalasia: the POEM procedure. Ann Surg. 2012;256(4):659–67.

Reoperative Antireflux Surgery

C. Daniel Smith

Introduction

Over the past several decades, antireflux surgery has promised to cure GERD and eliminate the need for antisecretory medications. Many studies have documented the effectiveness of antireflux surgery in correcting GERD and reducing or eliminating the need for antisecretory medication like proton pump inhibitors (PPIs) [1]. Additionally, PPIs have been found to be ineffective at completely controlling GERD symptoms in a significant number of patients, and new problems can develop in patients taking PPIs long-term, including an increased risk of hip fractures, C. difficile colitis, cardiac disease, and pneumonia [2–5]. With this, one would expect that antireflux surgery would be widely applied with very little need for a chapter focused on failure of antireflux surgery.

In fact, what has happened over the past few decades is that the use of antireflux surgery has declined and the use of antisecretories has risen. Despite the promise of an effective operation we have often delivered an ineffective antireflux operation or one that fails. Failure of antireflux surgery, defined as the need to perform another operation due to failure to control GERD, or to correct a new problem, often the result of the antireflux operation itself, ranges from 4 to 40 %[1, 6–20]. A failure rate with such a broad range suggests a few things. First, we have not standardized the patient selection, choice of operation, and surgical technique to deliver a reliable and predictable outcome. Additionally, this indicates that there will always be patients who fail their operation and will need remediation or a redo. Understanding the causes and patterns of failure, presenting symptoms and work-up, and approach for reoperative antireflux surgery can result in continued good outcomes from this intervention. This chapter will cover each of these aspects of reoperative antireflux surgery and offer an algorithm for management.

Need for Reoperation and Patterns of Failure

Before embarking on the details of how to identify, work-up, and manage a patient who might need reoperative antireflux surgery, it is first important to understand the causes of failure and recognize the patterns of failure. Understanding the nature and pattern of failure may help guide all aspects of the management of these patients.

Antireflux surgery comprises a large set of procedures (see Table 22.1). The concepts presented in this chapter can generalize to nearly all of these procedures. For the most part, esophagogastric fundoplication—either the total or partial fundoplication—comprise the majority of antireflux procedures performed today. Patterns of failure unique to some of the less common antireflux procedures including endoluminal techniques will be addressed toward the end of this chapter.

When considering why an antireflux operation has failed, broadly speaking, there are three reasons that an operation will fail to control a patient's symptoms and/or GERD.

1. Errors in work-up or patient selection
2. Errors in operative management
3. Natural history of the particular antireflux operation or condition being treated

If no. 1 and 2 above can be standardized, and the natural history of the operation and condition being managed is understood, then predictable outcomes should result. For example, from large series from high volume surgeons and centers, we know that in the setting of clinically and objectively confirmed GERD, with symptoms that are PPI responsive, normal esophageal motility, a body mass index less than 35, and no other confounding conditions, one would expect a 90 % likelihood that 10 years after surgery a patient

C.D. Smith, MD, FACS (✉)
Department of Surgery, Mayo Clinic Florida,
4500 San Pable Road, Jacksonville, FL 32224, USA
e-mail: smith.c.daniel@mayo.edu

L.L. Swanstrom and C.M. Dunst (eds.), *Antireflux Surgery*,
DOI 10.1007/978-1-4939-1749-5_22, © Springer New York 2015

will have continued control of their GERD, both objectively and symptomatically [1].

Regardless of which of the three reasons outlined above underlies the need for reoperation, defining and understanding the pattern of failure will guide subsequent management. One typically sees failure of a fundoplication in a few distinct patterns. These are outlined in Table 22.2 and Figs. 22.1 and 22.2. When considering these reasons for failure, hiatal hernia is the most common cause (44 % of cases). Wrap disruption or breakdown is the next leading cause accounting for 16 % of failures. Slipped wraps account for 11.7 % of failure, and finally, wraps improperly positioned at the time of their initial construction are found in 3.9 % of cases. Wrap or crural stenosis is a rare cause of failure and often times hard to determine as a primary etiology of failure.

If mesh was used at the initial operation, a distinctly different pattern of failure and management strategy is needed. This is discussed later in this chapter.

Presentation and Work-up

Early Versus Late Failure

Failure of an antireflux operation can occur immediately or many years later. Characterizing the failure as early or late is the beginning point in determining the possible reason for failure and will help guide a thoughtful investigation and subsequent management.

Table 22.1 Examples of antireflux procedures

Surgical fundoplication
360° Fundoplication (Nissen Fundoplication)
180° Posterior fundoplication (Toupet Fundoplication)
180° Anterior fundoplication (Dor Fundoplication)
Posterior gastropexy (Hill Procedure)
Transthoracic posterior plication (Belsey Procedure)
Endoluminal procedures
Radiofrequency application to LES (Stretta)
Transoral Incisionless Fundoplication (TIF)

Table 22.2 Patterns of failure

Wrap disruption or loosening
Wrap migration or slip
Hiatal herniation or re-herniation
Wrap or crural stenosis
Wrap too loose or misplaced at the initial operation

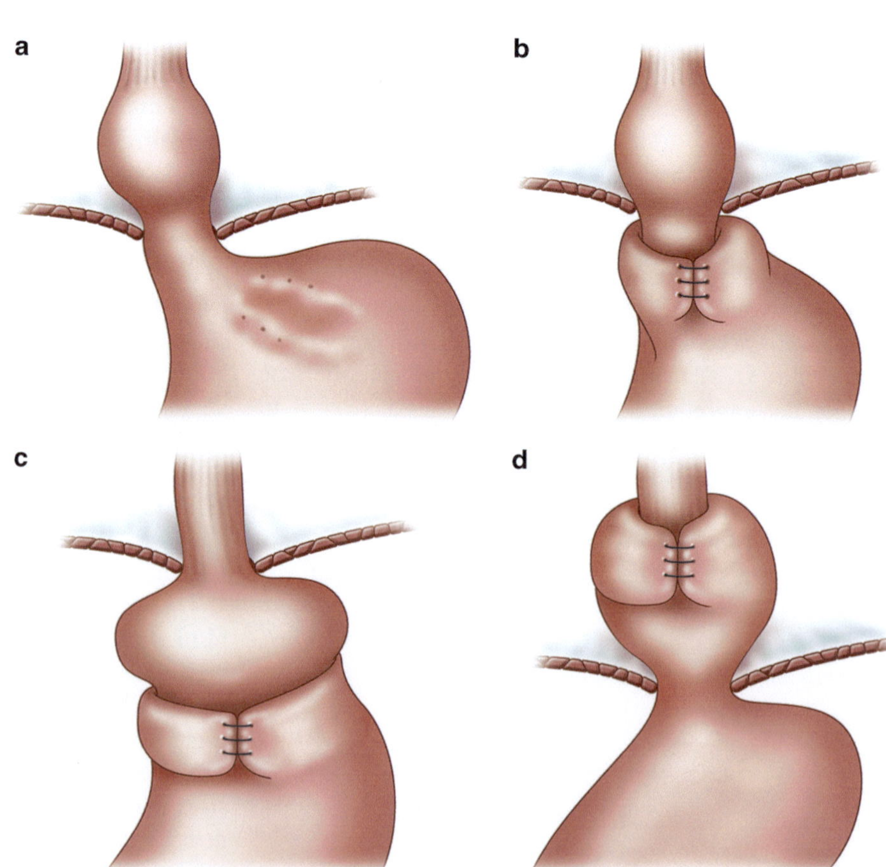

Fig. 22.1 Common anatomic patterns of antireflux surgery failure: (**a**) fundoplication disruption, (**b**) tight fundoplication or crural stenosis, (**c**) slipped fundoplication, (**d**) hiatal herniation

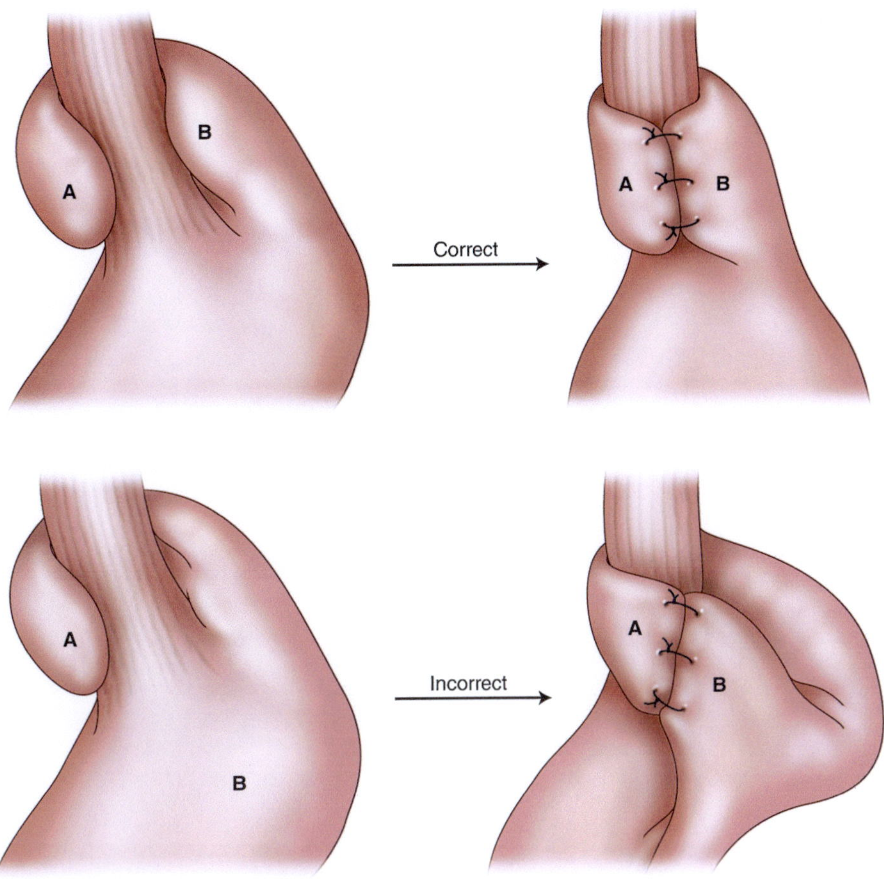

Fig. 22.2 Illustration of incorrectly created fundoplication compared to correct creation

Early Failure

Most commonly, early failure is the result of early postoperative nausea and vomiting, or some other trauma causing an abrupt rise in intra-abdominal pressure. The abrupt increase in intra-abdominal pressure that accompanies something like violent retching or a fall striking one's abdomen is thought to either tear stitches or tissue resulting in immediate wrap disruption or slip, or alternatively, breakdown of the cruroplasty and immediate herniation or the wrap or abdominal content above the diaphragm.

If a patient experiences such an event within a few days of surgery it is recommended to immediately obtain a contrast swallow, and if an anatomic abnormality is found to immediately return the patient to the operating room. Within the first few days from surgery it is usually an easy matter to re-wrap a disrupted or migrated wrap, or pull a herniated wrap back into the abdomen and redo a cruroplasty. Not uncommonly, if the crura have become disrupted, especially if a hiatal hernia repair accompanied the first procedure, a more advanced technique such as a remote diaphragm release to effect crural mobilization and mesh repair of the diaphragmatic defect may be needed (Figs. 22.3 and 22.4). If acute disruption occurs more than a few days after the operation, it is best to

wait 6–12 weeks before attempting to correct the anatomic problem. If one attempts to intervene sooner than this you are more likely to encounter dense adhesions and an extremely difficult dissection with accompanying risk of injury to the stomach, esophagus, or vagus nerve(s). Also, if attempting a redo in this early timeframe it is best to have considerable experience with reoperative antireflux surgery since these can be some of the most difficult redos to complete safely and attain good results.

Another more rare cause of immediate failure is a technical error during surgery such as a misplaced wrap, a tight cruroplasty, or a tight wrap. Technical failure at the time of surgery is typically not appreciated until months later when a pattern of unremitting pain, nausea, vomiting, or dysphagia that started immediately postoperatively is further investigated and an anatomic abnormality found. These reasons for failure are unlikely to be identified by the surgeon who performed the first operation, but rather, when a patient or the original surgeon seeks a second opinion. As a subsequent surgeon getting involved in a patient's care, while technical error as the reason for failure might be suspected, it is crucial to not opine as to this possibility since it cannot be known for certain, and patients may wrongfully attribute failure to an error

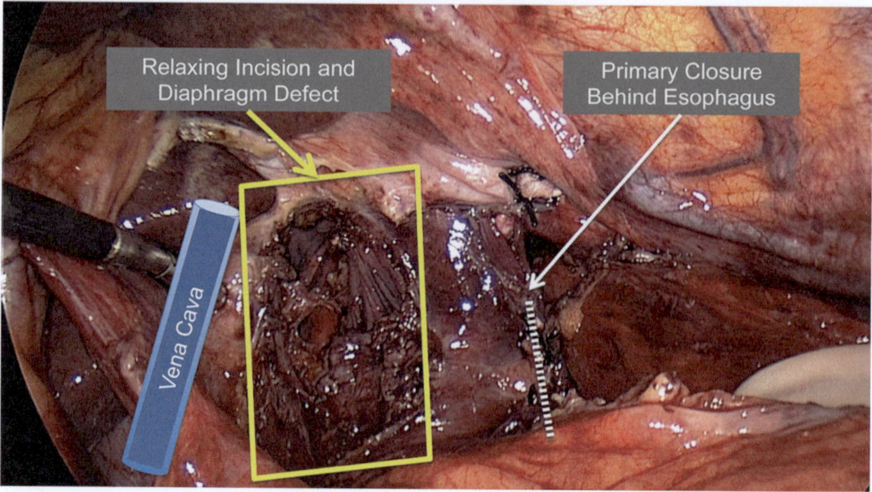

Fig. 22.3 Intraoperative photo depicting primary closure of esophageal hiatus with relaxing incision in diaphragm for hiatal reconstruction of large hiatal defect

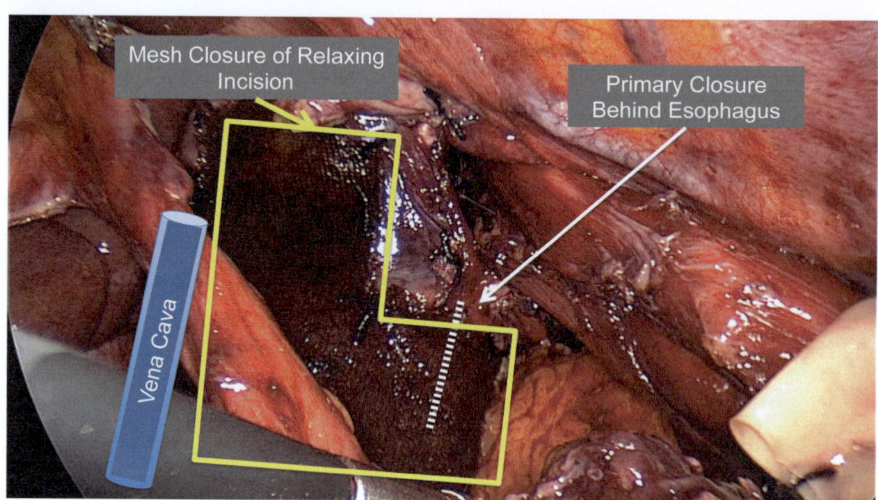

Fig. 22.4 Intraoperative photo depicting primary closure of esophageal hiatus with mesh patch of diaphragm relaxing incision

and pursue litigation. Only an undisputable and egregious error at the time of the first surgery would warrant such a path.

Finally, initial misdiagnosis or poor patient/procedure selection can lead to early failure. Unfortunately, there are still patients undergoing antireflux surgery without objective confirmation of GERD, misinterpretation of esophageal motility studies leading to wraps when achalasia is the diagnosis, and aggressive management of the esophageal hiatus in the absence of significant hiatal hernia, i.e., routine use of mesh hiatoplasty. In all cases of early failure, regardless of cause, if the problem is not found within a few days of the first operation, it is best to wait at least 3 months or longer before undertaking a redo.

Late Failure

More commonly, antireflux operations fail late with late failure defined as a patient who has had an initial good result with more than 90 days of resolution, or near resolution of symptoms, and no new foregut symptoms, who then develops recurrent or new symptoms. This definition is meant to isolate late failures from those that are immediate but have a later presentation. The majority of late failures are due either to wrap disruption, hiatal hernia, or to esophageal outlet issues from a restricted esophageal outlet (scarring, twisting, or crural stenosis).

Symptoms of Failure

Common symptoms of failure of an antireflux operation are outlined in Table 22.3. Of these, recurrent GERD is the most common (59 %), and dysphagia (31 %) the next most common. While these symptoms can occur with any or all of the patterns of failure, there are patterns of symptoms that correlate highly with a given mechanism of failure (Fig. 22.5). Gross anatomic abnormalities such as hiatal hernia or severe wrap/crural stenosis are more likely to present with symptoms related to poor esophageal transit and emptying. These symptoms commonly include dysphagia, chest pain, and regurgitation. The wrap that has loosened or come undone more commonly presents with recurrent GERD symptoms, often identical to those being experienced before the first antireflux procedure. Commonly this includes typical symptoms such as heartburn, regurgitation, and chest pain, but can also be more atypical symptoms like cough, laryngitis, or asthma. Again, the relationship and similarity of symptoms to those before the initial operation is strongly predictive of wrap disruption or loosening. Finally, the patient with a slipped wrap will often have a broad constellation of symptoms with more prevalence of nausea and epigastric pain than the other presentations. Overall, a favorable response to antisecretories and postural regurgitation can provide additional clues as to the possibility of wrap loosening or incompetence, while poor tolerance of foods of a more heavy consistency and weight loss can often predict hiatal herniation or esophageal outlet issues. Improvement with dilation also supports esophageal outlet restriction. Failure of symptoms to respond to any intervention including antisecretory medication or dilation is more likely with wrap slippage.

A confounding variable in presenting symptoms is the patient who will present with early postprandial bloating or meal induced diarrhea. In these cases one should be suspicious of dysfunctional gastric emptying as a result of vagal nerve injury or inflammation. Delayed gastric emptying and/or dumping can be a hallmark of vagal nerve injury and often is associated with antireflux surgery. This symptom complex in the absence of an obvious anatomic abnormality or a positive pH test should lead one to pursue further work-up rather than a redo antireflux operation. More surgery at the esophageal hiatus or gastroesophageal junction is unlikely to improve gastric function and may worsen the situation with potential vagal nerve injury and re-injury.

Work-up

When considering testing for suspected antireflux surgery failure, it helps to think about the investigations aimed at securing a diagnosis or reason for failure versus testing needed for planning a redo operation. An algorithm for the work-up of patients suspected to have failed a prior antireflux operation is shown in Fig. 22.6.

Establishing the Diagnosis

In pursuit of a diagnosis of failure, the work-up should start with an anatomic assessment. This usually includes an upper endoscopy (EGD) and contrast esophagram. Often, a contrast esophagram is all that is needed to identify the pattern of failure. Figure 22.7 depicts the esophagram findings corresponding to the various patterns of failure. Alternatively, an EGD may clearly show an anatomic abnormality, but since an upper endoscopy is often performed by a gastroenterologist who may not be familiar with the endoscopic findings of failure, we often find an esophagram the most helpful for the surgeon to interpret, or an endoscopy performed by a

Table 22.3 Common symptoms of antireflux surgery failure

Heartburn
Chest pain
Regurgitation
Dysphagia
Nausea
Bloating
Shortness of Breath (SOB)
Aspiration

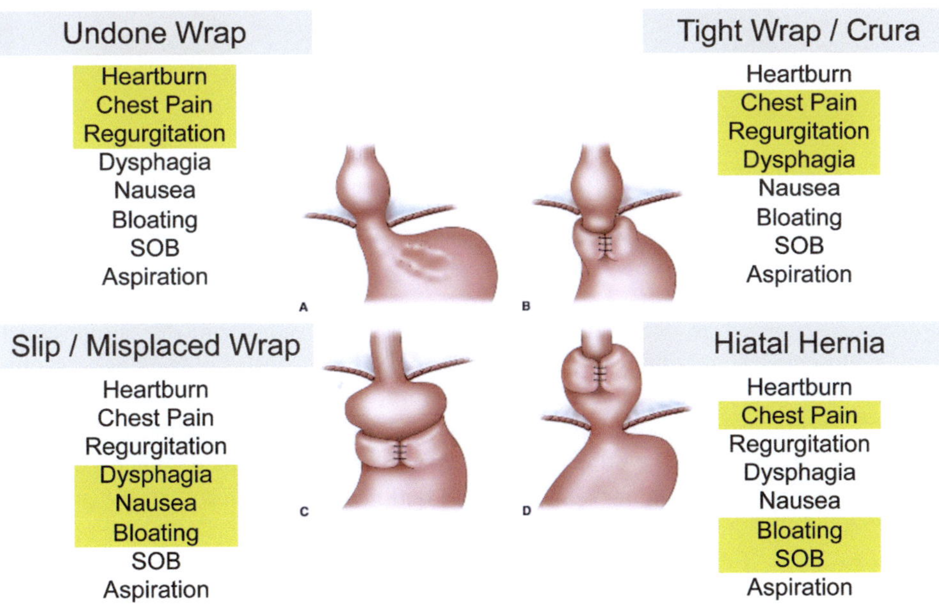

Fig. 22.5 Symptoms of antireflux surgery failure correlated with anatomic pattern of failure

Fig. 22.6 Flow chart of work-up for possible antireflux surgery failure

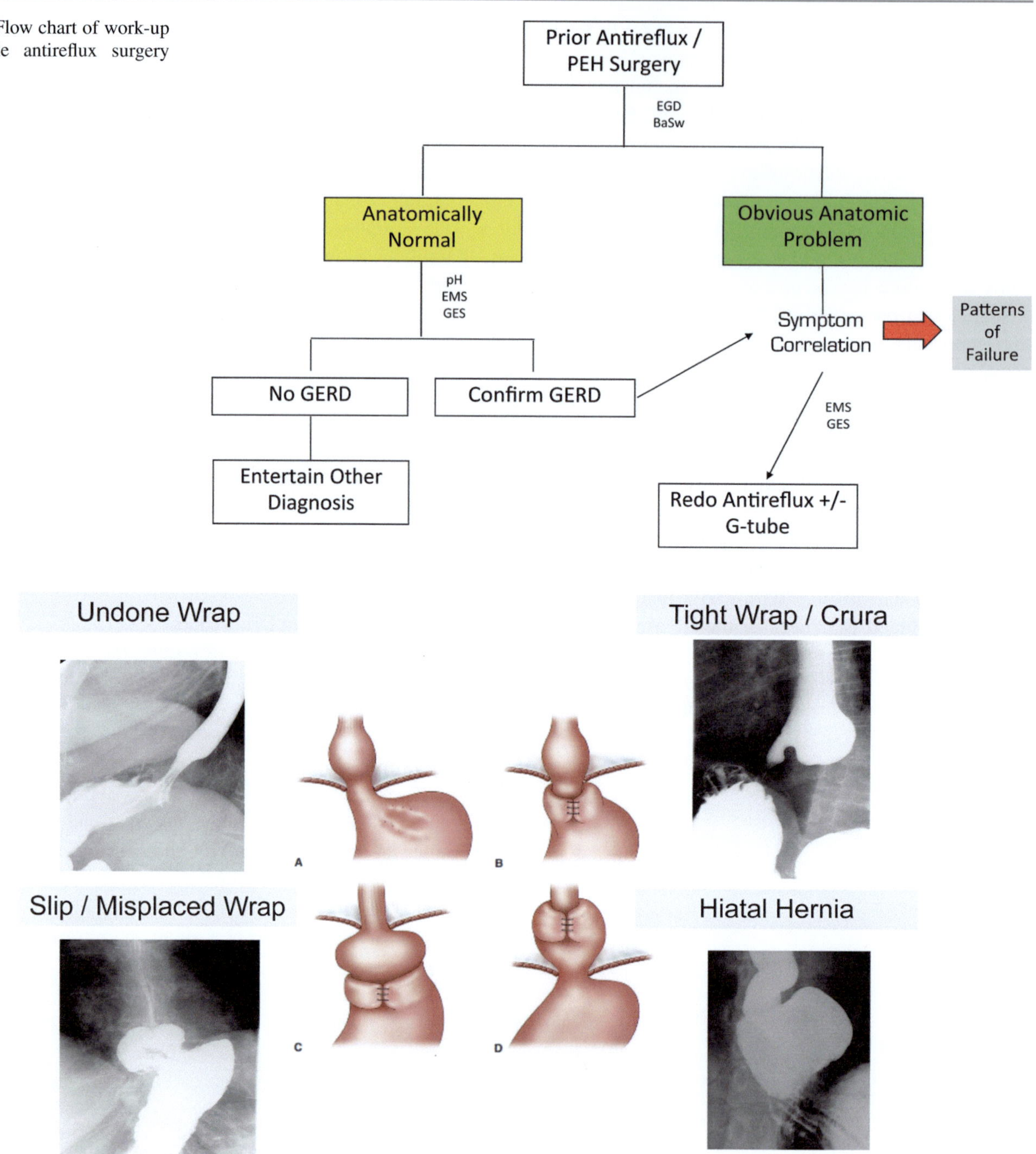

Fig. 22.7 Contrast swallow examples for each common anatomic pattern of failure

surgeon experienced in reoperative foregut surgery and upper endoscopy. If relying on endoscopy performed by someone other than the foregut surgeon it is helpful to have photos from the endoscopy available, especially retroflex views where abnormal findings are often most readily seen. The common endoscopic findings of failure are outlined in Table 22.4.

In many cases, if the presenting symptoms correlate with findings on an esophagram or EGD this is all that is needed to diagnosis failure and the need for reoperation. If these tests fail to identify an obvious anatomic cause for a patient's symptoms then further testing is required. If recurrent GERD is the dominant presentation then pH testing should be obtained. When pursuing pH testing it is critical to obtain this test with the patient off of all antisecretory medication. Increasingly, pH tests are being obtained while on medication, especially with the increased use of impedance pH testing. While this approach may reveal non-acid reflux,

Table 22.4 Endoscopic findings of failed antireflux operation

Viewing location	Findings (pattern of failure)
Retroflex view of distal esophagus	Gastric folds extending into wrap (slipped/misplaced fundoplication)
	Esophagogastric junction does not hug scope (loose or undone fundoplication)
	Gastric mucosa extending above hiatal indentation (hiatal hernia)
Forward view of distal esophagus	Narrowing that doesn't accept scope (tight wrap or crural stenosis)
	Esophagitis/esophageal ulcers (loose or undone fundoplication)
	Constriction on proximal stomach below constriction of wrap (hiatal hernia)
	Constriction of wrap distal to esophagogastric junction (slipped or misplaced wrap)

one should be very cautious about relying entirely on this test to decide about offering a reoperation. It is my strong recommendation that a pH off medication be obtained. If this confirms pathologic acid reflux the complexity of offering a redo based on the primary diagnosis of non-acid reflux can be avoided.

Planning for Operative Management

With a diagnosis of antireflux surgery failure secured, and a correctable pattern of failure identified, further testing may be indicated to help plan the most effective reoperative strategy. During a redo one must not only correct the primary anatomic problem, but also take steps to prevent another failure. This may include modifying the type of fundoplication or adjunct procedures to mitigate future complications that could lead to failure. The most common conditions associated with failure that need to be investigated are esophageal motility problems and impairment in gastric emptying. With this in mind, all patients should undergo an esophageal motility study and a gastric emptying study before being returned to an operating room for redo surgery.

Impairment in esophageal motility may indicate the need for a partial, 270° fundoplication, rather than a 360° fundoplication. Classically a partial fundoplication should be considered if normal esophageal peristalsis is present in less than 70 % of swallows, or esophageal body contraction pressure is less than 30 mmHg. A newer technique, high-resolution manometry (HRM), is providing a more detailed analysis of esophageal motor and propulsive function. The additional data collected with HRM often results in a diagnosis of "ineffective esophageal motility" (IEM) based on the Chicago classification of esophageal motility. This new label of IEM is poorly understood in the context of reoperative antireflux surgery. Until the clinical relevance of the IEM label is better understood, using the body pressure and percent peristalsis for decision-making about full or partial fundoplication is recommended.

Delayed gastric emptying may require the addition of a gastrostomy tube to provide gastric decompression in the early postoperative period thereby preventing gastric distension induced crural or wrap disruption, or performance of a concomitant pyloroplasty. Pyloroplasty is indicated for patients whose gastric ½ emptying time is greater than twice normal. Those with less severe delayed gastric emptying may respond to anatomic correction alone and thereby avoid the risk of long-term diarrhea that can occur after pyloroplasty.

A possible exception to obtaining an esophageal motility study is the patient with a large recurrent hiatal hernia. It can be very difficult to obtain a motility study in these patients due to the distorted esophageal anatomy, and interpreting the results can be difficult.

Operative Management

Reoperative antireflux surgery can be some of the more challenging foregut operations undertaken by a surgeon. Understanding the likely cause of failure aids in preoperative planning and approach, and intraoperative strategy. For example, if the cause of failure is hiatal hernia, especially recurrent hiatal hernia, one should be prepared to undertake an extensive mediastinal dissection of the esophagus to achieve adequate intra-abdominal esophageal length, even being prepared to perform a Collis gastroplasty for esophageal lengthening. When dealing with multiple prior failures, positioning for an open approach and possible thoracoabdominal incision is prudent. Alternatively, managing late failure for a wrap that has loosened would be unlikely to require extensive dissection or include direct thoracic access.

Operative Approach

For a skilled laparoscopic surgeon, almost all redos can be approached laparoscopically. Prior foregut surgery rarely results in adhesions or scarring making laparoscopic abdominal access impossible, and the magnification and facilitated exposure afforded by laparoscopy in the upper abdomen make a laparoscopic approach to these difficult cases preferred. I will in nearly all circumstances start laparoscopically. Early conversion to an open approach is more likely in the following situations:

- Multiple prior foregut procedures, especially prior open repairs
- Hiatal hernia with a significant amount of the stomach incarcerated in chest, especially if mesh was used in prior operations
- Prior operations that were complicated by postoperative leak, fistula, or early reoperation.

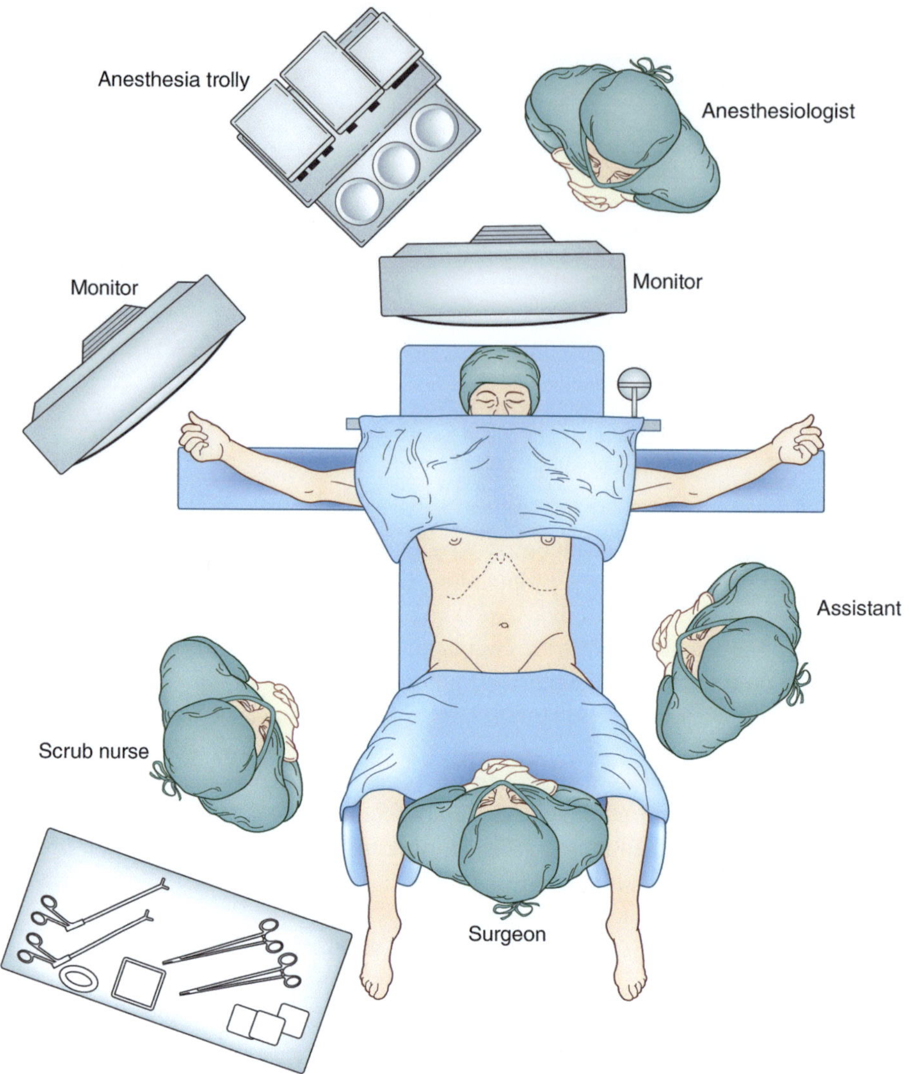

Fig. 22.8 Patient positioning for reoperative antireflux operation

In these situations where one may predict a higher likelihood of conversion, it is prudent to be prepared for not only an open approach, but also even a thoracoabdominal approach. Rather than position the patient for possible thoracoabdominal approach and compromise the initial laparoscopic approach (thoracoabdominal approach requires positioning the patient in semi-lateral decubitus position) I prefer to re-prep and drape if conversion to an open thoracoabdominal approach is needed.

In general, a split leg approach is used in nearly all foregut surgery (Fig. 22.8). If possible conversion to an open approach is anticipated, one arm should be tucked so that a table mounted retraction system can be secured at the patient's shoulder well away from the surgeons' standing position at the patient's side for open access.

Intraoperative Management

It is helpful to follow a standardized approach to reoperative antireflux surgery. Three essential elements are a part of every redo: (1) identification and exposure of relevant hiatal anatomy, (2) taking apart previous fundoplication and/or prior hiatal hernia repair, and 3) reconstruction of the esophageal hiatus and fundoplication. To achieve this, a thorough knowledge of foregut and peri-hiatal anatomy is essential since the anatomy is almost always obscured by adhesions and scarring that conceals and distorts the anatomy. Familiarity with tissue planes, both normal and those altered by previous surgery is critical. Due to this, early dissection is best effected in anatomically safe areas where the risk of significant injury is less likely. Progressing from known and recognized anatomy to unclear anatomy, starting with the safest area for dissection to the more hazardous, should result in developing the foregut and peri-hiatal anatomy without significant injury to the esophagus, stomach, crura, and surround structures. This is critical for preserving the integrity of the anatomy for subsequent reconstruction. The worse scenario one can encounter in reoperative antireflux surgery is injuring structures in the course of the dissection to identify anatomy and take apart the prior operation such that an adequate reconstruction is not possible. The goal of

Table 22.5 Sequence for successful hiatal dissection

- Start along greater curve of stomach
- Divide any remaining short gastric vessels (ideally none are encountered)
- Expose left crus from base through arch
- Enter mediastinum from left and posterior to hiatal content
- Dissect further proximal into mediastinum and from left to right along plane anterior to aorta until over spine
- Leave left side of hiatus and develop plane between anterior surface of stomach and undersurface of liver to find caudate lobe of liver
- Following lower edge of caudate lobe of liver, expose right crus from base to arch (often need to free wrap adhesions to right crus)
- Enter mediastinum from right and complete retroesophageal window
- Encircle esophagus with Penrose drain to manipulate and control esophagus during rest of mediastinal dissection and esophageal mobilization
- After hiatus completely dissected and esophagus mobilized, take down prior wrap by releasing anterior fusion/sutures and dissect wrap from esophagus
- Intraoperative endoscopy to identify location of squamocolumnar junction (adequate esophageal length) and wrap has been completely taken down (retroflexed view)

Table 22.6 Options for reconstructing gastroesophageal junction

Reconstruction option	Uses
360° fundoplication	Adequate fundus and normal esophageal motility
270° fundoplication	Poor esophageal motility or inadequate fundus for 360° fundoplication
No fundoplication	Tight wrap or hiatal stenosis with inadequate fundus for any fundoplication
Proximal divided gastroplasty/gastrectomy with Roux-en-y gastrojejunostomy	Recurrent GERD following multiple prior antireflux operations and/or no fundus for redo fundoplication with/without injury to gastric cardia/fundus during redo
Esophagogastric myotomy with/without partial fundoplication	Pseudoachalasia
Esophagectomy with gastric pull up or colon interposition	Severe pseudoachalasia with massive esophageal dilation
Roux-en-y esophagojejunostomy	Recurrent GERD following multiple prior antireflux operations and injury to gastric cardia or distal esophagus during redo

reoperative antireflux surgery is to undo the current anatomic aberrancy and then reconstruct correctly. Injuring the tissue during the initial dissection changes the goal from correction to salvage, something that is sometimes unavoidable, but should occur infrequently.

A sequence that allows early, safe identification of the peri-hiatal anatomy, thereby affecting early identification of the esophageal hiatus is outlined in Table 22.5.

In approaching the reconstruction of the esophageal hiatus and redoing the wrap, the reason for failure identified during takedown of the previous wrap should guide the technique of reconstruction. In general, the esophageal hiatal reconstruction should seek to minimize excessive tension on the crural repair. This can often be achieved by clearing the entire intra-abdominal surface of the right crus of any scar or adhesions out to the level of the inferior vena cava, decreasing the intra-abdominal insufflation pressure to 12 mmHg or less, and spacing sutures along the crura so that the depth of the sutures alternate to prevent the crura from splitting along the same bundle of muscle from dorsal to ventral. Alternating pledgeted mattress sutures with simple sutures often gathers sufficient tissue to implement an adequate primary repair. The wrap should be completed around an intraluminal calibrator to assure that the wrap effaces the esophagus circumferentially and is not excessively floppy, and the wrap is clearly at and above the gastroesophageal junction. Put simply, when the prior operation has been safely undone and the anatomy largely returned to its normal state, the operation should progress similar to a primary antireflux procedure. When this is done, the outcomes of reoperative antireflux surgery are very good (see section below). The key to being able to affect an outcome that is nearly comparable to a well-done primary antireflux operation relies on the proper diagnosis and work-up, and operative technique in taking down the prior operation.

At times, undoing the prior operation and returning normal anatomy is not possible. When undertaking these operations one must be prepared to alter the original reconstructive intent based on the final anatomy defined intraoperatively. There are a variety of options for reconstruction based on pre- and intra-operative findings (see Table 22.6). Expertise and experience with all of these techniques of reconstruction are essential if a surgeon is going to optimize outcomes with reoperative antireflux surgery.

Postoperative Care

Postoperative management after reoperative antireflux surgery mirrors the care of any foregut surgery patient. While often overlooked in standard teaching, a few aspects of postoperative care deserve highlighting. First, a preventable cause of antireflux surgery failure is early postoperative retching. The mechanical effect of retching can result in disruption of sutures or tissue comprising the cruroplasty and GEJ reconstruction (wrap or anastomosis), or movement or slippage of the appropriately positioned fundoplication and hiatal GEJ relationship. The two most common reasons for early postoperative retching are nausea and dietary indiscretion. To prevent these from occurring, patients should receive preemptive nausea control and anti-emetics, and be counseled carefully about maintaining a liquid and soft-food diet for at least one month after surgery. The anesthesia team should be engaged even before surgery to help effect anti-nausea precautions, and standing orders for an anti-emetic should be a part of the routine postoperative orders. Instructing patients to ingest only pourable liquids for the first week after surgery provides a simple rule to follow, and then providing a detailed menu of acceptable soft foods for another 3 weeks will help effect compliance with the postoperative diet.

Another area to address postoperatively is progression of activity and resumption of exercise. Again, too rapid advancement to activity that will result in increased intra-abdominal pressure can put sutures and the reconstructed anatomy at risk. A full 30 days of limiting lifting to no more than 30 pounds, and no vigorous exercise during this time provides simple guidelines for patients to follow. In cases where a more extensive dissection and reconstruction were necessary, a longer period of limited activity may be prudent.

Finally, setting appropriate expectations for patients with regard to their overall recovery, diet progression, and resolution of preoperative symptoms will help avoid the desire on a patient's part for early reintervention. For example, most commonly, dysphagia may linger for more than 4 weeks after a redo, and preparing patients for this likelihood will allow them to accept this more readily. A common occurrence when a patient complains of persistent dysphagia is to recommend an endoscopy and dilation. While early dilation may improve the dysphagia, it increases the risk of recurrent GERD eventual antireflux surgery failure, and therefore should be avoided if possible. We reserve dilation within the first 3 months after any antireflux operation for only those patients whose difficulty swallowing makes it hard to handle their own saliva or maintain hydration. In this situation we may reluctantly proceed to an endoscopy with careful dilation. All others are coached through this time, encouraging high-calorie liquids and even supplemental hydration in order to give the edema of the operation time to resolve and dysphagia to improve.

Outcomes of Reoperative Antireflux Surgery

Reoperative antireflux operations can be some of the most challenging foregut operations undertaken. While challenging and requiring advanced laparoscopic skill and foregut surgery expertise, the outcomes of these operations can be comparable to primary antireflux surgery, and in patients suffering with significant and debilitating symptoms, the operations can return patients to a nearly normal quality of life with low morbidity and virtually no mortality.

The most comprehensive summary of outcomes after reoperative antireflux surgery was compiled by van Beek and Soper and published in Surgical Endoscopy in 2011 [21]. Table 22.7 summarizes some of the findings in this paper and includes some more recent data.

Altogether, in the over 1,500 patients who comprised this summary, perioperative mortality was virtually zero, a significant finding considering the complexity of these operations. This is largely the result of the majority of reoperative foregut surgery being performed laparoscopically and by skilled and experienced surgeons. Not surprising, considering these are reoperations, intraoperative complications occurred in approximately 19 % of cases, with perforation of either the esophagus or stomach being the most common intraoperative complication, occurring in 14 % of cases and representing 76 % of the total intraoperative morbidity. Overall, 17 % of patients experienced a postoperative complication, again a very favorable outcome considering the redo nature of these operations. With an average follow-up of 18 months, the weighted success rate, on average, was 81 % (range, 65–100 %), and 82 % of patients were no longer dependent on PPIs at their most recent follow-up. Seventy-four percent of patients were "satisfied" with their outcome or would choose to have the procedure again.

From this literature review, one can conclude that the outcomes and complication rates of reoperative antireflux surgery are similar to those after primary antireflux surgery, and reoperative antireflux surgery is a viable treatment option for patients experiencing a recurrence of esophageal symptoms after an initial procedure.

The patient requiring multiple reoperations for failed antireflux surgery deserves special mention. Figure 22.9 summarizes the results from a large series of redo antireflux surgery highlighting the diminishing success with each subsequent redo [22] (see Fig. 22.10). When undertaking a fourth redo, the failure rate jumps for around 7 % to over

Table 22.7 Outcomes of reoperative antireflux surgery

Author	Date	Number of patients	Mortality	Morbidity (%)	Success (%)	Follow-up (mon)
Vignal [27]	2012	47	0	4.3	78	24
Musunuru [28]	2012	38	0	18.4	63	35
Frantzides [29]	2009	68	0	5.9	86	27
Smith [22]	2005	259	0	15.4	89	14
Khajanchee [30]	2007	176	0	9.8	75	9
Byrne [31]	2005	118	0	1.7	84	12
Legner [32]	2011	106	0	35.8	90	22
Dallemagne [33]	2011	129	0	7	83	75

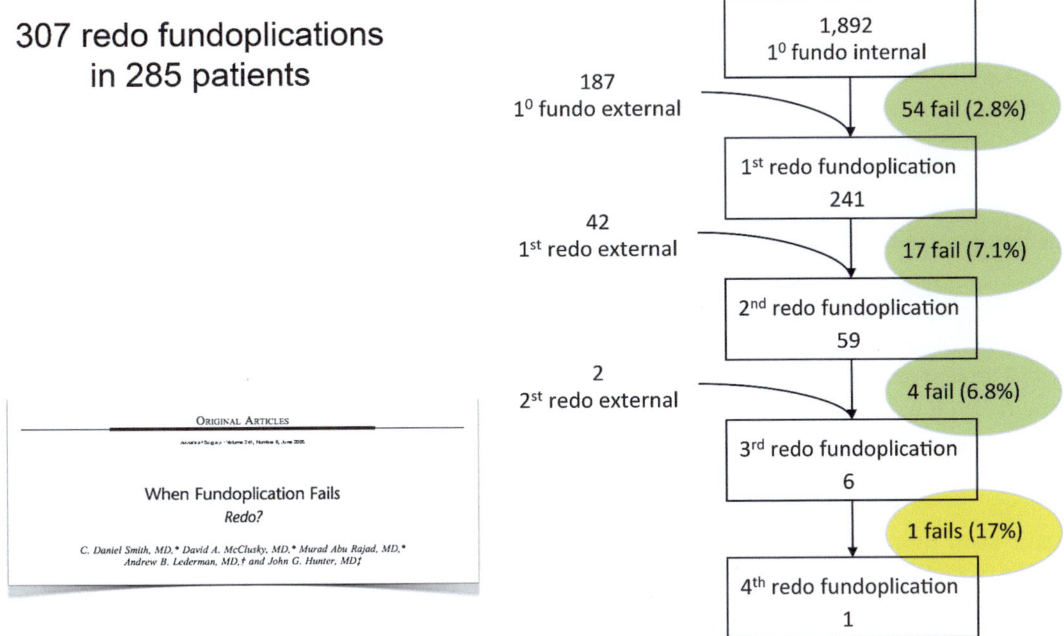

Fig. 22.9 Flow chart outlining results after multiple operations for antireflux surgery failure [22]

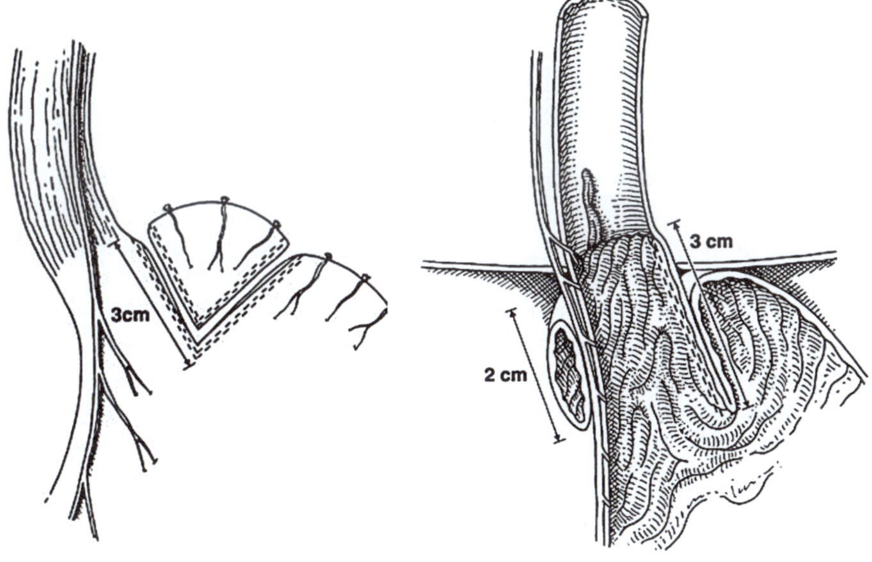

Fig. 22.10 (a) Proper performance of wedge gastrectomy to effect Collis gastroplasty for short esophagus, (b) correct placement of fundoplication on neo-esophagus created out of proximal 2–3 cm of gastric cardia

17 %. From this experience, we will rarely simply undertake a redo after three prior attempts, but rather, will abandon any attempt at redoing the primary operation, and instead, plan to perform a divided gastroplasty and Roux-en-Y reconstruction for recurrent severe GERD, an esophagogastric myotomy for pseudoachalasia or esophagectomy for severe pseudoachalasia with massively dilated esophagus, or an esophagojejunostomy for poor esophageal emptying with severe GEJ distortion, adding a gastrectomy for severe gastroparesis (see Table 22.6).

Special Circumstances

A few special circumstances deserve mention. When mesh has been used for hiatal reconstruction during primary antireflux surgery, the pattern of failure and management strategy is distinctly different than when no mesh has been used. Also, with hiatal hernia being the most common pattern of failure, the possibility of an underlying or acquired short esophagus must be considered. Each of these situations will require the surgeon undertaking a redo to be prepared to both recognize the special condition and manage in a way to minimize future operative failure. Finally, as endoluminal approaches to the management of GERD have been developed over the past 10–15 years, patients will fail these endoluminal procedures requiring remediation and redo procedures.

Mesh at the Esophageal Hiatus

Mesh at the esophageal hiatus presents a special problem, primarily due to the inflammation and scarring associated with mesh placed around or immediately behind the esophagus. This is true for both biological and synthetic mesh [23]. While the presentation of failure after mesh hiatal reconstruction can look like any other antireflux operation failure, patients with mesh are more likely to have more persistent and severe chest pain, dysphagia, or regurgitation. Barium swallow may show crural stenosis or a dilated esophagus, and endoscopy may reveal ulceration at the distal esophagus. There have been many cases reported in the literature of mesh erosion into the esophagus or GEJ.

The work-up in these situations remains the same for any suspected antireflux surgery failure. Similarly, the decisions regarding management are also nearly identical to what has already been outlined for antireflux surgery failure. One critical difference is the finding of mesh eroding into the lumen of the esophagus or stomach. When this is found, it is best to attempt endoscopic removal by attempting pulling any loose or extruding mesh to see if it will break free, and cutting off any excess within the lumen. Surgery should be delayed until the mesh extrudes, and serial EGDs are indicated to follow the extrusion process. Operating when the mesh has eroded into the bowel is certain to require a resection to manage the defect left if mesh is removed surgically. Many patients have been managed over months and even years with eroded mesh awaiting extrusion without significant complications. An exception would be the patient who has a free perforation or uncontrollable sepsis due to mesh erosion.

When performing a redo in the face of prior mesh, the likelihood of effecting a true redo of the initial operation is decreased. Dense adhesions, distorted anatomy, and partial thickness mesh erosion may require bowel resection thereby limiting the ability to redo a fundoplication. When no mesh has been used, a full or partial fundoplication is possible in 78 % of cases. In contrast, when mesh has been used, a fundoplication is possible in only 50 % of cases [24].

Recurrent Hiatal Hernia and Short Esophagus

Occasionally, the crura cannot be closed behind the esophagus without excessive tension. This is especially true in reoperative cases where scarring from the prior repair can make the tissue more rigid and firm, and less likely to come together without tension. If after placing a few crural stitches, the tension for primary closure leads to the crura fraying, it is my preference to perform a relaxing incision through the diaphragm just to the left of the vena cava leaving a cuff of tissue along the left edge of the vena cava (Fig. 22.3). This relaxing incision allows the crura to be closed primarily behind the esophagus, and then a mesh patch is placed to cover the resulting diaphragm defect along the vena cava (Fig. 22.4). This places tissue immediately behind the esophagus and prevents mesh from lying directly behind the esophagus where there is risk of scarring and erosion of the mesh into the gastroesophageal junction. Another consideration for recurrent hiatal hernia is esophageal lengthening using a Collis gastroplasty to prevent tension from a short esophagus pulling the wrap and stomach back up through the hiatus and into the mediastinum (Fig. 22.3). While infrequently needed, familiarity with this technique is essential for the surgeon undertaking redo antireflux surgery. An incorrectly performed Collis, or one that attempts to gain more than 2–3 cm of esophageal length may decrease hiatal hernia recurrence, but increases the risk of dilation of the neo-esophagus and acid pooling above the wrap [25].

Redo After Prior Endoluminal Antireflux Procedure

Over the past 15 years there have been several endoluminal antireflux procedures developed and introduced for use. All of these promise a less invasive technique for mechanically augmenting the LES and effecting GERD control. All of the devices and techniques introduced have failed to achieve results comparable to the more widely accepted laparoscopic techniques, and many of the companies who have developed these technologies are no longer in business. For the most part, lack of durability and efficacy has limited the use of these techniques to select patients. While infrequently used, there are patients who have undergone endoluminal antireflux procedures that have failed and are in need or reoperative antireflux surgery. Fortunately, most of the endoluminal techniques do not prevent future laparoscopic antireflux procedures. Table 22.8 outlines the more commonly used endoluminal procedures and options for management when they fail.

Finally, the best management strategy for failed antireflux procedures is to minimize the likelihood of failure. Table 22.9 details a standardized technique for laparoscopic antireflux surgery that has proven very effective over the years and minimizes the likelihood of failure [26].

Table 22.8 Reoperation after endoluminal antireflux failure

Endolumenal procedure	Redo options/difficulty
Transoral Incisionless Fundoplication (TIF), esophyx	360° or 270° fundoplication/potentially difficult with scarring and need to remove fixation devices
Radiofrequency energy delivery to LES, stretta	360° fundoplication/similar to first time antireflux surgery with virtually no scarring
GEJ plication, NDO	360° fundoplication/similar to first time antireflux surgery with virtually no scarring
GEJ plication, endocinch	360° fundoplication/similar to first time antireflux surgery with virtually no scarring
Co-polymer injection into GEJ, enteryx	360° fundoplication/potentially difficult with mediastinal scarring and inflammation

GEJ, gastroesophageal junction; *LES*, lower esophageal sphincter

Table 22.9 Standard technique for antireflux surgery success

- Full hiatal dissection (reduce and resect any hiatal hernia sac)
- Adequate esophageal mobilization—3–4 cm of esophagus below diaphragm
- Divide all short gastric vessels (be sure to mobilize fundus posteriorly to find and divide any high posterior vessel(s)
- Resect any epiphrenic fat (careful to not undermine the anterior vagus)
- Determine esophageal length and location of EGJ (use endoscopy if unsure)
- Careful handling of crura during dissection and closure
- Decrease pneumoperitoneum to unload the diaphragm during closure
- Anterior crural stitch if large hiatal defect
- Calibrate wrap (assure the fundus is in contact with the esophagus circumferentially–you can make a wrap too loose)
- Use gastrostomy tube for gastric decompression if large hiatal hernia or excessive manipulation of stomach/area of vagal nerves
- Avoid postoperative nausea (use pre-emptive anti-emetics)

EGJ, esophagogastric junction

References

1. Broeders JA, Roks DJ, Ahmed Ali U, et al. Laparoscopic anterior 180-degree versus Nissen fundoplication for gastroesophageal reflux disease: systematic review and meta-analysis of randomized clinical trials. Ann Surg. 2013;257(5):850–9.
2. Voelker R. Proton pump inhibitors linked to fracture risk. JAMA. 2010;304(1):29.
3. Kuehn BM. Reflux drugs linked to C. difficile-related diarrhea. JAMA. 2012;307(10):1014.
4. Cayla G, Hulot JS, O'Connor SA, et al. Clinical, angiographic, and genetic factors associated with early coronary stent thrombosis. JAMA. 2011;306(16):1765–74.
5. Giuliano C, Wilhelm SM, Kale-Pradhan PB. Are proton pump inhibitors associated with the development of community-acquired pneumonia? A meta-analysis. Expert Rev Clin Pharmacol. 2012; 5(3):337–44.
6. Teixeira JP, Moreira LM, Flores A, Ribeiro C. Durability of long-term outcome of laparoscopic Nissen – comparison of the results at 5 and 10 years after surgery. Hepatogastroenterology 2012;59(120): 2428–31.
7. Rosemurgy A, Paul H, Madison L, et al. A single institution's experience and journey with over 1000 laparoscopic fundoplications for gastroesophageal reflux disease. Am Surg. 2012;78(9):917–25.
8. Oelschlager BK, Ma KC, Soares RV, Montenovo MI, Munoz Oca JE, Pellegrini CA. A broad assessment of clinical outcomes after laparoscopic antireflux surgery. Ann Surg. 2012;256(1):87–94.
9. Engstrom C, Cai W, Irvine T, et al. Twenty years of experience with laparoscopic antireflux surgery. Br J Surg. 2012;99(10):1415–21.
10. Broeders JA, Roks DJ, Draaisma WA, et al. Predictors of objectively identified recurrent reflux after primary Nissen fundoplication. Br J Surg. 2011;98(5):673–9.
11. Watson DI, Devitt PG, Smith L, Jamieson GG. Anterior 90 partial vs Nissen fundoplication–5 year follow-up of a single-centre randomised trial. J Gastrointest Surg. 2012;16(9):1653–8.
12. Salminen P, Hurme S, Ovaska J. Fifteen-year outcome of laparoscopic and open Nissen fundoplication: a randomized clinical trial. Ann Thorac Surg. 2012;93(1):228–33.
13. Koch OO, Kaindlstorfer A, Antoniou SA, Asche KU, Granderath FA, Pointner R. Laparoscopic Nissen versus Toupet fundoplication: objective and subjective results of a prospective randomized trial. Surg Endosc. 2012;26(2):413–22.
14. Khatri K, Sajid MS, Brodrick R, Baig MK, Sayegh M, Singh KK. Laparoscopic Nissen fundoplication with or without short gastric vessel division: a meta-analysis. Surg Endosc. 2012;26(4): 970–8.
15. Cao Z, Cai W, Qin M, Zhao H, Yue P, Li Y. Randomized clinical trial of laparoscopic anterior 180 partial versus 360 Nissen fundoplication: 5-year results. Dis Esophagus. 2012;25(2):114–20.
16. Broeders JA, Roks DJ, Jamieson GG, Devitt PG, Baigrie RJ, Watson DI. Five-year outcome after laparoscopic anterior partial versus Nissen fundoplication: four randomized trials. Ann Surg. 2012;255(4):637–42.
17. Aye RW, Swanstrom LL, Kapur S, et al. A randomized multiinstitution comparison of the laparoscopic Nissen and Hill repairs. Ann Thorac Surg. 2012;94(3):951–7. discussion 7–8.
18. Dallemagne B, Perretta S. Twenty years of laparoscopic fundoplication for GERD. World J Surg. 2011;35(7):1428–35.
19. Wileman SM, McCann S, Grant AM, Krukowski ZH, Bruce J. Medical versus surgical management for gastro-oesophageal reflux disease (GORD) in adults. Cochrane Database Syst Rev. 2010;3, CD003243.
20. Smith CD. Surgical therapy for gastroesophageal reflux disease: indications, evaluation, and procedures. Gastrointest Endosc Clin N Am. 2009;19(1):35–48, v–vi.
21. van Beek DB, Auyang ED, Soper NJ. A comprehensive review of laparoscopic redo fundoplication. Surg Endosc. 2011;25(3):706–12.
22. Smith CD, McClusky DA, Rajad MA, Lederman AB, Hunter JG. When fundoplication fails: redo? Ann Surg. 2005;241(6):861–9. discussion 9–71.
23. Stadlhuber RJ, Sherif AE, Mittal SK, et al. Mesh complications after prosthetic reinforcement of hiatal closure: a 28-case series. Surg Endosc. 2009;23(6):1219–26.
24. Parker M, Bowers SP, Bray JM, et al. Hiatal mesh is associated with major resection at revisional operation. Surg Endosc. 2010;24(12): 3095–101.
25. Lin E, Swafford V, Chadalavada R, Ramshaw BJ, Smith CD. Disparity between symptomatic and physiologic outcomes following esophageal lengthening procedures for antireflux surgery. J Gastrointest Surg. 2004;8(1):31–9. discussion 8–9.
26. Morgenthal CB, Lin E, Shane MD, Hunter JG, Smith CD. Who will fail laparoscopic Nissen fundoplication? Preoperative prediction of long-term outcomes. Surg Endosc. 2007;21(11):1978–84.
27. Vignal JC, Luc G, Wagner T, Cunha AS, Collet D. Re-operation for failed gastro-esophageal fundoplication. What results to expect? J Visc Surg. 2012;149(1):e61–5.

28. Musunuru S, Gould JC. Perioperative outcomes of surgical procedures for symptomatic fundoplication failure: a retrospective case–control study. Surg Endosc. 2012;26(3):838–42.
29. Frantzides CT, Madan AK, Carlson MA, et al. Laparoscopic revision of failed fundoplication and hiatal herniorraphy. J Laparoendosc Adv Surg Tech A. 2009;19(2):135–9.
30. Khajanchee YS, O'Rourke R, Cassera MA, Gatta P, Hansen PD, Swanstrom LL. Laparoscopic reintervention for failed antireflux surgery: subjective and objective outcomes in 176 consecutive patients. Arch Surg. 2007;142(8):785–901. discussion 791–2.
31. Byrne JP, Smithers BM, Nathanson LK, Martin I, Ong HS, Gotley DC. Symptomatic and functional outcome after laparoscopic reoperation for failed antireflux surgery. Br J Surg. 2005;92(8): 996–1001.
32. Legner A, Tsuboi K, Bathla L, Lee T, Morrow LE, Mittal SK. Reoperative antireflux surgery for dysphagia. Surg Endosc. 2011;25(4):1160–7.
33. Dallemagne B, Arenas Sanchez M, Francart D, et al. Long-term results after laparoscopic reoperation for failed antireflux procedures. Br J Surg. 2011;98(11):1581–7.

Side Effects of Fundoplications and How to Deal with Them

Bernard Dallemagne

Introduction

The results of the surgery of gastro-esophageal reflux are irrefutable. Multiple clinical studies have shown its effectiveness to control pathological gastro-esophageal reflux. Comparisons with a suitable medical treatment regularly demonstrated its superiority and even, in the less favorable studies, its equivalence [1–4]. If surgery is effective in controlling reflux, it nevertheless generates side effects that are reported by a majority of the patients [5–8]. Typically, these side effects are dysphagia, to varying degrees, a difficulty or inability to belch and, in corollary, a tendency to abdominal bloating and flatulence. They have a mechanical origin, related to a hyper-competence of the antireflux barrier. To reduce them, changes to the architecture of the valve have been proposed, from a completely circular valve to varying degrees of partial valves [9]. The importance and impact of the side effects on the quality of life of patients depend on proper selection of patients, technical quality of the surgical procedure, and on the physiological principles of antireflux procedures. They are generally more severe in the immediate postoperative course and decrease in the long course, either because the antireflux mechanism weakens, or because of addiction or adaptation of the body of the patient, or by a phenomenon of psychological habituation [6, 10]. Nevertheless they can be extremely disabling in some patients, and can pose therapeutic problems. In general, the management strategy will be either conservative management, endoscopy, or further. The most appropriate strategy varies according to the individual patient and the particular problem, and for this reason it must be tailored to the specific situation.

B. Dallemagne, MD (✉)
NHC – University Hospital of Strasbourg, Digestive and Endocrine Surgery, 1 place de l'Hopital, Strasbourg 67000, France
e-mail: Bernard.dallemagne@ircad.fr

Antireflux Barrier and Fundoplication

The antireflux barrier corresponds to the Gastro-Esophageal Junction (GEJ), which is a complex anatomical zone whose functionality is dependent on the intrinsic lower esophageal sphincter (LES), the muscles of the diaphragm (extrinsic), the integrity of the phreno-esophageal ligament and the persistence of the angle of His (gastric flap valve).

Current understanding of gastroesophageal reflux makes a distinction between LES relaxation and GEJ opening, the latter being essential for reflux to occur [11]. The opening of the GEJ when swallowing, or during TLESR episodes, is the result of relaxation of the LES (internal component) and focal inhibition of the pillars of the diaphragm during inspiration (external component) [12, 13]. This results in a significant reduction of the intraluminal GEJ pressure. In addition to relaxation, there is a proximal migration of the GEJ, more important during TLESR than swallowing [11, 14]. The proximal movement may be a means by which the gastric flap valve is overcome and the GEJ lumen opens in order to allow the air to escape. Studies have shown that most episodes of belching occurred during TLESRs [15].

Reduction of hiatus hernia and re-approximation of the diaphragmatic pillars, restoration of intra-abdominal length of the esophagus, re-creation of the flap valve of the esophagus, mechanical compression of the esophagus can, either isolated or combined, lead to an increased pressure at the level of the GEJ, a decreased incidence of transient lower esophageal sphincter relaxations and incomplete GEJ relaxation on swallowing or during transient sphincter relaxation, which are the hypothetical mechanisms of efficacy of a fundoplication [16–18].

With regard to the effect of fundoplication on LES pressure and relaxation, there are conflicting data about whether it increases basal LES pressure by exerting a mechanical compressive effect on the LES [19, 20]. Jiang et al. did not find any significant change in basal LES pressure after fundoplication in an animal model and concluded that the effects of fundoplication were not related to the compressive effects of surgical

L.L. Swanstrom and C.M. Dunst (eds.), *Antireflux Surgery*,
DOI 10.1007/978-1-4939-1749-5_23, © Springer New York 2015

wrap [21]. Fundoplication reduces cranial displacement and relaxation of the LES in response to axial stretch and vagal nerve stimulation [19]. Diminution of cranial displacement of LES after fundoplication surgery was also reported by Kahrilas et al. [21]. They suggest also that the major contribution in terms of pressure is provided by the re-calibration of the hiatal opening and the restoration of the contact of the diaphragmatic pillars with the GEJ, the fundoplication essentially ensuring the length of the subdiaphragmatic zone of high-pressure [22]. The effect of the cruroplasty adds to the repositioning and the strengthening of the lower esophageal sphincter by the fundoplication. These concepts are important because they explain the variability of the results obtained by different operators, which close more or less the hiatal opening and create valves of variable length [23].

More recently, a new technology based on impedance planimetry allows to study the dynamics of the GEJ, and in particular its distensibility [24]. Years ago, Harris et al. identified that sphincters do not necessarily need to contract tightly to be competent, and their work suggested that resistance to distension by measurement of radial force should be the prime determinant of sphincteric strength [25]. This parameter appears more appropriate than the simple measures of intraluminal pressure, as it is provided by manometry, and takes into account the Cross Sectional Area of opening of the junction in response to intraluminal controlled parameters of distension. This allows measuring the resistance to the opening of the junction and better reflects the physiological reality. Kwiatek et al. have demonstrated, using this technology, that the less distensible zone of the GEJ is the hiatal orifice, in healthy individuals and after fundoplication, that the distensibility of the hiatus was significantly higher during the post-deglutition relaxation, but was reduced after fundoplication, and that, after fundoplication, patients have a more reduced distensible segment than controls [26]. These results confirm the data of post-operative manometry showing a reduction in the capacity of relaxation of the high pressure zone after surgery [16, 27–29].

Dysphagia

Dysphagia is a common side effect of fundoplication, reported between 10 and 90 %, to varying degrees, for which there may be several reasons [30, 31]. The two components of the GEJ competency and distensibility, the diaphragm and the lower esophageal sphincter, are modified during fundoplication, and may, alone or in a combined manner, modify the flow through the GEJ. This increased resistance at the GEJ is inevitable and usually the esophagus adapts its propulsive power, provided that it has sufficient reserves [27–29, 32–34].

The relationship between GEJ transit and symptoms of dysphagia is still incompletely understood. Theoretically, GEJ transit depends on several mechanical parameters including viscosity of the bolus, the pressure gradient across the GEJ, and the resistance to flow across the GEJ. GEJ transit after fundoplication is associated with an elevated intrabolus pressure. This pressure, built up during the time between arrival of the front of the bolus at the GEJ and the actual opening of the GEJ, is required to physically open the GEJ during swallow induced LES relaxation. Scheiffer et al. reported that postoperative dysphagia scores do not relate to manometric parameters but are related to the transit time of both liquid and solid boluses across the GEJ [35]. The reduced GEJ transit efficacy is due to the increased outflow resistance evident from the narrowed and elongated hiatal passage likely due to a reduced GEJ compliance limiting GEJ opening. Common factors of GEJ transit in several studies are impaired GEJ relaxation [27, 36] and minimal diameter of opening of the GEJ [37, 38]. Recent studies of the distensibility of the GEJ with impedance planimetry showed that the least distensible locus (narrowest cross-sectional area) within the GEJ was consistently found at the hiatus in patients who have had Nissen fundoplication [26, 35]. These findings emphasize the importance of the functional balance between intrinsic and extrinsic contractile components of the GEJ in modulating trans-sphincter flow—a balance that is difficult to normalize with surgery. A reduction in the prevalence of dysphagia after fundoplication has been achieved through modifications to operative technique [23, 39, 40].

Too tight a crural repair, too tight or twisted a fundoplication, too long a valve, cause dysphagia. In addition, a malposition or a displacement of the valve of fundoplication (slippage) can lead also to dysphagia. This anomaly is usually associated with recurrent reflux as one of the components of the GEJ, the LES, is not or is no more corrected.

Management

Acute Postoperative Dysphagia

In a small number of patients acute dysphagia occurs in the first 1–2 days following surgery and should be distinguished from the usual postoperative dysphagia experienced by most patients. A swallow X-ray should be performed. If the exam shows contrast passing into the stomach, albeit slowly, and a correct sub-diaphragmatic position of the antireflux valve and stomach, a conservative approach can usually be followed, and swallowing will usually improve over the ensuing few days (see Fig. 23.1).

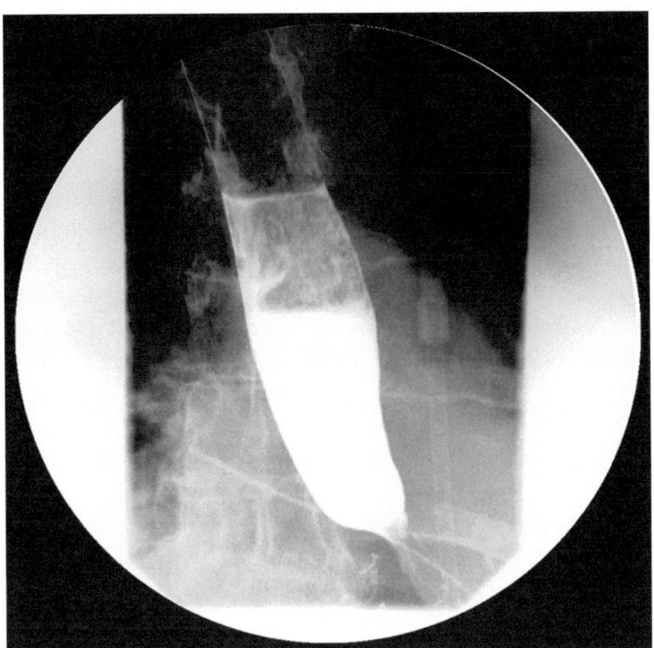

Fig. 23.1 Steroids can possibly accelerate recovery. However, if no contrast passes into the stomach, urgent intervention is necessary. The choice of method is between endoscopy and dilatation versus surgery. In some patients endoscopy and the passage of a large (17 mm or larger) Savary type bougie over a guide wire is followed by improved swallowing, and further intervention is not needed. However, if this fails, it is usually straightforward to undertake a further laparoscopic procedure within the first post-operative week

Persistent Dysphagia

Although dysphagia occurs in all patients in the early postoperative period following fundoplication, the majority of patients are able to swallow normally at late follow-up. A small number of patients experience dysphagia which is persistent and sufficiently severe to require further operative intervention.

Our attitude is to carefully monitor patients during the first 3 months, with a careful evaluation of the evolution of dysphagia and weight monitoring. Endoscopic dilation is proposed in the case of severe grade dysphagia. It is repeated in the case of partial response. Persists of dilatation, dysphagia recurs quickly, a new radiological assessment is carried out looking for any expansion of the lower esophagus, and persisting narrowing of the GEJ, which testifies to the importance of the obstacle to the evacuation. If this is the case, a re-intervention is programmed. The most common causes of this complication are a tight closure of the pillars of the diaphragm, or a too-tight valve. If there is no sign of suffering of the esophagus and the state of nutrition is maintained, the conservative attitude can be continued on the basis of the importance of discomfort described by the patient. A fairly common cause of this persistent dysphagia, without worrying radiological sign, is the "twisted" fundoplication. This technical error is usually associated with the technique of Nissen without mobilization of gastric fundus and consists in a phenomenon of rotation (twist) of the esophagus on its axis, caused by a tension of the gastric fundus. Response to dilatation is usually very low, and reoperation is habitually necessary.

Late Onset Dysphagia

The later onset of dysphagia in the postoperative course is usually caused by an anatomical change of the antireflux mechanism, the valve and/or the cruroplasty. Usually these anatomical abnormalities are easily detected by radiology or endoscopy. Intrathoracic migration of the valve, slippage of the valve on the stomach, diaphragmatic fibrosis and paraesophageal hernia are the most common causes, and all can be corrected only by a surgical approach [41–44].

Postoperative Gas-Related Symptoms

The normal mechanism of ventilation of the stomach occurs mainly during transient relaxations of LES, not associated with swallowing. They are caused by gastric distension which provokes a vagovagal reflex leading to a steep drop in the pressure of the LES [45]. Concomitantly, coordinated events inhibit the contraction of the pillars of the diaphragm and cause a longitudinal contraction of the esophagus and aboral displacement of the LES. This mechanism may overcome the gastric valve effect and allow draining air through the GEJ. Fundoplication, essentially ensuring the length of the subdiaphragmatic zone of high-pressure, reduces cranial displacement and relaxation of the LES in response to axial stretch and vagal nerve stimulation [19], thereby air venting. Both partial and 360° fundoplication alter the belching pattern by reducing gastric belches and increasing supra-gastric belches [46]. The first serve to vent ingested air from the stomach, whereas the latter are esophageal belches that do not allow air ventilation from the stomach. Consequently, fundoplication reduces air venting, which causes gas-related symptoms. Postoperative gas-related symptoms are demonstrated to be common after fundoplication.

The so-called gas bloat syndrome is characterized by abdominal bloating, epigastric pain, and difficulty belching. Frequent bowel movements and excessive flatus may be related symptoms. In the long-term, decreased belching ability, increased rectal flatulence and bloating were reported by up to 70, 95.5, and 79.2 % patients, respectively [47]. However, there is a very high variability in the definition and how to quantify this problem. In addition, incidence of post-fundoplication symptoms should be compared with the preoperative incidence of the same symptoms. "Wind-related" symptoms may appear, improve or disappear following laparoscopic fundoplication, confirming that some of these symptoms are part of the spectrum of reflux symptomatology [48–51]. In a recent randomized trial comparing Nissen fundoplication and medical therapy, bloating and flatulence were reported by 40 vs 28 %, and 57 vs 40 %, respectively [52]. In a similar randomized trial, heartburn, regurgitation, and belching were reported less frequently in the group randomized to surgery than among those randomized to medication, with no significant differences in 'difficulty swallowing,' 'wind from the bowel,' and nausea [51]. Moreover, some patients with gastro-esophageal reflux develop the habit of air-swallowing [48]. This entails subconscious repetitive swallowing, presumably in response to the regurgitation of gastric content into the esophagus. Long-term sequential follow-up study demonstrated a significant reduction in the incidence of dysphagia and flatulence, in contrast to the results for abdominal bloating [6]. There was no significant difference in the incidence of side effects between partial and total fundoplication [6, 53].

Some authors suggest that the relative risk of one of these problems occurring is in part determined by the type of fundoplication performed. The incidence of these side effects are discordant, some reporting lower rates for partial fundoplication, others reporting similar rates [6, 40, 46, 54]. The rates of inability to belch (7.8 vs. 15.7 %) and gas bloating (22.5 vs. 35.9 %) by a recent meta-analysis comparing 270° and 360° fundoplication [40, 55] and the prevalence of increased flatulence were also similar to the results of the only randomized trial that compared increased flatulence after 270° and 360° LPF (67.2 vs. 74.6 %) [47]. Long-term follow-up of partial anterior vs Nissen did not demonstrate any difference after 10–15 years [6, 56].

Despite this disparity in reports, the treatment of "wind-related" side effects, when troublesome for the patient, is difficult. Implementing changes in diet and allowing sufficient time for "wind-related" symptoms to improve will result in a satisfactory outcome in many patients.

There are few published reports describing the outcome of endoscopic or surgical revision primarily for troublesome "wind-related" side effects. Indication for surgical redo is considered in 4–5 % of patients [42, 57]. Conversion to a lesser degree of fundoplication was associated with a good outcome in the small numbers of patients in one study [58]. These results were not confirmed in others reports [44, 59].

Other Side Effects

Early satiety, nausea, vomiting and bloating and diarrhea are recognized side effects of anti-reflux surgery.

They can be part of the gas-bloat syndrome, resulting from the inability to vent gas from the stomach to the esophagus, they can also be caused by alterations in gastric emptying or result from vagal injury. Gastric emptying becomes normal or accelerated after surgery in the majority of patients with symptoms suggesting a delay in gastric emptying (20–40 % of patients with GERD) [60–62]. Yet, if severe, this delay may contribute to reflux or promote reflux disease and was identified as a factor for unsatisfactory results after antireflux surgery [63]. Some surgeons combine fundoplication with gastric drainage, commonly pyloroplasty, when pathological delayed gastric emptying has been objectified [64–66]. Postoperative gastroparesis can also be caused by eso-gastric surgery (19 %) and vagal damage [67]. Actual incidence of vagal damage after antireflux surgery is completely unknown [68]. Vagus dysfunction, measured indirectly by the response of plasma PP to insulin-induced hypoglycemia, has been identified in 10 % of patients after partial fundoplication, without impact on gastric emptying and symptomatology [60, 68]. The vast majority of patients show signs of gastroparesis during the first 3 to 6 months after surgery, in the form of early satiety, bloating, and flatulence. After 1 year, these symptoms have improved 90 % of the patients [69]. The finding of postoperative symptoms suggesting delayed gastric emptying among patients with antireflux operations followed for >1 year was usually associated with delayed gastric emptying pre-operatively [70]. The impact of vagal dysfunction/injury on the side effects can be extrapolated from the experience of reoperation after failed fundoplication/recurrent hiatal hernia. Indeed, redo procedures require extensive dissection at the gastroesophageal junction due to major anatomic disturbances and may lead to vagal nerve injury. In this particular context, delayed gastric emptying appears not as a significant complication [42, 57]. Moreover, uni- or bilateral vagotomy is performed by some surgeons to increase the length of the esophagus in case of short esophagus. No impact on gastric emptying was observed in a series of 150 patients operated for complex para-esophageal hernias and hiatal hernia recurrence [71].

The primary objectives in gastroparesis treatment are decreasing symptoms and improving nutrition. The severity of gastroparesis dictates management. Mild to moderate gastroparesis can be managed medically with dietary modifications, nutritional supplements, pro-motility agents, and anti-emetics.

A spasm of pylorus may be the cause of gastroparesis. Endoscopic treatment (dilatation balloon or intrasphincteric injection of botulinum toxin) can be discussed. Pneumatic dilation results remain uncertain. In addition, studies did not highlight clear therapeutic benefit of intrasphincteric injection of botulinum toxin [72]. Gastric electrical stimulation demonstrated significant subjective and objective improvement up to 10 years after device placement in patients with severe gastroparesis [73].

Surgical indications remain exceptional. In major gastric stasis, with daily symptoms and important nutritional impact, a surgical treatment should be discussed only when all other options have failed. If the motor disorder is strictly limited to the stomach, partial or subtotal gastrectomy may be considered [74].

New onset diarrhea may occur in up to 33 % of post-fundoplication cases and is typically mild, low in volume, and worse after meals [75, 76]. The cause of post-fundoplication diarrhea is thought to be a result of vagal injury, small bowel bacterial overgrowth, rapid gastric emptying, and reduced gastric relaxation or exacerbation of underlying irritable bowel syndrome, and attributing diarrhea to a specific etiology can be quite difficult. Reports noted that as many as 33–66 % of patients who underwent antireflux surgery had pre-existing irritable bowel syndrome and stressed the value of obtaining a comprehensive preoperative gastrointestinal history in patients undergoing laparoscopic antireflux surgery [75, 77]. Diarrhea responds favorably to antimotility drugs, antibiotics for small bowel overgrowth, or cholestyramine [67]. Severe or uncontrollable diarrhea occurred in the minority of patients [78]. Surgical procedures should be reserved for patients presenting with complex clinical situations, mixing gas-bloating, altered gastric emptying or dumping syndrome, in whom medical treatment fails [77, 78].

References

1. Anvari M, Allen C, Marshall J, Armstrong D, Goeree R, Ungar W, et al. A randomized controlled trial of laparoscopic Nissen fundoplication versus proton pump inhibitors for treatment of patients with chronic gastroesophageal reflux disease: one-year follow-up. Surg Innov. 2006;13(4):238–49.
2. Lundell L, Miettinen P, Myrvold HE, Hatlebakk JG, Wallin L, Engström C, et al. Comparison of outcomes twelve years after antireflux surgery or omeprazole maintenance therapy for reflux esophagitis. Clin Gastroenterol Hepatol. 2009;7(12):1292–8.
3. Mahon D, Rhodes M, Decadt B, Hindmarsh A, Lowndes R, Beckingham I, et al. Randomized clinical trial of laparoscopic Nissen fundoplication compared with proton-pump inhibitors for treatment of chronic gastro-oesophageal reflux. Br J Surg. 2005;92(6):695–9.
4. Mehta S, Bennett J, Mahon D, Rhodes M. Prospective trial of laparoscopic Nissen fundoplication versus proton pump inhibitor therapy for gastroesophageal reflux disease: seven-year follow-up. J Gastrointest Surg. 2006;10(9):1312–7.
5. Triponez F, Dumonceau J-M, Azagury D, Volonte F, Slim K, Mermillod B, et al. Reflux, dysphagia, and gas bloat after laparoscopic fundoplication in patients with incidentally discovered hiatal hernia and in a control group. Surgery. 2005;137(2):235–42.
6. Dallemagne B, Weerts J, Markiewicz S, Dewandre JM, Wahlen C, Monami B, et al. Clinical results of laparoscopic fundoplication at ten years after surgery. Surg Endosc. 2006;20(1):159–65.
7. Anvari M, Allen C. Postprandial bloating after laparoscopic Nissen fundoplication. Can J Surg. 2001;44(6):440–4.
8. De Beaux AC, Watson DI, O'Boyle C, Jamieson GG. Role of fundoplication in patient symptomatology after laparoscopic antireflux surgery. Br J Surg. 2001;88(8):1117–21.
9. Broeders JA, Mauritz FA, Ahmed Ali U, Draaisma WA, Ruurda JP, Gooszen HG, et al. Systematic review and meta-analysis of laparoscopic Nissen (posterior total) versus Toupet (posterior partial) fundoplication for gastro-oesophageal reflux disease. Br J Surg. 2010;97(9):1318–30.
10. Fein M, Bueter M, Thalheimer A, Pachmayr V, Heimbucher J, Freys S, et al. Ten-year outcome of laparoscopic antireflux surgery. J Gastrointest Surg. 2008;12(11):1893–9.
11. Pandolfino JE, Zhang QG, Ghosh SK, Han A, Boniquit C, Kahrilas PJ. Transient lower esophageal sphincter relaxations and reflux: mechanistic analysis using concurrent fluoroscopy and high-resolution manometry. Gastroenterology. 2006;131(6):1725–33.
12. Kahrilas PJ, Wu S, Lin S, Pouderoux P. Attenuation of esophageal shortening during peristalsis with hiatus hernia. Gastroenterology. 1995;109(6):1818–25.
13. Mittal RK, Rochester DF, McCallum RW. Sphincteric action of the diaphragm during a relaxed lower esophageal sphincter in humans. Am J Physiol. 1989;256(1 Pt 1):G139–44.
14. Lee YY, Whiting JGH, Robertson EV, Derakhshan MH, Wirz AA, Smith D, et al. Kinetics of transient hiatus hernia during transient lower esophageal sphincter relaxations and swallows in healthy subjects. Neurogastroenterol Motil. 2012;24(11):990–9.
15. Wyman JB, Dent J, Heddle R, Dodds WJ, Toouli J, Downton J. Control of belching by the lower oesophageal sphincter. Gut. 1990;31(6):639–46.
16. Ireland AC, Holloway RH, Toouli J, Dent J. Mechanisms underlying the antireflux action of fundoplication. Gut. 1993;34(3):303–8.
17. Lundell L, Myers JC, Jamieson GG. The effect of antireflux operations on lower oesophageal sphincter tone and postprandial symptoms. Scand J Gastroenterol. 1993;28(8):725–31.
18. Johnsson F, Holloway RH, Ireland AC, Jamieson GG, Dent J. Effect of fundoplication on transient lower oesophageal sphincter relaxation and gas reflux. Br J Surg. 1997;84(5):686–9.
19. Jiang Y, Sandler B, Bhargava V, Mittal RK. Antireflux action of Nissen fundoplication and stretch-sensitive mechanism of lower esophageal sphincter relaxation. Gastroenterology. 2011;140(2):442–9.
20. Pandolfino JE, Curry J, Shi G, Joehl RJ, Brasseur JG, Kahrilas PJ. Restoration of normal distensive characteristics of the esophagogastric junction after fundoplication. Ann Surg. 2005;242(1):43–8.
21. Kahrilas PJ, Lin S, Spiess AE, Brasseur JG, Joehl RJ, Manka M. Impact of fundoplication on bolus transit across esophagogastric junction. Am J Physiol. 1998;275(6 Pt 1):G1386–93.
22. Kahrilas PJ, Lin S, Manka M, Shi G, Joehl RJ. Esophagogastric junction pressure topography after fundoplication. Surgery. 2000;127(2):200–8.
23. DeMeester TR, Bonavina L, Albertucci M. Nissen fundoplication for gastroesophageal reflux disease. Evaluation of primary repair in 100 consecutive patients. Ann Surg. 1986;204(1):9–20.
24. McMahon BP, Rao SSC, Gregersen H, Kwiatek MA, Pandolfino JE, Drewes AM, et al. Distensibility testing of the esophagus. Ann N Y Acad Sci. 2011;1232(1):331–40.
25. Harris LD, Pope CE. "Squeeze" vs. resistance: an evaluation of the mechanism of sphincter competence*. J Clin Invest. 1964;43(12):2272–8.
26. Kwiatek M, Kahrilas P, Soper N, Bulsiewicz W, McMahon B, Gregersen H, et al. Esophagogastric junction distensibility after fundoplication assessed with a novel functional luminal imaging probe. J Gastrointest Surg. 2010;14(2):268–76.
27. Mathew G, Watson DI, Myers JC, Holloway RH, Jamieson GG. Oesophageal motility before and after laparoscopic Nissen fundoplication. Br J Surg. 1997;84(10):1465–9.
28. Marjoux S, Roman S, Juget-Pietu F, Robert M, Poncet G, Boulez J, et al. Impaired postoperative EGJ relaxation as a determinant of post laparoscopic fundoplication dysphagia: a study with

high-resolution manometry before and after surgery. Surg Endosc. 2012;26(12):3642–9.

29. Myers J, Jamieson G, Sullivan T, Dent J. Dysphagia and gastro-esophageal junction resistance to flow following partial and total fundoplication. J Gastrointest Surg. 2012;16(3):475–85.

30. Negre JB. Post-fundoplication symptoms. Do they restrict the success of Nissen fundoplication? Ann Surg. 1983;198(6):698–700.

31. Catarci M, Gentileschi P, Papi C, Carrara A, Marrese R, Gaspari AL, et al. Evidence-based appraisal of antireflux fundoplication. Ann Surg. 2004;239(3):325–37.

32. Ghosh SK, Pandolfino JE, Rice J, Clarke JO, Kwiatek M, Kahrilas PJ. Impaired deglutitive EGJ relaxation in clinical esophageal manometry: a quantitative analysis of 400 patients and 75 controls. Am J Physiol Gastrointest Liver Physiol. 2007;293(4):9.

33. Myers JC, Jamieson GG, Sullivan T, Dent J. Dysphagia and gastro-esophageal junction resistance to flow following partial and total fundoplication. J Gastrointest Surg. 2012;16(3):475–85.

34. Bais JE, Wijnhoven BP, Masclee AA, Smout AJ, Gooszen HG. Analysis and surgical treatment of persistent dysphagia after Nissen fundoplication. Br J Surg. 2001;88(4):569–76.

35. Scheffer RC, Samsom M, Haverkamp A, Oors J, Hebbard GS, Gooszen HG. Impaired bolus transit across the esophagogastric junction in postfundoplication dysphagia. Am J Gastroenterol. 2005;100(8):1677–84.

36. Scheffer RC, Samsom M, Frakking TG, Smout AJ, Gooszen HG. Long-term effect of fundoplication on motility of the oesophagus and oesophagogastric junction. Br J Surg. 2004;91(11):1466–72.

37. Kahrilas PJ, Lin S, Spiess AE, Brasseur JG, Joehl RJ, Manka M. Impact of fundoplication on bolus transit across esophagogastric junction. Am J Physiol. 1998;275(6 Pt 1):G1386–93.

38. Kwiatek MA, Kahrilas PJ. Physiology of the LES. Dis Esophagus; 2011.

39. Broeders JA, Roks DJ, Ahmed Ali U, Watson DI, Baigrie RJ, Cao Z, et al. Laparoscopic anterior 180-degree versus Nissen fundoplication for gastroesophageal reflux disease: systematic review and meta-analysis of randomized clinical trials. Ann Surg. 2013;257(5):850–9.

40. Broeders JAJL, Mauritz FA, Ahmed Ali U, Draaisma WA, Ruurda JP, Gooszen HG, et al. Systematic review and meta-analysis of laparoscopic Nissen (posterior total) versus Toupet (posterior partial) fundoplication for gastro-oesophageal reflux disease. Br J Surg. 2010;97(9):1318–30.

41. Hunter JG, Smith CD, Branum GD, Waring JP, Trus TL, Cornwell M, et al. Laparoscopic fundoplication failures: patterns of failure and response to fundoplication revision. Ann Surg. 1999;230(4):595–604. discussion –6.

42. van Beek DB, Auyang ED, Soper NJ. A comprehensive review of laparoscopic redo fundoplication. Surg Endosc. 2011;25(3):706–12.

43. Furnee EJ, Draaisma WA, Broeders IA, Gooszen HG. Surgical reintervention after failed antireflux surgery: a systematic review of the literature. J Gastrointest Surg. 2009;13(8):1539–49.

44. Dallemagne B, Arenas Sanchez M, Francart D, Perretta S, Weerts J, Markiewicz S, et al. Long-term results after laparoscopic reoperation for failed antireflux procedures. Br J Surg. 2011;98(11):1581–7.

45. Shi G, Pandolfino JE, Joehl RJ, Brasseur JG, Kahrilas PJ. Distinct patterns of oesophageal shortening during primary peristalsis, secondary peristalsis and transient lower oesophageal sphincter relaxation. Neurogastroenterol Motil. 2002;14(5):505–12.

46. Broeders JA, Bredenoord AJ, Hazebroek EJ, Broeders IA, Gooszen HG, Smout AJ. Reflux and belching after 270 degree versus 360 degree laparoscopic posterior fundoplication. Ann Surg. 2012;255(1):59–65.

47. Kellokumpu I, Voutilainen M, Haglund C, Farkkila M, Roberts PJ, Kautiainen H. Quality of life following laparoscopic Nissen fundoplication: assessing short-term and long-term outcomes. World J Gastroenterol. 2013;19(24):3810–8.

48. Bredenoord AJ, Weusten BLAM, Timmer R, Smout AJPM. Air swallowing, belching, and reflux in patients with gastroesophageal reflux disease. Am J Gastroenterol. 2006;101(8):1721–6.

49. Anvari M, Allen C. Postprandial bloating after laparoscopic Nissen fundoplication. Can J Surg. 2001;44(6):440–4.

50. Oelschlager BK, Ma KC, Soares RV, Montenovo MI, Munoz Oca JE, Pellegrini CA. A broad assessment of clinical outcomes after laparoscopic antireflux surgery. Ann Surg 2012; **Publish Ahead of Print**: 10.1097/SLA.0b013e318254f7fe.

51. Grant AM, Cotton SC, Boachie C, Ramsay CR, Krukowski ZH, Heading RC, et al. Minimal access surgery compared with medical management for gastro-oesophageal reflux disease: five year follow-up of a randomised controlled trial (REFLUX). BMJ. 2013;346:f1908.

52. Galmiche J-P, Hatlebakk J, Attwood S, Ell C, Fiocca R, Eklund S, et al. Laparoscopic antireflux surgery vs esomeprazole treatment for chronic GERD. JAMA. 2011;305(19):1969–77.

53. Fein M, Bueter M, Sailer M, Fuchs KH. Effect of cholecystectomy on gastric and esophageal bile reflux in patients with upper gastrointestinal symptoms. Dig Dis Sci. 2008;53(5):1186–91.

54. Broeders JA, Roks DJ, Ahmed Ali U, Watson DI, Baigrie RJ, Cao Z, et al. Laparoscopic anterior 180-degree versus Nissen fundoplication for gastroesophageal reflux disease: systematic review and meta-analysis of randomized clinical trials. Ann Surg. 2013.

55. Booth MI, Stratford J, Jones L, Dehn TC. Randomized clinical trial of laparoscopic total (Nissen) versus posterior partial (Toupet) fundoplication for gastro-oesophageal reflux disease based on preoperative oesophageal manometry. Br J Surg. 2008;95(1):57–63.

56. Broeders JA, Broeders EA, Watson DI, Devitt PG, Holloway RH, Jamieson GG. Objective outcomes 14 years after laparoscopic anterior 180-degree partial versus Nissen fundoplication: results from a randomized trial. Ann Surg. 2012.

57. Symons NRA, Purkayastha S, Dillemans B, Athanasiou T, Hanna GB, Darzi A, et al. Laparoscopic revision of failed antireflux surgery: a systematic review. Am J Surg. 2011;202(3):336–43.

58. Byrne JP, Smithers BM, Nathanson LK, Martin I, Ong HS, Gotley DC. Symptomatic and functional outcome after laparoscopic reoperation for failed antireflux surgery. Br J Surg. 2005;92(8):996–1001.

59. Safranek PM, Gifford CJ, Booth MI, Dehn TC. Results of laparoscopic reoperation for failed antireflux surgery: does the indication for redo surgery affect the outcome? Dis Esophagus. 2007;20(4):341–5.

60. Lindeboom MY, Ringers J, van Rijn PJ, Neijenhuis P, Stokkel MP, Masclee AA. Gastric emptying and vagus nerve function after laparoscopic partial fundoplication. Ann Surg. 2004;240(5):785–90.

61. Bais JE, Samsom M, Boudesteijn EA, van Rijk PP, Akkermans LM, Gooszen HG. Impact of delayed gastric emptying on the outcome of antireflux surgery. Ann Surg. 2001;234(2):139–46.

62. Hinder RA, Stein HJ, Bremner CG, DeMeester TR. Relationship of a satisfactory outcome to normalization of delayed gastric emptying after Nissen fundoplication. Ann Surg. 1989;210(4):458–64.

63. Rebecchi F, Allaix ME, Giaccone C, Morino M. Gastric emptying as a prognostic factor for long-term results of total laparoscopic fundoplication for weakly acidic or mixed reflux. Ann Surg. 2013;258(5):831–6.

64. Khajanchee YS, Dunst CM, Swanstrom LL. Outcomes of Nissen fundoplication in patients with gastroesophageal reflux disease and delayed gastric emptying. Arch Surg. 2009;144(9):823–8.

65. Masqusi S, Velanovich V. Pyloroplasty with fundoplication in the treatment of combined gastroesophageal reflux disease and bloating. World J Surg. 2007;31(2):332–6.

66. Farrell TM, Richardson WS, Halkar R, Lyon CP, Galloway KD, Waring JP, et al. Nissen fundoplication improves gastric motility in patients with delayed gastric emptying. Surg Endosc. 2001;15(3):271–4.

67. Lin DC, Chun CL, Triadafilopoulos G. Evaluation and management of patients with symptoms after anti-reflux surgery. Dis Esophag. 2013: n/a-n/a.

68. Balaji NS, Crookes PF, Banki F, Hagen JA, Ardill JE, DeMeester TR. A safe and noninvasive test for vagal integrity revisited. Arch Surg. 2002;137(8):954–9.

69. Frantzides CT, Carlson MA, Zografakis JG, Moore RE, Zeni T, Madan AK. Postoperative gastrointestinal complaints after laparoscopic Nissen fundoplication. JSLS. 2006;10(1):39–42.

70. Lundell LR, Myers JC, Jamieson GG. Delayed gastric emptying and its relationship to symptoms of "gas float" after antireflux surgery. Eur J Surg. 1994;160(3):161–6.

71. Oelschlager B, Yamamoto K, Woltman T, Pellegrini C. Vagotomy during hiatal hernia repair: a benign esophageal lengthening procedure. J Gastrointest Surg. 2008;12(7):1155–62.

72. Arts J, Holvoet L, Caenepeel P, Bisschops R, Sifrim D, Verbeke K, et al. Clinical trial: a randomized-controlled crossover study of intrapyloric injection of botulinum toxin in gastroparesis. Aliment Pharmacol Ther. 2007;26(9):1251–8.

73. McCallum RW, Lin Z, Forster J, Roeser K, Hou Q, Sarosiek I. Gastric electrical stimulation improves outcomes of patients with gastroparesis for up to 10 years. Clin Gastroenterol Hepatol. 2011;9(4):314–9.

74. Jones MP, Maganti K. A systematic review of surgical therapy for gastroparesis. Am J Gastroenterol. 2003;98(10):2122–9.

75. Klaus A, Hinder RA, DeVault KR, Achem SR. Bowel dysfunction after laparoscopic antireflux surgery: incidence, severity, and clinical course. Am J Med. 2003;114(1):6–9.

76. Richter JE. Gastroesophageal reflux disease treatment: side effects and complications of fundoplication. Clin Gastroenterol Hepatol. 2013;11(5):465–71.

77. Swanstrom L, Wayne R. Spectrum of gastrointestinal symptoms after laparoscopic fundoplication. Am J Surg. 1994;167(5):538–41.

78. Ukleja A, Woodward TA, Achem SR. Vagus nerve injury with severe diarrhea after laparoscopic antireflux surgery. Dig Dis Sci. 2002;47(7):1590–3.

79. Stein HJ, Feussner H, Siewert JR. Failure of antireflux surgery: causes and management strategies. Am J Surg. 1996;171(1):36–9.

Mehran Anvari

Antireflux surgery, once limited to patients with refractory disease, has now become an appropriate therapy for many patients through the introduction of minimally invasive technology. Although the use of laparoscopic fundoplication is now common practice, and many short-term studies have proven procedural effectiveness [1, 2], the long-term outcomes are under-reported and variable [3, 4]. The limitations in the effectiveness of medical treatment of reflux necessitate the use of surgical intervention in a significant proportion of chronic gastroesophageal reflux disease (GERD) sufferers. Surgical revision can correct the functional incompetence of the lower esophageal sphincter (LES), an unattainable outcome by medical intervention alone. Fundoplication, whether conducted by laparoscopic or open technique, is still a surgical procedure, which carries some, albeit small risks. Predictors for successful outcomes must be considered, including a lower body mass index (BMI), younger age, typical reflux symptoms, and absence of significant psychological factors. Generally, the long-term outcomes of antireflux surgery are good, particularly with appropriate patient selection. Results of re-operative procedures of fundoplication do not have equivalent rates of success as the primary but are still adequate.

Evolution of Antireflux Surgery

The first surgical repair of hiatal hernia was illustrated by Angelo Soresi in 1919, with a technique to reduce the hernia and open the diaphragm [5]. Years later, Harrington reported a similar procedure, emphasizing the importance of closing the hernia opening with suturing to the abdominal wall [6, 7]. A transthoracic technique was then published by Sweet [8] involving the crushing of the phrenic nerve, folding and suturing of the hernial sac, and narrowing of the hiatus using a heavy silk suture into the diaphragm. These early surgical attempts were focused on hernia reduction and hiatal closing, without repair to the LES and were therefore often unsuccessful in reducing symptoms of GERD.

The relation of GERD to hiatal hernia was established in 1951 by Allison and Barrett. Allison advocated that the crural sling procedure would prevent GERD [9]. His approach involved reducing the hiatal hernia, dividing the phrenoesophageal ligament, with suture fixation of the diaphragmatic sling [10, 11]. Unfortunately, his surgical technique resulted in poor long-term success, with a high rate of recurrence (49 %) [9]. Barrett asserted that restoration of the cardio-esophageal angle was crucial for the successful treatment of GERD [12].

Belsey focused on intra-abdominal esophagus length, and believed a length of 4–5 cm should be restored to prevent reflux [13]. He devised a partial fundoplication involving a 270° wrap of the stomach around the distal esophagus and cardia, reducing the tissue into the abdomen [13]. Hill developed a similar partial technique, closing the hiatus, and re-establishing the 180° mucosa-mucosal fold at the esophagogastric junction [13]. Rudolf Nissen used a modified fundoplication procedure involving a resection of the cardia to treat an esophageal ulcer in 1939, which remarkably resulted in reduced GERD symptoms. He later revised and published his technique in the mid 1950s, omitting the resection, but maintaining division of the gastrohepatic ligament, and the wrapping of the fundus of the stomach 360-degrees around the lower esophagus with reinforcement [14, 15]. The procedure resulted in reported complications such as dysphagia, gas, bloating, and a slipped wrap. Modifications over the years have altered the technique to include repair of the crura, reinforcement of the LES closure, narrowing the esophageal hiatus, division of the short gastric vessels, and mobilization of the gastric fundus.

Disclosure: This work was not externally funded; the author has not received any financial support.

M. Anvari, MBBS, PhD, FRCSC, FACS (✉)
Department of Surgery, St. Joseph's Healthcare Hamilton,
50 Charlton Avenue East, Hamilton, ON, Canada L8N 4A6
e-mail: anvari@mcmaster.ca

L.L. Swanstrom and C.M. Dunst (eds.), *Antireflux Surgery*,
DOI 10.1007/978-1-4939-1749-5_24, © Springer New York 2015

The "floppy Nissen fundoplication" was a modification introduced to enlarge the diameter of the fundus wrap, resulting in a symptom resolution rate of 97 % [16]. Improvements were specifically noted in gas bloating with this revised technique. DeMeester additionally modified the procedure by shortening the fundoplication length and dividing the short gastric vessels for complete mobilization of the fundus with positive 10 years results of 91 % symptom resolution and significant reduction of dysphagia (from 21 to 3 %) [13, 17]. Modifications to the procedure were made to allow for a partial fundoplication, initially recommended for patients with poor esophageal motility [18, 19].

With the advent of proton pump inhibitors (PPIs), which were shown to be clinically superior to histamine H2 receptor antagonists, the open surgical treatment of GERD became infrequent. Regular access to an effective, rapid symptom relieving medication shifted the balance of GERD treatment towards medical therapy once again. The conventional open approach to antireflux surgery was associated with a number of complications including large abdominal or thoracic scars, wrap disruption or migration, splenic injury, and a 25 % recurrence of GERD in 5 years [20].

The introduction of laparoscopic surgery presented advantages of reduced physical impact, shorter recovery time, reduced scarring, and lower complication rates. The first description of laparoscopic Nissen fundoplication (LNF) was published in 1991 [21]. LNF has since been established as a safe procedure with morbidity and mortality rates well below those reported for traditional open surgery. Viljakka et al. (1997 as cited in Peters et al. 2009) found complication rates of 14 % with LARS and 24 % with OARS during a 32-year analysis of antireflux procedures [22]. Similarly, in a Netherlands randomized antireflux surgery study, early complications were reported in 11 % of laparoscopic procedures and 22 % of open [23].

Postoperative Complications

Postoperative complications, including dysphagia, nausea, gas bloating, recurrent reflux symptoms, diarrhea, vomiting and early satiety, occur at rates of approximately 3.5–14 % [24]. These symptoms are often short-lived, reported in the first few weeks following surgery, requiring therapy in only a small percentage of patients (>5 %) [25]. Other early complications include pneumothorax (up to 2 %), vascular injury, paraesophageal hiatus herniation (up to 7 %), pulmonary embolism, perforation of the gastrointestinal tract (1 %), migration of the wrap, and death [26] (Table 24.1).

The rate of conversion from laparoscopic to open is similar to that of other disciplines. A 10-year randomized trial conducted by Broeders et al. reported a rate of 7.6 % [27],

Table 24.1 Reported complication rates with laparoscopic Nissen

Complication	Early	Late
Death	0.09	0.001
Conversion to open	0–10 %	
Reoperation	<0.1 %	3–10 %
Side effects (dysphagia, bloating, nausea, etc.)	20–60 %	5–10 %

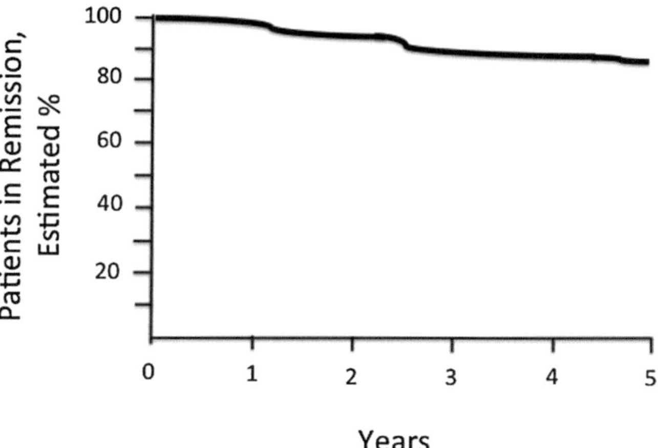

Fig. 24.1 Five-year outcomes of standardized laparoscopic Nissen fundoplication showing excellent durability. Data adapted from the LOTUS trial [31]

similar to a rate of 7.3 % cited in a meta-analysis by Catarci et al. [28], and a rate of 6.3 % reported by Peters et al. [22] in a meta-analysis of RCTs. These rates fall in line with those reported nationally for conversion from laparoscopic to open cholecystectomy (5–10 %) [29] and for laparoscopic hysterectomy (0–19 %, mean 3.5 %) [30].

Mortality rates are low for antireflux surgery, even more so for laparoscopic procedures (0.2 % open versus 0.09 % LARS) [28]. The failure rate of laparoscopic fundoplication at 5 years follow-up is reported at 5–13 %, depending on whether failure is defined by subjective symptomatic failure or objective evidence [20].

Long-Term Outcomes of Laparoscopic Antireflux Surgery

Although studies show that the short-term outcomes of laparoscopic antireflux surgery (LARS) for the treatment of GERD are good, the long-term results are variable. LNF provides effective management of reflux symptoms, achieving long-term relief including heartburn and regurgitation in 84–97 % of patients [20]. Recent data demonstrates excellent heartburn and regurgitation control 5 years after standardized laparoscopic Nissen fundoplication [31] (Figs. 24.1 and 24.2). After 10 years, control of reflux symptoms was observed in 89.5 %

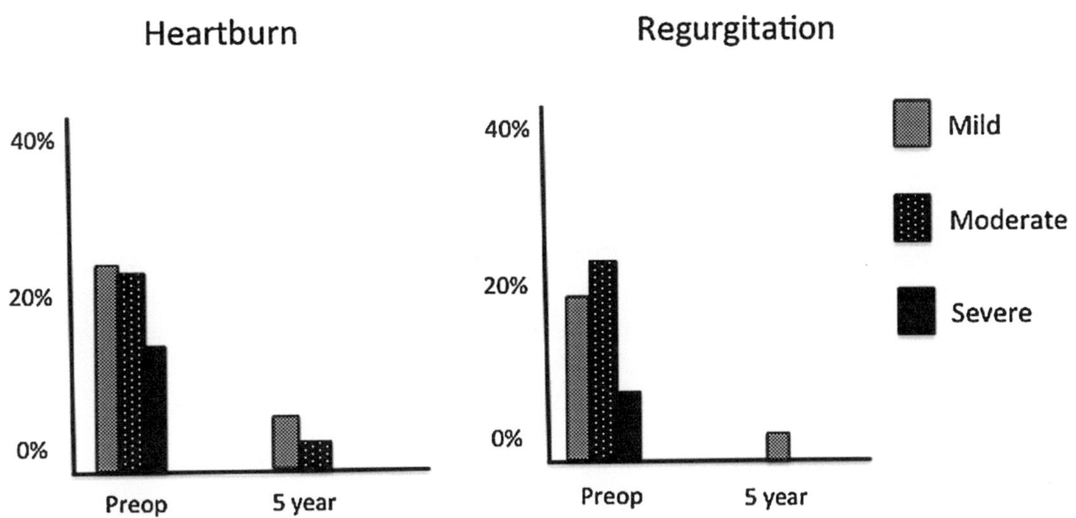

Fig. 24.2 Comparison of control of typical symptoms before and 5 years after laparoscopic Nissen fundoplication. Data adapted from the LOTUS trial [31]

Table 24.2 Symptom relief after Nissen fundoplication at 20 years

Symptom	Heartburn (%)	Regurgitation (%)	Dysphagia (%)
Open Nissen [34]	72	60	72
Lap Nissen [35]	74	90	71

of LNF patients, with PPI antacid medications being used by only 8.4 % of patients [32]. Long-term outcomes from the University of Washington revealed that the majority of patients showed a maintained improvement or resolution of symptoms including heartburn (90 %), regurgitation (92 %), and dysphagia (75 %) at 69 months, however lesser improvements were observed with symptoms of hoarseness (69 %) and cough (69 %) [33].

A long-term post-surgical analysis conducted by Luostarinen et al. [34] found good results in patients 20 years after open antireflux surgery in most patients, with positive outcomes dependent on the condition of the fundic wrap. A reflux symptom resolution rate of 60 % was reported, with the incidence of dysphagia and heartburn being directly correlated with defective wraps, which were found in 28 % of patients [34] (Table 24.2).

While short-term outcomes of LARS are good, with an average of 85–95 % of patients experiencing excellent control of GERD symptoms [36, 37], long-term evidence suggests that these benefits diminish over time [3, 4]. A study evaluating LARS outcomes found better results at 5 years with resolution of significant reflux symptoms in 93 % of the patients, while at 10 years, 89.5 % of the patients were symptom free [32]. Valiati et al. [24] similarly revealed a short-term reflux recurrence rate of 3–4 % within 2 years of laparoscopic fundoplication, and 8 % long-term rate within 7 years.

Dysphagia

In an effort to provide the necessary structural integrity, the crural closure and fundoplication wrap procedure tightens the carida, which can result in dysphagia in some patients. Rates of dysphagia are variably reported (0–24 % in first few months post-surgery) and generally decrease with time (3–5 % long-term follow-up) [24]. A long-term study of LARS by Oelschlager et al. [33] concluded that after a median follow-up of 69 months, dysphagia symptoms were improved in 78 % of patients and resolved in 67 %. When medical treatment is compared, an RCT comparing esomeprazole to LARS reported symptoms at 5 year of 5 and 11 % for dysphagia, and 28 and 40 % for bloating (for the esomeprazole and LARS groups respectively) [38].

Although not statistically significant, the incidence of postoperative dysphagia was found to be greater in patients who had poorly controlled reflux and regurgitation. Data from multiple long-term studies from a literature review by Valiati et al. [24] summarized that the rate of persistent dysphagia is approximately 2–8 %. The occurrence of dysphagia is related to the type of fundoplication procedure, with total fundoplication associated with higher incidence rates. Surgeon experience is also thought to play a role in the prevalence of the complication.

Heartburn, Regurgitation, and Bloating

Long-term relief of heartburn and regurgitation can be achieved with laparoscopic fundoplication in 84–97 % of patients [20, 39]. A long-term study of LARS indicated that after a median follow-up of 69 months, heartburn symptoms were improved in 90 % of patients and resolved in 67 % [33]. A longer-term study with 10-year follow-up reported the percentage of patients with no or mild heartburn as 94.9 % following LNF [27].

Comparison of medical treatment to LARS for the management of reflux symptoms results in good control in both groups. A randomized trial comparing esomeprazole to LARS reported GERD symptoms at 5 years follow-up of: 16 and 8 % for heartburn, 13 and 2 % for acid regurgitation (for the esomeprazole and LARS groups, respectively) [38]. Heartburn free days were calculated in a randomized controlled trial comparing LNF to medical therapy (PPIs). The surgical group improved significantly with a mean of 1.35 more heartburn free days per week than the medical group (95 % CI) [40]. A study of 288 LARS patients revealed patients had considerably improved symptoms of regurgitation, with improvement in 92 % of patients at 5 years follow-up, and resolution in 70 % [33].

Reported incidence of gas bloating, abdominal distension, and flatulence are common following fundoplication. During a 10-year study of LARS, Dallemagne et al. [32] found the rate of flatulence decreased significantly over time, but abdominal distension and bloating increased with time. Valiati et al. [24] also report a steady increase in gas bloating and epigastric pain over time with a rate of 2.2 and 2.8 % <2 years and 3.9 and 4.9 % at >2 years.

Patient Satisfaction

Patient-reported outcomes assess the patient's experience and are reported in terms of health-related quality of life, current health state, and patient satisfaction. A high rate of patient satisfaction is reported following laparoscopic fundoplication, ranging from 80 [31] to 96.5 % [20]. A randomized trial found a high satisfaction rate for LARS of 90 % [20], similarly, a 15 year RCT found a rate of 91.7 % [75].

When surgical treatment is compared to pharmacological therapy, an RCT using the VAS score to report overall patient satisfaction found significant improved symptom control at 3 years for the surgical group, whereas the medical group reported maintained scores (82.60–81.95 for the PPI group versus 81.79–92.67, $P=0.0072$ for the LNF group) [39]. Contini and Scarpignato [41] highlight that patient satisfaction is correlated with improvement in quality of life and resolution of symptoms, while the use of antireflux medication does not influence the rate of satisfaction significantly. Broeders et al. [27] found that quality of life scores increased following LNF with a mean increase of 25.8 % at 10 years. It is understood that numerous patient-related factors can contribute to and affect quality of life and satisfaction scores following LARS, however subjective degree of symptoms is not a reliable indicator of objective reflux.

Antireflux Medication Utilization Following Surgery

The use of PPIs is the primary treatment for GERD [42], however many patients still experience recurrent symptoms, with a failure rate of up to 40 % [43]. The need for antireflux medication following fundoplication is often used as an outcome measure for success. Some studies show an increase of acid-suppressing medication use following antireflux surgery to a rate of 15–22 % [24, 27, 44–47].

Conversely, some long-term trials have found a large percentage of LNF patients achieving relief of reflux symptoms no longer requiring acid-suppressing medications (72.2 %) [27]. A study by Papasavas et al. [48] found the use of PPI medication decreased from 84.4 % preoperatively to 18.7 with 82.7 % free of routine pharmacological treatment (PPIs, H-2 receptor blockers, and antacids for GERD symptoms) at 2 years follow-up. Draaisma et al. [49] indicate similar results at 5 years follow-up, with 13.9 % LNF patients requiring continued use of antireflux medications.

The reasons for frequent use of antireflux medication postoperatively must be explored, as abnormal esophageal acid is not always correlated with postoperative pharmacotherapy [49–51]. Antireflux medications are frequently prescribed in our current health care system, for a variety of GI presentations. Salminen [20] found that although 18.7 % of patients were taking PPI medication at 2 years post-surgery, GERD symptoms scores, as assessed using the Jamieson symptom scoring system, revealed that 82 % of patients improved from severe to mild reflux symptoms. Papasavas et al. [48] found that at 2 years LNF, PPI therapy was required by 10 % of patients for typical GERD symptoms, and 8.7 % were using PPIs for other reasons, such as Barrett's esophagus, "sensitive" stomach, and irritable bowel syndrome. A study by Oelschlager et al. [33] withdrew antireflux medications from post antireflux surgery patients for 2 weeks to investigate GERD symptoms, and found that symptoms did not change significantly during the absence of medication (as cited in Oelschlager et al. [33]). The use of pharmacotherapy for alternate or unnecessary reasons after fundoplication can distort results when outcomes of surgical failure are analyzed by medication use; therefore it is not an efficient measure for procedure efficacy.

Failure Rates and Reoperation

In some cases the fundoplication can unwrap or the sutured connection may become unsecured. Contributing factors of wrap displacement include insufficient adhesions, inadequate closure of the diaphragmatic crura, and a short esophagus and/or insufficient esophagus mobilization.

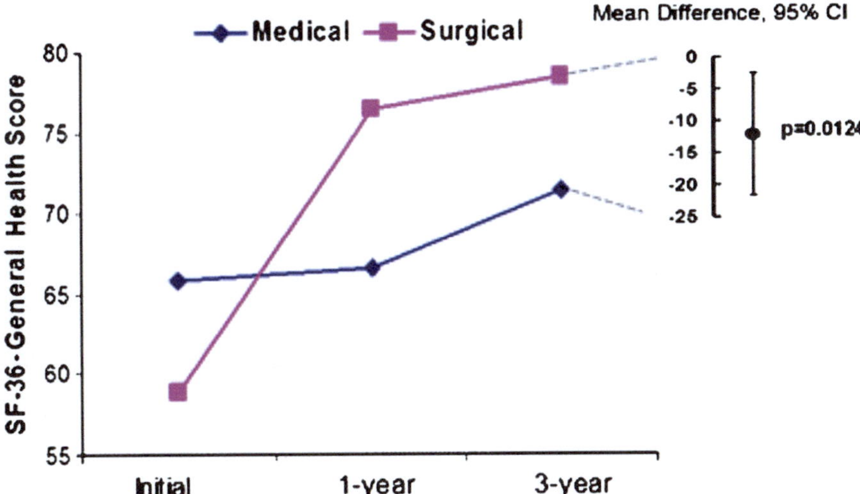

Fig. 24.3 Quality of Life scores with medical and surgical management of GERD [39]

Reoperation, when required, can be especially challenging, resulting in poorer outcomes than initial fundoplication.

A common outcome metric for the efficacy of antireflux surgery is the requirement of revisional surgery which occurs at a rate of around 3–7 %. A study at the University of Washington reports a reoperation rate of 3 % following LARS, for reasons of gastric perforation, acute herniation, and revision for chronic problems such as dysphagia or recurrent GERD [33]. A revision rate of 4 % was found in a study evaluating LARS 10 year's post-surgery, attributed to recurrent reflux symptoms and persistent dysphagia [32]. Another study found that 2.8 % of patients required redo fundoplication, many due to mechanical failure of the wrap (61 % transdiaphragmatic wrap herniation) [52]. The second procedure was successful for 93 % of patients [52]. Higher rates of reoperation were found in a study by Kelly et al. [53] of LNF outcomes at 10 years, with surgical revision required for 17 % of patients (6 % for recurrent hiatus hernia, 6 % for dysphagia, 4 % for recurrent reflux, and 0.04 % for postoperative bleeding from a short gastric vessel).

The results of re-fundoplication are often inferior to those of the initial procedure. A study by Salminen et al. [54] reported a morbidity rate of 21 %, a mortality rate of 1.4 %, and reoperation rate of 16 % following fundoplication revision. Complications of re-fundoplication include recurrent hiatus hernia (70 % [55]) and hollow viscus injury (22 % [55], 21.8 % [52]). The level of surgical expertise and the need for proper patient selection are important factors for success not only for the initial surgery, but perhaps even more emphatically for re-intervention.

Comparing LARS to Long-Term PPI Therapy

For patients with severe GERD symptoms, medical management continues to be the first treatment, however, evidence suggests that symptom control should be re-evaluated, and LNF considered as an alternative or follow-up treatment for those with poor or moderate control. Uncertainty remains as to whether antireflux surgery is effective for treating patients with poor response to PPIs. A study by Anvari et al. [56] investigated patients with poorly and well-controlled GERD following laparoscopic fundoplication, finding that GERD patients who responded poorly to PPI therapy experienced significantly improved physical and mental health QoL scores following surgical intervention. The study confirmed that response to PPI therapy does not impact surgical treatment, and all patients should experience good results following laparoscopic fundoplication.

Randomized trials comparing antireflux surgery to optimized medical therapy have concluded LNF to be superior in terms of symptom control and quality of life. An RCT of 104 patients compared long-term, symptomatically stable, medically controlled patients to laparoscopic Nissen fundoplication [39]. All patients had chronic GERD symptoms requiring long-term therapy prior to enrollment, with a minimum of 1-year PPI therapy, with continued expected need. Greater improvement was shown in the surgical group with patients experiencing a mean of 1.35 more heartburn free days per week than medical management patients and a more significant improvement in symptom scores using the global visual analog scale (VAS) from a mean of 81.79 at baseline to 92.67 ($P=0.0072$). Greater improvement was also found in Quality of life scores (Short Form 36) with a mean difference of -12.19 ($P=0.0124$) at 3 years (Fig. 24.3) [39]. The study concluded that although similar GERD symptom scale results were found with both LNF and PPI therapy, surgical treatment offered benefits of an increase in heartburn free days, improved VAS score, and lowered the esophageal acid exposure to the normal range for this group [39].

The LOTUS trial evaluated optimized esomeprazole therapy compared to LARS in GERD patients across 11 European countries [31]. A total of 554 patients were randomized in this open, parallel-group trial, with 372 patients completing the 5-year follow-up [31]. Remission rates were evaluated at this time, defined as the need for acid suppressive therapy in the surgical group, and inadequate symptom control after dose adjustment in the medical group, and were reported as 92 % (95 % CI, 89–96 %) in the esomeprazole group and 85 % (95 % CI, 81–90 %) in the LARS group ($P=0.048$) [31]. This study similarly to the Anvari and Allen trial [39] previously mentioned found a greater prevalence and severity of heartburn in the medical group with 16 % in the esomeprazole group and 8 % in the LARS ($P=0.14$), as well as 13 and 2 % for acid regurgitation ($P<0.001$) [31]. The medical group reported a lower incidence of dysphagia with 5 versus 11 % ($P=0.001$), and slightly decreased rates of bloating and flatulence than the surgical group [31].

Evidence has shown that antireflux surgery is an effective treatment for patients with poor response to standard PPI treatment. A prospective randomized study of 183 patients, compared LNF and PPI therapy, and further explored the medically managed patients, offering LNF following 12 months of pharmacotherapy treatment [57]. Although both LNF and PPI therapy were found to provide effective long-term treatment of GERD, a cohort of patients (54 patients) in the medical arm achieved only moderate benefit and chose to undergo laparoscopic Nissen fundoplication. These patients experienced further relief from symptoms, with a mean DeMeester symptom score at baseline of 3.3, 2.3 at 12 months (with PPI therapy only) and 0.8 at a median of 6.9 years follow-up (post LNF) with a significant change in score from 12 months ($P<0.01$) [57]. Similar findings were discovered in a trial evaluating the effectiveness of laparoscopic Nissen–Rossetti fundoplication in patients with GERD who are poorly responsive to standard PPI therapy. Thirty-five patients with persistent pathological esophageal acid and/or bilirubin exposure underwent LARS, and significant improvement was found in their symptom scores 1-year post-surgery when compared to standard PPI treatment [58].

Many studies correlate long-term PPI use with increased fracture risk. Although PPIs have a very favorable safety profile, potential long-term effects of chronic acid suppression on the absorption of vitamins and nutrients and increased occurrence of osteoporosis-related bone fractures are now raising concern and awareness [59]. While it has been proven that both optimal PPI therapy and laparoscopic Nissen fundoplication are effective treatments for GERD, surgery offers additional benefit for those who have only partial symptomatic relief from pharmacotherapy, and reduces any risk associated with long-term PPI use. Laparoscopic Nissen fundoplication has the potential to become an alternative long-term therapy for GERD, particularly in patients requiring extended use of PPIs.

Predictors of Success

The success of antireflux surgery depends heavily on patient selection. Patients with a good response to medical therapy without complicated disease have been shown to have superior outcomes following antireflux surgery [60, 61]. Patients who have been identified with clinical testing as having pathological acid reflux are more likely to respond well to surgical treatment than those with unknown or complicated diagnoses. Campos et al. [61] conducted a multivariate analysis to analyze predictive factors of LNF outcomes, finding three predictive factors of successful outcome: an abnormal 24-h pH score, the presence of typical symptoms of gastroesophageal reflux, and a significant improvement in symptoms with acid suppression therapy prior to surgery.

When predicting successful long-term outcomes of reflux surgery, sex, age, obesity, history of psychiatric illness and the presence of dysphagia pre-surgery are all indicators. Although symptoms of dysphagia often improve after fundoplication, the incidence of pre-surgical dysphagia negatively influences clinical outcome. Univariate regression analysis conducted by Oeschlager et al. [33] found that male patients, of younger age, presenting with heartburn, were much more likely to have successful outcomes of LARS, whereas preoperative dysphagia, airway manifestations, bloating, and defective esophageal motility were negative predictive factors. A study by Morgenthal et al. [62] found that preoperative morbid obesity (BMI > 35 kg/m^2) was associated with LNF failure, while obesity was not (BMI 30–34.9 kg/m^2). A history of psychiatric illness trended toward a failed outcome, but did not reach statistical significance ($P=0.06$) [62]. Similarly a regression analysis completed by Irino et al. [63] concluded that a BMI > 25 kg/m^2 and age >60 years were significant factors negatively affecting scores of postoperative GERD specific QOL.

Many authors have suggested clinical presentations of large hiatal hernias, atypical symptoms, the presence of Barrett's esophagus and esophagitis, and a defective LES lead to increased failure rates and poor outcomes of fundoplication, though these opinions are not expressed consistently throughout the literature [19, 62]. Procedural variations such as division of the SGVs, degree of the wrap, and technology may play a minimal role in the success of surgical treatment (Table 24.3).

Surgeon Experience

It has been reported that the rate of laparoscopic fundoplication complications lowers with increased surgeon expertise. Salimen et al. [64] indicate that adverse outcomes are more likely during the first 20 cases a surgeon performs. The authors studied the relation between surgeon experience and outcomes and found that higher rates of conversion (2.2 versus 4.4 %), early complication (3.5 and 7.6 %, $P=0.0892$), and reported dysphagia at 6 months (7.4 versus 16.1 %, $P=0.0115$) resulted following procedures performed by surgeons with less experience, than those with substantial experience [64]. Similarly, Watson et al. [65] found that rates of complication, reoperation, and conversion were higher following antireflux surgery for the first 20 cases performed by each surgeon, generally decreasing with increased experience. Complication rates decreased by 20 %, reoperation rates 22 % and conversion rates 13 % from outcomes of the first 20 cases to the rate associated with 251–280 cases of experience (see Fig. 24.1). The authors concluded that

surgeon supervision should be available for inexperienced LARS surgeons during the first 20 procedures to reduce complications and adverse outcomes [65] (Fig. 24.4).

Obesity

GERD is more prevalent among the morbidly obese, as obesity is a risk factor for the development of GERD [66, 67]. Few studies have examined the correlation of BMI in relation to outcomes of antireflux surgery, and the results have been conflicting.

It is a commonly believed that obesity contributes to poor ARS outcomes due to increased intra-abdominal pressure and fat causing increased incidence of complications such as hiatal herniation. Although there is evidence that preoperative morbid obesity is associated with LNF failure, many clinical trials have determined that obesity does not affect surgical outcomes. The prospective study by Anvari and Bamehriz [68] of 70 morbidly obese LNF patients resulted in one postoperative complication (1.4 %), a transhiatal herniation of the stomach, with one reoperation required. Both the morbidly obese group and the normal-weight group experienced a significant decrease in the esophageal acid exposure time, and an increase in LES pressures, a significant decrease in percent acid reflux in 24-h testing, and a significant improvement in GERD symptom score [68].

Similarly, Chisholm et al. [69] determined BMI did not influence outcomes. Winslow et al. [70] also found similar improvement of GERD symptoms and reduction of reflux medications at long-term follow-up for obese and non-obese

Table 24.3 Suggested factors affecting good outcomes of antireflux surgery

Predictor of positive outcome	Predictor of poor outcome
Good response to PPI	No response to PPI
Typical symptoms	Atypical symptoms
High volume practice	Low volume practice
No/small Hiatal Hernia	Large Hiatal Hernia
Male gender	Female gender
No Barrett's	Barrett's
Normal weight	Obesity
Normal motility	Poor motility
No esophagitis	Active esophagitis
Mentally healthy	Psychiatric co-morbidity
First time surgery	Re-operative surgery

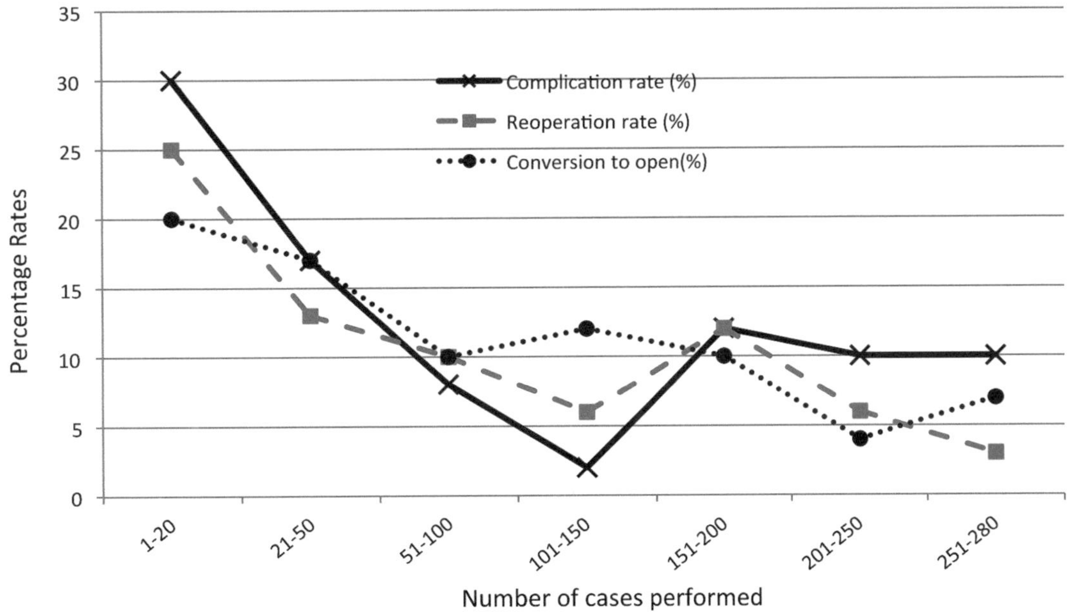

Fig. 24.4 The effect of surgeon experience with LARS on outcomes [65]

patients. Patients with higher BMI levels have similar post-surgical outcomes to those of normal weight with equivalent symptom improvement and patient satisfaction following ARS indicating that obesity should not be a contraindication to the surgical treatment of reflux.

Other studies have shown contradicting results. A retrospective study by Perez et al. [71] found the rate of recurrence increased with obesity: 2.5 % for normal weight patients, 8 % for overweight patients, and 31.3 % for obese patients. Similarly, a retrospective review by Hahnloser et al. [76] found that 31 % of patients with a BMI of >30 kg/m² experienced complications (intraoperative and postoperative) following LNF versus 12 % of patients with a BMI <30 kg/m². These studies confirm the predictive indicators of success of LNF mentioned previously, relating preoperative morbid obesity and obesity as significant factors negatively affecting the outcomes of antireflux surgery.

As global obesity rates reach epidemic proportions the issue of obesity and the surgical treatment of GERD escalates. Bariatric surgical procedures used to treat morbid obesity have also proven to be effective in the secondary treatment of GERD [72, 73]. The decrease in GERD symptoms is significant, with heartburn decreasing from 87 to 22 %, and related medication use reducing from 44 to 9 % for PPI use after Roux-en-Y gastric bypass [74]. The effective treatment of both obesity and GERD concurrently is therefore a practice to be further analyzed.

Patient Selection for Antireflux Surgery

Preoperative patient evaluation and selection is imperative to successful antireflux surgery. Esophageal motility and 24-h ph studies have improved the process of selecting appropriate patients. Reflux symptoms can be the result of other conditions such as acid peptic disease, cholelithiasis, and irritable bowel syndrome. Pre-procedural endoscopy should be utilized to rule out other complications such as Barrett's esophagus and esophagitis, and to document esophageal anatomy. To confirm diagnosis of reflux, 24-h acid monitoring should be tested.

Conclusion

Reduction and elimination of reflux symptoms are the main goals of any treatment approach for GERD. Laparoscopic fundoplication has shown to be safe and effective in the control of reflux symptoms. Short-term results of LARS are good, and long-term results are variable, with benefits shown to diminish over time. A high rate of patient satisfaction is reported following LARS, with low rates of revision and reoperation. Antireflux medication use post-surgery is reported at different rates, but the reason for use must be further investigated, and unnecessary use has been widely accounted.

LARS is an effective option for the treatment of GERD. Patients should be selected appropriately with consideration of presenting symptoms and complications. ARS should be performed by surgeons with sufficient training and expertise to ensure successful treatment.

Acknowledgement The author wishes to acknowledge the significant contribution of Ruth Breau in the preparation of this chapter.

References

1. Anvari M, Allen C. Laparoscopic Nissen fundoplication: two-year comprehensive follow-up of a technique of minimal paraesophageal dissection. Ann Surg. 1998;227(1):25–32.
2. Trus TL, Laycock WS, Waring JP, Branum GD, Hunter JG. Improvement in quality of life measures after laparoscopic antireflux surgery. Ann Surg. 1999;229(3):331–6.
3. Lundell L, Miettinen P, Myrvold HE, et al. Continued (5-year) followup of a randomized clinical study comparing antireflux surgery and omeprazole in gastroesophageal reflux disease. J Am Coll Surg. 2001;192(2):172–9. discussion 179–181.
4. Spechler SJ, Lee E, Ahnen D, et al. Long-term outcome of medical and surgical therapies for gastroesophageal reflux disease: follow-up of a randomized controlled trial. JAMA. 2001;285(18):2331–8.
5. Soresi AL. Diaghragmatic hernia: it's unsuspected frequency: it's diagnosis: technic for radical cure. Ann Surg. 1919;69(3):254–70.
6. Harrington SW. Diaphragmatic hernia. Arch Surg. 1928;16:386–415.
7. Harrington SW. The surgical treatment of the more common types of diaphragmatic hernia: esophageal hiatus, traumatic, pleuroperitoneal hiatus, congenital absence and foramen of Morgagni: report of 404 cases. Ann Surg. 1945;122:546–68.
8. Sweet RH. Diaphragmatic hernia. In: Sweet RH, editor. Thoracic surgery. Philadelphia: WB Saunders; 1950. p. 316–34.
9. Ellis Jr FH. The Nissen fundoplication. Ann Thorac Surg. 1992;54(6):1231–5.
10. Allison PR. Reflux esophagitis, sliding hiatal hernia and anatomy of repair. Surg Gynecol Obstet. 1951;92:419–31.
11. Allison PR. Hiatus hernia (a 20 year retrospective survey). Ann Surg. 1973;178:273–6.
12. Barrett NR. Hiatus hernia. Br J Surg. 1954;42:231–43.
13. Christian DJ, Buyske J. Current status of antireflux surgery. Surg Clin North Am. 2005;85(5):931–47.
14. Nissen R. A simple operation for control of reflux esophagitis. Schweiz Med Wochenschr. 1956;18:86.
15. Nissen R. Gastropexy and "fundoplication" in surgical treatment of hiatal hernia. Am J Dig Dis. 1961;6:954–61.
16. Donahue PE, Samuelson S, Nulus LM, et al. The floppy Nissen fundoplication. Effective long term control of pathologic reflux. Arch Surg. 1985;120:663–7.
17. Demeester TR, Bonavina L, Albertucci M. Nissen fundoplication for gastroesophageal reflux disease. Evaluation of primary repair in 100 consecutive patients. Ann Surg. 1986;204:9–20.
18. Jobe BA, Wallace J, Hansen PD, et al. Evaluation of laparoscopic Toupet fundoplication as a primary repair for all patients with medically resistant gastroesophageal reflux. Surg Endosc. 1997;11:1080–3.
19. Horvath KD, Jobe BA, Herron DM, et al. Laparoscopic Toupet fundoplication is an inadequate procedure for patients with severe reflux disease. J Gastrointest Surg. 1999;3:583–91.

20. Salminen P. The laparoscopic Nissen fundoplication – a better operation? Surgeon. 2009;7(4):224–7.

21. Dallemagne B, Weerts JM, Jehaes C, Markiewicz S, Lombard R. Laparoscopic Nissen fundoplication: preliminary report. Surg Laparosc Endosc. 1991;1(3):138–43.

22. Peters MJ, Mukhtar A, Yunus RM, Khan S, Pappalardo J, Memon B, Memon MA. Meta-analysis of randomized clinical trials comparing open and laparoscopic anti-reflux surgery. Am J Gastroenterol. 2009;104(6):1548–61.

23. Bais JE, Bartelsman JF, Bonjer HJ, Cuesta MA, Go PM, Klinkenberg-Knol EC, van Lanschot JJ, Nadorp JH, Smout AJ, van der Graaf Y, Gooszen HG. Laparoscopic or conventional Nissen fundoplication for gastro-oesophageal reflux disease: randomised clinical trial. The Netherlands Antireflux Surgery Study Group. Lancet. 2000;355(9199):170–4.

24. Valiati W, Fuchs KH, Valiati L, Freys SM, Fein M, Maroske J, Tigges H, Thiede A. Laparoscopic fundoplication – short- and long-term outcome. Langenbecks Arch Surg. 2000;385(5):324–8.

25. Biertho L, Sebajang H, Allen C, Anvari M. Does laparoscopic Nissen fundoplication lead to chronic gastrointestinal dysfunction? Surg Endosc. 2006;20(9):1360–3.

26. Watson DI, Jamieson GG. Antireflux surgery in the laparoscopic era. Br J Surg. 1998;85(9):1173–84.

27. Broeders JA, Rijnhart-de Jong HG, Draaisma WA, Bredenoord AJ, Smout AJ, Gooszen HG. Ten-year outcome of laparoscopic and conventional Nissen fundoplication: randomized clinical trial. Ann Surg. 2009;250(5):698–706.

28. Catarci M, Gentileschi P, Papi C, Carrara A, Marrese R, Gaspari AL, Grassi GB. Evidence-based appraisal of antireflux fundoplication. Ann Surg. 2004;239(3):325–37.

29. Livingston EH, Rege RV. A nationwide study of conversion from laparoscopic to open cholecystectomy. Am J Surg. 2004; 188(3):205–11.

30. Twijnstra AR, Blikkendaal MD, van Zwet EW, Jansen FW. Clinical relevance of conversion rate and its evaluation in laparoscopic hysterectomy. J Minim Invasive Gynecol. 2013;20(1):64–72.

31. Galmiche JP, Hatlebakk J, Attwood S, Ell C, Fiocca R, Eklund S, Långström G, Lind T, Lundell L, LOTUS Trial Collaborators. Laparoscopic antireflux surgery vs esomeprazole treatment for chronic GERD: the LOTUS randomized clinical trial. JAMA. 2011;305(19):1969–77.

32. Dallemagne B, Weerts J, Markiewicz S, Dewandre JM, Wahlen C, Monami B, Jehaes C. Clinical results of laparoscopic fundoplication at ten years after surgery. Surg Endosc. 2006;20(1):159–65.

33. Oelschlager BK, Quiroga E, Parra JD, Cahill M, Polissar N, Pellegrini CA. Long-term outcomes after laparoscopic antireflux surgery. Am J Gastroenterol. 2008;103(2):280–7.

34. Luostarinen M, Isolauri J, Laitinen J, Koskinen M, Keyriläinen O, Markkula H, Lehtinen E, Uusitalo A. Fate of Nissen fundoplication after 20 years. A clinical, endoscopical, and functional analysis. Gut. 1993;34(8):1015–20.

35. Robinson BJ, Ahmed M Sharata, MD, Maria A, Cassera BS, Christy M, Dunst, MD, Kevin M, Reavis MD, Lee L, Swanstrom LL. 20 years later: laparoscopic fundoplication durability, Surg Endosc. 2014; submitted for publication.

36. Eubanks T, Omelanczuk P, Richards C, et al. Outcomes of laparoscopic antireflux procedures. Am J Surg. 2000;179:391–5.

37. Peters J, DeMeester T, Crookes P, et al. The treatment of gastroesophageal reflux disease with laparoscopic Nissen fundoplication: a prospective evaluation of 100 patients with "typical" symptoms. Ann Surg. 1998;228:40–50.

38. Anvari M, Allen C. Five-year comprehensive outcomes evaluation in 181 patients after laparoscopic Nissen fundoplication. J Am Coll Surg. 2003;196(1):51–7.

39. Anvari M, Allen C, Marshall J, Armstrong D, Goeree R, Ungar W, Goldsmith C. A randomized controlled trial of laparoscopic Nissen fundoplication versus proton pump inhibitors for the treatment of patients with chronic gastroesophageal reflux disease (GERD): 3-year outcomes. Surg Endosc. 2011;25(8):2547–54.

40. Zaninotto G, Molena D, Ancona E. A prospective, multicenter study on laparoscopic treatment of gastroesophageal reflux in Italy: type of surgery, conversions, complications and early results. Surg Endosc. 2000;14:282–8.

41. Contini S, Scarpignato C. Evaluation of clinical outcome after laparoscopic antireflux surgery in clinical practice: still a controversial issue. Minim Invasive Surg. 2011;2011:725472.

42. The American Gastroenterological Association Institute Medical Position Panel. American Gastroenterological Association medical position statement on the management of gastroesophageal reflux disease. Gastroenterology. 2008;135:1383–91.

43. Narsule CK, Wee JO, Fernando HC. Endoscopic management of gastroesophageal reflux disease: a review. J Thorac Cardiovasc Surg. 2012;17.

44. Salminen PT, Hiekkanen HI, Rantala AP, et al. Comparison of long-term outcome of laparoscopic and conventional Nissen fundoplication: a prospective randomized study with an 11-year follow-up. Ann Surg. 2007;246:201–6.

45. Yang H, Watson DI, Lally CJ, et al. Randomized trial of division versus nondivision of the short gastric vessels during laparoscopic Nissen fundoplication: 10-year outcomes. Ann Surg. 2008; 247:38–42.

46. Mardani J, Lundell L, Lonroth H, et al. Ten-year results of a randomized clinical trial of laparoscopic total fundoplication with or without division of the short gastric vessels. Br J Surg. 2008; 96:61–5.

47. Cai W, Watson DI, Lally CJ, et al. Ten-year clinical outcome of a prospective randomized clinical trial of laparoscopic Nissen versus anterior 180(degrees) partial fundoplication. Br J Surg. 2008; 95:1501–5.

48. Papasavas PK, Keenan RJ, Yeaney WW, Caushaj PF, Gagné DJ, Landreneau RJ. Effectiveness of laparoscopic fundoplication in relieving the symptoms of gastroesophageal reflux disease (GERD) and eliminating antireflux medical therapy. Surg Endosc. 2003; 17(8):1200–5.

49. Draaisma WA, Rijnhart-de Jong HG, Broeders IA, Smout AJ, Furnee EJ, Gooszen HG. Five-year subjective and objective results of laparoscopic and conventional Nissen fundoplication: a randomized trial. Ann Surg. 2006;244(1):34–41.

50. Jenkinson AD, Kadirkamanathan SS, Scott SM, et al. Relationship between symptom response and oesophageal acid exposure after medical and surgical treatment for gastro-oesophageal reflux disease. Br J Surg. 2004;91:1460–5.

51. Lord RV, Kaminski A, Oberg S, et al. Absence of gastroesophageal reflux disease in a majority of patients taking acid suppression medications after Nissen fundoplication. J Gastrointest Surg. 2002;6:3–9.

52. Smith CD, McClusky DA, Rajad MA, Lederman AB, Hunter JG. When fundoplication fails: redo? Ann Surg. 2005;241(6):861–9.

53. Kelly JJ, Watson DI, Chin KF, Devitt PG, Game PA, Jamieson GG. Laparoscopic Nissen fundoplication: clinical outcomes at 10 years. J Am Coll Surg. 2007;205(4):570–5.

54. Salminen P, Gullichsen R, Ovaska J. Subjective results and symptomatic outcome after fundoplication revision. Scand J Gastroenterol. 2008;43(5):518–23.

55. Bathla L, Legner A, Tsuboi K, Mittal S. Efficacy and feasibility of laparoscopic redo fundoplication. World J Surg. 2011;35(11): 2445–53.

56. Anvari M, Allen C. Surgical outcome in gastro-esophageal reflux disease patients with inadequate response to proton pump inhibitors. Surg Endosc. 2003;17(7):1029–35.

57. Mehta S, Bennett J, Mahon D, Rhodes M. Prospective trial of laparoscopic Nissen fundoplication versus proton pump inhibitor

therapy for gastroesophageal reflux disease: seven-year follow-up. J Gastrointest Surg. 2006;10(9):1312–6.

58. Brillantino A, Schettino M, Torelli F, Marano L, Porfidia R, Reda G, Grassia M, Braccio B, Di Martino N. Laparoscopic Nissen–Rossetti fundoplication is a safe and effective treatment for both acid and bile gastroesophageal reflux in patients poorly responsive to proton pump inhibitor. Surg Innov. 2011;18(4):387–93.

59. Ito T, Jensen RT. Association of long-term proton pump inhibitor therapy with bone fractures and effects on absorption of calcium, vitamin B12, iron, and magnesium. Curr Gastroenterol Rep. 2010;12(6):448–57.

60. Csendes A. Multivariate analysis of factors predicting outcome after laparoscopic Nissen fundoplication. J Gastrointest Surg. 2000;4:650–7.

61. Campos GM, Peters JH, DeMeester TR, Oberg S, Crookes PF, Tan S, DeMeester SR, Hagen JA, Bremner CG. Multivariate analysis of factors predicting outcome after laparoscopic Nissen fundoplication. J Gastrointest Surg. 1999;3(3):292–300.

62. Morgenthal CB, Lin E, Shane MD, Hunter JG, Smith CD. Who will fail laparoscopic Nissen fundoplication? Preoperative prediction of long-term outcomes. Surg Endosc. 2007;21(11):1978–84.

63. Irino T, Takeuchi H, Ozawa S, Saikawa Y, Oyama T, Hiraiwa K, Yoshikawa T, Kitajima M, Kitagawa Y. Age and body mass index: significant predictive factors for successful laparoscopic antireflux surgery. Surg Today. 2010;40(12):1137–43.

64. Salminen P, Hiekkanen H, Laine S, Ovaska J. Surgeons' experience with laparoscopic fundoplication after the early personal experience: does it have an impact on the outcome? Surg Endosc. 2007; 21(8):1377–82.

65. Watson DI, Baigrie RJ, Jamieson GG. A learning curve for laparoscopic fundoplication. Definable, avoidable, or a waste of time? Ann Surg. 1996;224(2):198–203.

66. Varela JE, Hinojosa MW, Nguyen NT. Laparoscopic fundoplication compared with laparoscopic gastric bypass in morbidly obese patients with gastroesophageal reflux disease. Surg Obes Relat Dis. 2009;5(2):139–43.

67. Ruhl CE, Everhart JE. Overweight, but not high dietary fat intake, increases risk of gastroesophageal reflux disease hospitalization: the NHANES I epidemiologic follow-up study. First National Health and Nutrition Examination Survey. Ann Epidemiol. 1999;9:424–35.

68. Anvari M, Bamehriz F. Outcome of laparoscopic Nissen fundoplication in patients with body mass index > or = 35. Surg Endosc. 2006;20(2):230–4.

69. Chisholm JA, Jamieson GG, Lally CJ, Devitt PG, Game PA, Watson DI. The effect of obesity on the outcome of laparoscopic antireflux surgery. J Gastrointest Surg. 2009;13(6):1064–70.

70. Winslow ER, Frisella MM, Soper NJ, Klingensmith ME. Obesity does not adversely affect the outcome of laparoscopic antireflux surgery (LARS). Surg Endosc. 2003;17(12):2003–11.

71. Perez AR, Moncure AC, Rattner DW. Obesity adversely affects the outcome of antireflux operations. Surg Endosc. 2001;15(9): 986–9.

72. Perry Y, Courcoulas AP, Fernando HC, et al. Laparoscopic Rouxen-Y gastric bypass for recalcitrant gastroesophageal reflux disease in morbidly obese patients. JSLS. 2004;8:19–23.

73. Westling A, Ohrvall M, Gustavsson S. Roux-en-Y gastric bypass after previous unsuccessful gastric restrictive surgery. J Gastrointest Surg. 2002;6:206–11.

74. Frezza EE, Ikramuddin S, Gourash W, et al. Symptomatic improvement in gastroesophageal reflux disease (GERD) following laparoscopic Roux-en-Y gastric bypass. Surg Endosc. 2002;16(7): 1027–31.

75. Salimen P, Hurme S, Ovaska J. Fifteen-year outcome of laparoscopic and open Nissen fundoplicaiton: a randomized clinical trial. Ann Thorac Surg. 2012 Jan;93(1):228–33.

76. Hahnloser D, Schumacher M, Cavin R, Cosendey B, Petropoulos P. Risk factors for complications of laparoscopic Nissen fundoplication. Surg Endosc. 2002 Jan;16(1):43–7.

Index